JOURNAL OF PROSTHODONTICS
ON COMPLEX RESTORATIONS

JOURNAL OF PROSTHODONTICS ON COMPLEX RESTORATIONS

Edited by

NADIM Z. BABA, DMD, MSD, FACP

DAVID L. GUICHET, DDS, FACP

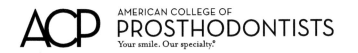

WILEY Blackwell

Published by John Wiley & Sons, Inc., Hoboken, New Jersey.
Published simultaneously in Canada.

For general information on our other products and services or for technical support, please contact our Customer Care Department within the United States at (800) 762-2974, outside the United States at (317) 572-3993 or fax (317) 572-4002.

Wiley also publishes its books in a variety of electronic formats. Some content that appears in print may not be available in electronic formats. For more information about Wiley products, visit our web site at www.wiley.com.

Library of Congress Cataloging-in-Publication Data:

Names: Baba, Nadim Z., editor. | Guichet, David L., editor. | American
  College of Prosthodontists, issuing body.
Title: Journal of prosthodontics on complex restorations / edited by Nadim Z.
  Baba, David L. Guichet.
Other titles: Journal of Prosthodontics.
Description: Hoboken, New Jersey : John Wiley & Sons Inc. : American College
  of Prosthodontists, [2016] | Compilation of articles from Journal of
  Prosthodontics. | Includes bibliographical references and index.
Identifiers: LCCN 2016019941| ISBN 9781119274490 (cloth) | ISBN 9781119274582
  (epub) | ISBN 9781119274575 (Adobe PDF)
Subjects: | MESH: Prosthodontics—methods | Dental Restoration,
  Permanent—methods | Collected Works
Classification: LCC RK651 | NLM WU 500 | DDC 617.6/9—dc23 LC record available at https://lccn.loc.gov/2016019941

Cover image: Courtesy of Nadim Z. Baba and David L. Guichet

Cover design: Wiley

Printed in the United States of America.

10 9 8 7 6 5 4 3 2 1

CONTENTS

v

PREFACE

Patients often present with a myriad of complex dental restorative challenges. Prosthodontists, restorative dentists, and other team members are called upon to solve these dilemmas. In most instances, established protocols are available. Often more imaginative techniques are applied in the manufacture and the delivery of complex restorations including nontraditional workflows and new CAD/CAM solutions. Examples of this are the advances in 3D manufacturing technology, which has come of age along with dental digital design software and machinable high-strength esthetic materials.

As new information, materials, and techniques have become available, contributors to the *Journal of Prosthodontics* have shared their developments. These authors have endeavored to position their work in the context of traditional approaches to enable the reader to draw on the historical standards and differentiate the new from the tried and true. This book is a collection of notable works on the subject of complex dental restorations.

The editors have identified six areas where significant developments have taken place in the arena of complex dental restorations. The selected articles illustrate either highly refined, traditional techniques or highlight the use of new, innovative processes. These articles represent the best application of techniques available for patients requiring complex dental restorations. The foundational principles of successful prosthodontic rehabilitations serve as a framework against which all of these articles have been evaluated.

The six areas include management of maxillofacial defects using CAD/CAM technology; management of tooth wear; management of congenital disorders; management of orthodontic/prosthodontic patients; management of patients with surgical and prosthodontic challenges; and management of completely edentulous patients using new ceramic materials.

The American College of Prosthodontists has undertaken numerous initiatives advancing knowledge in the field of complex dental restorations including digital dental rehabilitation. These include updates at the ACP Annual Session, the Prosthodontic Review Course, and the ACP Digital Dentistry Symposium, as well as efforts to support the integration of CAD/CAM technology into dental education and create a new curriculum in digital dentistry.

These initiatives are part of a strong foundation being established by the American College of Prosthodontists as it leads this arena of dentistry into the future. Together with these efforts, this compilation serves to advance scientific knowledge in the field of fundamental prosthodontics, digital dentistry, and complex dental restorations.

NADIM Z. BABA, DMD, MSD, FACP
DAVID L. GUICHET, DDS, FACP

ACKNOWLEDGMENTS

The editors would like to thank the authors whose work is collected in this volume dedicated to the restoration of complex patient situations. We wish to express our appreciation to Dr. David Felton, editor-in-chief, and Dr. Radi Masri, associate editor-in-chief of the *Journal of Prosthodontics*, for their trust in choosing us to edit this book. We take the opportunity to thank Mr. Mark Heiden for his professionalism, help, and guidance during the preparation of this book, as well as Ms. Alethea Gerding for her work as Managing Editor of the *Journal of Prosthodontics*. We extend our thanks to Ms. Nancy Deal Chandler and the ACP executive committee for their support in bringing this book to life.

PART I

MANAGEMENT OF MAXILLOFACIAL DEFECTS USING CAD/CAM TECHNOLOGY

1

COMPARATIVE ACCURACY OF FACIAL MODELS FABRICATED USING TRADITIONAL AND 3D IMAGING TECHNIQUES

Ketu P. Lincoln, dmd,[1] Albert Y. T. Sun, phd, cswa,[2] Thomas J. Prihoda, phd,[3] and Alan J. Sutton, dds, ms, facp[4]

[1]Department of Graduate Prosthodontics, USAF, Joint Base San Antonio-Lackland, San Antonio, TX
[2]Department of Mechanical Engineering, National Taipei University of Technology, Taipei, Taiwan
[3]Department of Pathology, University of Texas Health Science Center, San Antonio, TX
[4]Department of Restorative Dentistry, University of Colorado School of Dental Medicine, Aurora, CO

Keywords
Moulage; facial prosthetics; 3D imaging; 3D models; dental materials; stereolithography; rapid prototyping.

Correspondence
Alan Sutton, 13045 E. 17th Ave Ste F845, Aurora, CO 80045. E-mail: Alan.sutton@ucdenver.edu

The authors deny any conflicts of interest.

Accepted June 14, 2015

Published in *Journal of Prosthodontics* September 2015

doi: 10.1111/jopr.12358

ABSTRACT

Purpose: The purpose of this investigation was to compare the accuracy of facial models fabricated using facial moulage impression methods to the three-dimensional printed (3DP) fabrication methods using soft tissue images obtained from cone beam computed tomography (CBCT) and 3D stereo-photogrammetry (3D-SPG) scans.

Materials and Methods: A reference phantom model was fabricated using a 3D-SPG image of a human control form with ten fiducial markers placed on common anthropometric landmarks. This image was converted into the investigation control phantom model (CPM) using 3DP methods. The CPM was attached to a camera tripod for ease of image capture. Three CBCT and three 3D-SPG images of the CPM were captured. The DICOM and STL files from the three 3dMD and three CBCT were imported to the 3DP, and six testing models were made. Reversible hydrocolloid and dental stone were used to make three facial moulages of the CPM, and the impressions/casts were poured in type IV gypsum dental stone. A coordinate measuring machine (CMM) was used to measure the distances between each of the ten fiducial markers. Each measurement was made using one point as a static reference to the other nine points. The same measuring procedures were accomplished on all specimens. All measurements were compared between specimens and the control. The data were analyzed using ANOVA and Tukey pairwise comparison of the raters, methods, and fiducial markers.

Results: The ANOVA multiple comparisons showed significant difference among the three methods ($p < 0.05$). Further, the interaction of methods versus fiducial markers also showed significant difference ($p < 0.05$). The

CBCT and facial moulage method showed the greatest accuracy.

Conclusions: 3DP models fabricated using 3D-SPG showed statistical difference in comparison to the models fabricated using the traditional method of facial moulage and 3DP models fabricated from CBCT imaging. 3DP models fabricated using 3D-SPG were less accurate than the CPM and models fabricated using facial moulage and CBCT imaging techniques.

Craniofacial dysmorphology (CD) is the study of structural defects caused by trauma, treatment of neoplasms, or congenital anomalies characterized by complex irregularities in the shape and configuration of facial soft tissue structures.[1] Patients with CD may undergo extensive surgical procedures, including the fabrication of facial prostheses to restore an extraoral maxillofacial defect.[2] The facial prostheses are not functional, but provide the patient with an esthetic result for psychological and social acceptance.[3–6]

Anthropometry is a way to assess changes in facial soft tissue over time through line measurements between two landmarks.[7] The challenge has been to identify landmarks and plot them accurately in the three planes of space, in order to describe the dimensions of the face.[8] Traditionally, direct anthropometry was done using calipers. This assessment was a reliable and inexpensive method for data collection of surface measurements.[4] However, there were several limitations, including technician training, direct patient contact requiring extensive time to make multiple measurements, patient compliance to sit in one position, inability to archive information, difficulty attaining several measurements as tissue undergoes changes with time, and finally comparing tissue changes with accurate landmark location.[9]

Making a facial moulage impression was, and still is, another means for 3D facial structure capture, analysis, and documentation. This method has been used successfully for almost 100 years, dating back to World War I.[10] Currently, various impression materials like alginate, poly(vinyl siloxane), and reversible hydrocolloid are used to create a facial moulage. The facial moulage method can be time consuming, and soft tissue deformation is a significant problem. Furthermore, it is difficult to obtain accurate impressions of certain defects involving the orbit where the periorbital tissue displaces easily.[11] The casts made from the impressions are fragile and require large physical storage space, and it is extremely difficult to communicate physical data to other providers in distant locations.[12] Also, archival preoperative casts may not be available for many patient treatments due to storage limitation.

Several types of 3D imaging systems have been created in the past three decades, including cone beam computed tomography (CBCT) and 3D stereophotogrammetry (3D-SPG). Both methods are noninvasive and allow for archival of data and virtual models that can subsequently be used for comparison purposes.

Computed tomography (CT), and more specifically CBCT, is currently used to capture soft tissue surface images because it is accurate and repeatable for anthropometric measurements.[7] Collimating the X-ray beam decreases the radiation exposure dose, and the scan time is 10 to 70 seconds.[13] The dose of radiation ranges between 60 and 1000 µSv versus medical grade CT of the mandible, which ranges from 1320 to 3324 µSv.[13–15] More recent studies have generated 3D facial soft tissue surface computer models from image data captured by CBCT. Linear anthropometric measurements on computer models using CBCT software proved reliable and as accurate as the traditional direct method.[7] The data and virtual models are easily archived without physical storage requirements and can provide pre- and postoperative information for skeletal or soft tissue comparisons.[13]

3D-SPG is a newer technique/method for craniofacial surface imaging that allows for the capture evaluation of the external surface of a subject. The method creates a 3D image reconstructed from multiple digital images taken at different angles simultaneously. The resultant image is a collection of points positioned along an x, y, and z coordinate system. These points can be identified as landmarks, then used for subsequent analysis.[9] Reports indicate that 3D-SPG is reliable and accurate for determining the location of landmarks and interlandmark craniofacial distances.[16,17] The advantages include minimal artifact production due to short image capture time (approximately 1.5 ms), ability to archive and compare subject images, three-point (x, y, z) coordinate format of locating tissue landmarks, high resolution, and no radiation. Software programs are available to identify landmarks and calculate anthropometric measurements.[18] In addition, the error in the location of a landmark when using 3D-SPG is less than 1 mm.[19]

The use of 3D-SPG has a great potential for use in the military. During World War II, the Korean War, and the Vietnam War, the mean incidence of head, face, and neck injury (HNFI) was approximately 16%. A recent study looked at the characteristics and causes of HFNIs sustained by US military forces during the stability and support phase of Operation Iraqi Freedom (OIF-II). The number of HFNIs increased to 39%, and of these injuries, 65% were injuries to the face.[20] A more recent study showed a comprehensive analysis of craniomaxillofacial battle injuries sustained by military members evacuated to level III-V military treatment facilities to be 42.2% HNFIs.[21] The reason for the notable increase in the past decade is an increase in survival rate due to improvement in body armor, battlefield medicine, tactically placed medical units, and quick evacuation tactics.

Both CBCT and 3D-SPG use computer-aided design (CAD) software to facilitate the design of soft tissue surface images and virtual models. With rapid prototyping (RP), information from the CAD software can be used along with computer-aided manufacturing (CAM) to fabricate 3D physical models. Image data from CBCT and 3D-SPG scans translated into the digital imaging and communication in medicine (DICOM) file format, which are converted to a CAM file format to produce a 3D model using RP methods and equipment.

One RP method used in the medical and dental field is 3D printing (3DP). This process uses a polyjet selectively depositing fine powder polymer droplets evenly along a piston and liquid binder. Additional layers are added as the piston powder bed and cured model is lowered layer by layer. The resolution accuracy is 100 μm for one-dimensional features and 300 μm for 3D features.[11] The 3D printed models are accurate to 0.016 mm (Objet Eden 260V; Stratasys Ltd., Minneapolis, MN), and the build time is at a rate of 1 cm of height per hour.[22]

The 3D models are useful for surgical planning, creation of surgical templates, and fabrication of craniofacial prostheses and custom implants used in craniofacial reconstruction.

The accuracy of the RP models has been measured by software calculations,[23-25] digital calipers,[18] and more recently the use of a coordinate measurement machine (CMM). The CMM can provide accurate location of x, y, and z coordinate reference points. This device is very useful in locating the same landmark on various models and therefore accurate in determining any error in model production.

RP techniques are proving beneficial in the treatment planning, diagnosis, surgical assistance, prosthesis fabrication and postassessment of patients with craniofacial anomalies, facial trauma, and structural defects caused by neoplasms; however, further studies need to be done to evaluate the precise fit of models fabricated from soft tissue imaging. The purpose of this investigation was to compare the accuracy of facial models fabricated using facial moulage impression methods to the 3DP fabrication methods using soft tissue images obtained from CBCT and 3D-SPG.

MATERIALS AND METHODS

One human form was obtained from a two-pod 3D-SPG surface imaging system and software system (3dMDface; 3dMD, Atlanta, GA). The scanned image was saved as an Standard Triangulation Language (STL) file and uploaded into the modeling software program (Geomagic Freeform Modeling Plus; Geomagic, Wilmington, MA) to create the virtual model. The virtual model was used to design the control phantom model (CPM). Five millimeter diameter spheres were built into the model to mark the following ten landmarks on the facial soft tissue: Glabella, Nasion, Pronasale, right and left Orbitale, right and left Frontale, right and left Cheilion, and Pogonion (Fig 1.1A).[4,5,7,9,26,27] The

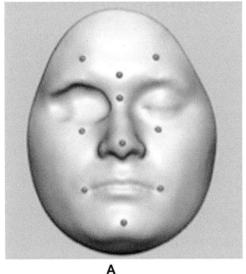
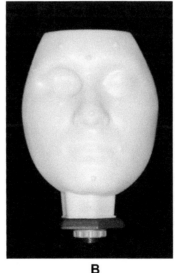
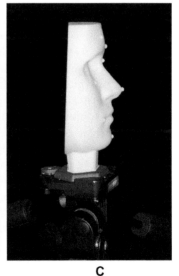

A   **B**   **C**

FIGURE 1.1   (A) Virtual model with landmarks. (B) Printed control phantom model (CPM) frontal view. (C) CPM lateral view.

virtual master model was processed using 3DP software (Objet Studio; Stratasys Ltd., Minneapolis, MN), and the physical CPM was created using 3DP (Objet Eden 260V; Stratasys Ltd.) (Figs 1.1B and 1.1C).

The CPM was used to create three facial moulage experimental gypsum dental stone models using reversible hydrocolloid (Polyflex Duplicating Material; Dentsply International, York, PA). Reversible hydrocolloid at room temperature was heated to its liquefaction temperature to convert the gel to the sol condition.[28] The reversible hydrocolloid was applied to the CPM using a synthetic brush (Synthetic brush #16; Dentsply). Cotton gauze ($2\,in^2$) was embedded in the solidifying reversible hydrocolloid to reinforce the material and allow for the attachment to dental stone. Athin consistency of dental stone (Mounting Stone ISO type 3; Whip Mix Corp., Louisville, KY) was applied over the reversible hydrocolloid and gauze in a uniform half-inch thickness to fabricate an external tray. The ratio of the dental stone to filtered water was 900 g to 170 ml. Once the stone set, the impression was removed from the master model and poured in type IV dental stone (Silky Rock, Whip Mix Corp.) (Fig 1.2A).[29] The ratio of type IV dental stone to filtered water was 600 g to 138 ml. Each of the resultant three stone models was labeled accordingly (Fig 1.2B).

To position the CPM for CBCT capture, a tripod measurement base assembly was fabricated using a tripod screw platform with acrylic resin (Ortho Acrylic Resin; Great Lakes Orthodontics, Tonawanda, NY) (Fig 1.3).[30] The CBCT system (Kodak 9500 Cone Beam 3D System; Carestream Health, Inc., Rochester, NY) was calibrated following the manufacturer's instructions. The CPM was stabilized on the tripod, and a total of three images were made individually and labeled one through three (Fig 1.4). The images were saved as DICOM files and copied onto a disc for use with the RP system.

The same tripod base assembly for the CPM was used to obtain the 3D-SPG images (3dMDface). The system was calibrated according the manufacturer's instructions.[31] The tripod with CPM was positioned at a 15° anterior tilt to capture an image with minimal shadowing (Fig 1.5). A total of three images were made individually and labeled one through three. These images were saved as STL files and saved onto a disc for use with the RP system.

The DICOM images and STL files from the CBCT and 3dMD, respectively, were used to create the virtual models using computer software. A DICOM segmentation program (MIMICS 12.1; Materialise Dental, Plymouth, MI) was used to identify the CPM and generate a surface model (in STL format) from the series of CBCT images (Fig 1.6). The six STL files were aligned, and a common base was designed and merged to the 3D surface of each of the scans. Then, using 3DP (Objet Eden 260V) six individual models were fabricated prior to measurement procedures (Fig 1.7).

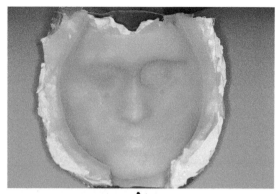

A

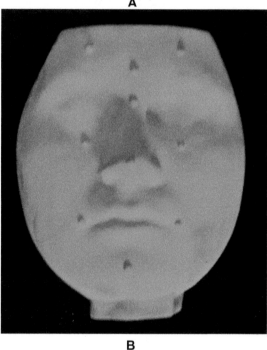

B

FIGURE 1.2 (A) Reversible hydrocolloid impression. (B) Stone model.

The printed RP models and gypsum stone models were measured for accuracy by three individual raters using a CMM (Faro, Lake Mary, FL). A 3 mm ball probe stylus was placed on the surface of each fiducial marker, and a discrete point cloud was recorded into Geomagic Studio as the measuring software interface. Each cloud data set was interpreted as a sphere feature on the model. The scans resulted in a collection of point cloud data representing the feature location in space relative to each of the other spheres (Figs 1.7 and 1.8).

The software was then used to calculate a best-fit sphere for each of the point cloud groups. Three sphere centers (1, 2, and 10) were used to define a reference plane. New points were defined by projecting each of the sphere centers to the reference plane in a direction normal to the plane (Fig 1.9).

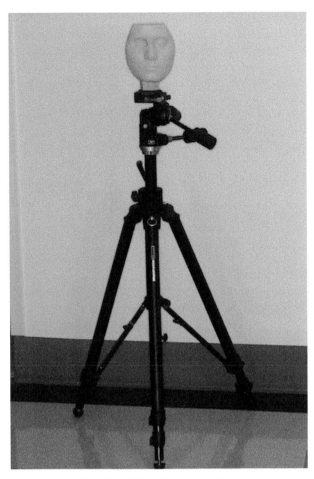

FIGURE 1.3   Tripod assembly.

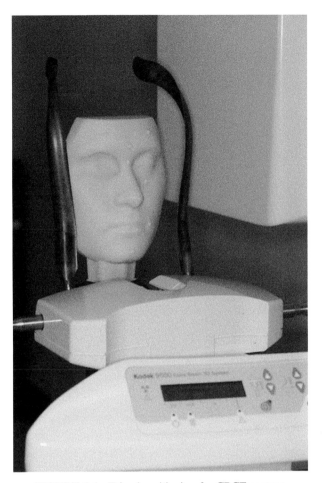

FIGURE 1.4   Tripod positioning for CBCT capture.

Nine projected points were then measured against the projected point #3 on the same model. The following 3D Distance Formula was used where $i = 1, 2, 4, \ldots, 10$ and $j = 3$.

$$\sqrt{(x_i - x_j)^2 + (y_i - y_j)^2 + (z_i - z_j)^2}$$

This procedure was accomplished for each landmark on the CPM model and compared to the same measurements obtained on the facial moulage stone reproductions and the printed models.

Statistical Analysis

Vertical distances from point #3 were analyzed. First, the master distances were averaged over the three raters at each point. Then, for each rater on CBCT (CT), 3D-SPG (OP), and stone (ST) the vertical distance from point #3 was subtracted from the master mean of the three raters and divided by the master mean and multiplied by 100 to obtain a percent difference from the master for each rater and each point of the other three methods. The percent differences were analyzed with ANOVA for repeated measures, since the raters repeatedly measured each point from each of the cast methods.

The three raters were compared, the three methods were compared, and the nine points were compared. Since all distances were relative to point #3, those values were always zero, and that point was not included in the analysis. In addition, the two-way interaction of method and points was analyzed. Interactions with the rater factor were the denominators for the F-tests in the ANOVA for repeated measures. Tukey's comparison was done for pairwise comparisons of means following the ANOVA. Residuals of the ANOVA were calculated and plotted to verify they had a near normal bell-shaped curve and that their variance was similar over the range of predicted values.

RESULTS

The percent difference of each of the three methods (CT, OP, ST) from the control mean relative to point 3 for each method is shown in Figure 1.10. The ANOVA was done and is displayed in Table 1.1. The method (meth) by point (pt)

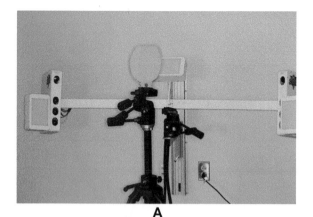

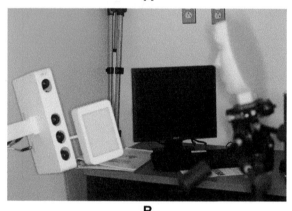

FIGURE 1.5   (A) Tripod positioning of CPM for 3dMD capture. (B) 15° anterior tilt position of CPM.

source was significant. Therefore, a comparison was done with the three methods to the control and each method to each other. Multiple comparisons showed the raters were not different. Pairwise comparisons of the methods were different with OP not having as small a percentage error as the other two methods, while the other two had similar percent error overall (Tables 1.2 and 1.3). Overall, OP showed statistically significant difference ($p < 0.05$) in comparison to the CT and ST; however, Figure 1.10 shows the greatest difference localized to points #1, 2, and 5. The OP data for the other points are similar to the CT and ST findings.

DISCUSSION

The impression technique for making facial models has been used for many years, but a major disadvantage is soft tissue deformation caused by the direct contact of the impression material to the facial soft tissue. Holberg et al reported that making an alginate impression of the face produced between 1 and 3 mm of soft tissue deformation in varying areas.[32] Germec-Cakan et al found significant differences between clinical and facial plaster cast measurements explained by distortion related to the impression material.[12] In this study, the CPM was made from a rigid resin material. When a facial moulage was made of the CPM, there were no signs of deformation, which would normally be seen in a patient. Therefore, the results at each point showed very minimal percentage difference in comparison to the CPM.

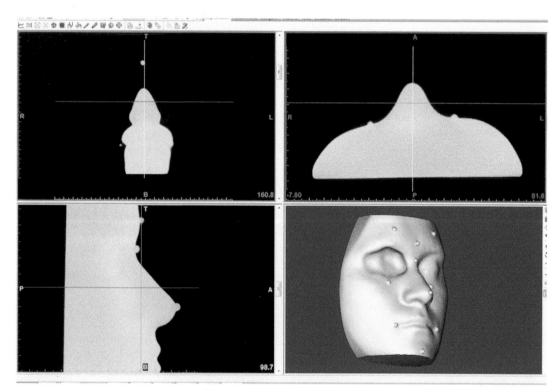

FIGURE 1.6   Mimics DICOM segmentation.

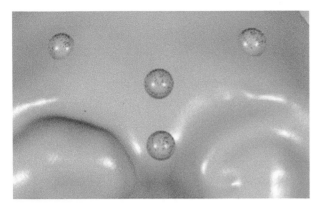

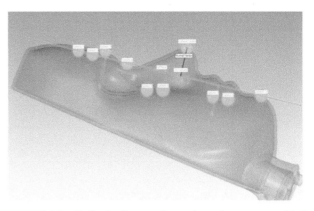

FIGURE 1.9   Defined reference plane using sphere centers of 1, 2, and 10.

Numerous studies have shown that imaging done by CT, and more specifically CBCT, is currently used to capture hard and soft tissue surface images because of its accuracy, reliability, and repeatability for anthropometric measurements.[33–35] Fourie et al compared linear measurements derived from 11 soft tissue landmarks on seven cadaver heads made directly using digital calipers to CBCT-based computer-generated models. Their results showed surface detail of the soft tissue images was insufficient; however, overall, the data proved to be reliable and accurate.[7] Once again, the CPM was a rigid resin form without soft tissue-like surfaces. The results showed that CT data were not significantly different from the CPM measurements and confirmed that CT-generated models were reliable and accurate.

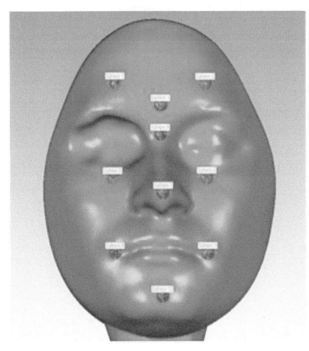

FIGURE 1.8   Point cloud data of spheres 1 to 10.

3D-SPG imaging provides accurate detail of surface texture, contour, and color. Many studies have been done comparing 3D-SPG imaging to direct anthropometry resulting in repeatable, precise, and accurate measurements.[16,36,37] Additional studies by Weinberg et al and Wong et al showed an increase in accuracy and precision of landmark location with labeling prior to image capture.[5,9] In a study done by Plooij et al, midline landmarks were precisely generated compared to pair landmarks, especially if the interlandmark distance increased.[17] In the present study, spherical landmarks were created in the CPM that were reproducible using impression material and the two imaging techniques. Capturing the landmarks was an important factor to calculate the linear measurements and make comparisons of accuracy.

In all of these studies involving CT or 3D-SPG computer-generated images, 3D imaging software was used to calculate linear measurements, which were compared to direct anthropometric measurements. Caliper measurements can be subjective and therefore the accuracy and reliability of the data may be questionable.[38] In the present study, a CMM was used to decrease the subjectivity found in using digital calipers. In Taft et al's study,[39] stainless steel spheres (5.00 ± 0.005 mm in diameter) were secured on a dry cadaver skull in seven locations. Point locations of the spheres were measured by placing the CMM ball probe on the points of interest, thus improving accuracy and reliability. Also, because the spheres were used as fiducial markers, a mean centroid location was identified for each sphere, and the distance between two points was then determined. In this study, a CMM in conjunction with computer software was used to calculate a best-fit sphere for each of the landmarks. There were three raters who collected point cloud data at each sphere, and a rater pairwise comparison showed no significant difference among the raters. The CMM proved to be reliable and accurate in this study.

Both CBCT and 3D-SPG image files can be imported into CAD/CAM software to create an RP model. The accuracy of the RP models have been studied by measuring distances

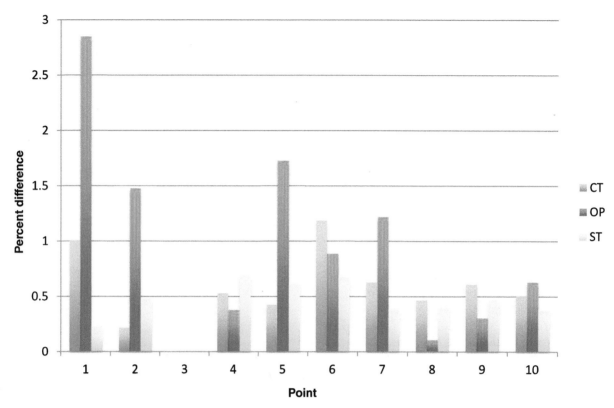

FIGURE 1.10 Percent difference from control mean relative to point 3.

between landmarks on 3D phantom models and comparing those points with measurements calculated through the CT software.[23–25] In this study 3DP models were fabricated using the DICOM images and STL files from the CBCT and 3dMD, respectively; however, instead of using computer software to make the measurements for the CBCT and 3DMD, the CMM was the constant measuring tool for the stone and the 3DP models.

The accuracy of RP models fabricated to replace hard tissue has been studied with skull models and is used in

TABLE 1.1 ANOVA Table for Percent Difference from Master Mean

Source	DF	Sum of Squares	Mean Square	F value	$Pr > F$
Rater	2	0.53050924	0.26525462	1.60	0.2169
Meth	2	5.03638366	2.51819183	59.86	0.0010
Meth × rater	4	0.16827539	0.04206885	0.25	0.9048
Pt	8	7.17435054	0.89679382	5.05	0.0029
Pt × rater	16	2.83916780	0.17744799	1.07	0.4169
Meth × pt	16	13.47849934	0.84240621	5.09	< 0.0001
Residual	32	5.29215010	0.165379691		
Corrected total	80	34.51933608			

TABLE 1.2 Rater Pairwise Comparison: Tukey Comparison

		p-Values	
Rater	Difference Percentage Mean	versus 2	versus 3
1	0.61600732	0.1984	0.4865
2	0.81106176		0.8187
3	0.74416230		

Table 1.3 Method Pairwise Comparison: Tukey Comparison

		p-Values	
Method	Difference Percentage Mean	versus OP	versus ST
CT	0.62195799	0.0030	0.1357
OP	1.06703386		0.0010
ST	0.48223953		

reconstructive craniofacial surgeries.[33,39] However, many craniofacial anomalies also involve the facial soft tissue, requiring accurate dimensional measurements to fabricate prosthetics. Studies have been done using CT scans to create casts from the RP models for facial prosthesis engineering.[40–43] Few studies have evaluated the precise fit of prostheses fabricated from RP models manufactured from soft tissue imaging obtained by 3D-SPG.[18] This investigation was limited because a rigid resin model was used as a control.

According to this investigation, 3DP models fabricated using 3D-SPG showed statistical difference compared to the models fabricated using the traditional method of facial moulage and 3DP models fabricated from CBCT imaging. Major discrepancies stemmed from points #1 and 2 (Fig 1.10). The greater difference of the optical scan point values in comparison to those of the models made from CBCT imaging and facial moulage at the other points may be because a two-pod system was used and the 15° anterior angulation of the control during 3dMD image capture.

Percentage differences of the individual points on all three methods in comparison to the control, points #4, 8, 9, and 10 were not statistically significant differences from the CBCT and stone method. Thus, 3D-SPG is a viable option for RP production of facial models, especially in situations where it is not feasible to use CBCT imaging. Many patients with craniofacial dysmorphologies undergo numerous surgeries in a short period of time, and the 3D-SPG method would eliminate radiation exposure from CT. Additionally, the short image capture time would be extremely beneficial for patients with the inability to be still for the time it takes to make a CBCT. Comparative growth studies could be accomplished using this technology, and if necessary, RP models could be engineered to help with treatment needs. The incorporation of this technology is beneficial for the facial reconstruction process because of its high efficiency, the ability to provide accurate facial surface detail, and the overall treatment planning information obtained for patients. The ability to archive images further helps with the treatment process and analysis of any subsequent changes in the soft tissue.

The 3D-SPD method can also be used in conjunction with CBCT.[44] The accurate hard tissue image obtained from a CBCT can be referenced to a 3D-SPG scan providing detailed images relating the hard tissue with soft tissue for analysis prior to orthognathic surgery. Furthermore, it is difficult to capture an image using 3D-SPG in a defect area where undercuts are present, and the image captured through a CBCT may help define the boundaries of the defect. This merging of hard and soft tissue images can be extremely beneficial in viewing, treatment planning, and fabricating an accurate prosthesis for a craniofacial defect.

In addition, military members suffering from HFNIs present to medical and dental clinics with facial dysmorphologies, such as missing ears, requiring facial prostheses. In the past, these patients required creation of models of the area of deformity by using previous 2D photographs, an impression of family member anatomical replicas, or a prosthesis fabricated by an anaplastologist to replicate the lost tissue. Now, with 3D-SPG and CBCT images, recreation of missing tissue can be accomplished by banked images, images of family members, or even custom-created anatomic forms. Furthermore, images of military members could be obtained and archived prior to entering a military conflict. If the military member should sustain any HFNI, then the archive image can be referenced to create a model in the fabrication of a more accurate facial prosthesis.

Future Directions

There were limitations to this study. First, the CPM was made from a rigid resin material. When a facial moulage was made of the CPM, there were no signs of deformation, which would normally be seen in a patient. Also, a CT image does capture hard tissue detail accurately but lacks in soft tissue detail. 3D-SPG imaging provides a 3D viewing ability to see soft tissue color and texture detail. Therefore, future studies should be done using a patient with a craniofacial defect, and all three methods should be reinvestigated. Also, investigation of five-pod 3D-SPG systems may provide a more accurate 3D image. Finally, it may be beneficial to investigate the accuracy of 3D-SPG in conjunction with CBCT imaging to fabricate facial models.

CONCLUSION

This investigation was based on an innovative research setting creating facial models using a two-pod 3D-SPG imaging system, and a CBCT imaging method, then comparing the accuracy of these models to the traditional facial moulage impression model fabrication technique.

Within the limitations of this investigation, the following conclusions could be made:

1. 3DP models fabricated using 3D-SPG showed statistical difference in comparison to the models fabricated using the traditional method of facial moulage and 3DP models fabricated from CBCT imaging.
2. 3DP models fabricated using 3D-SPG were less accurate in comparison to the CPM and models fabricated using facial moulage and CBCT imaging techniques.
3. Models fabricated using CBCT imaging and facial moulage showed no statistical difference and proved to be accurate in comparison to the CPM.

ACKNOWLEDGMENTS

A special thanks to Mrs. Nancy Hansen, CDT, CCA, BS, and Mr. Alain Carballeyra, BS, for their support.

REFERENCES

1. Merriam-Webster Dictionary. [Internet]. Merriam-Webster, Incorporated; 2013. Dysmorphology; Accurate; Precision. [cited 2013 Feb 10]. Available from: http://www.merriam-webster.com.

2. Eckert SE, Desjardins RP: Prosthetic considerations. In Branemark PI (ed): *Osseointegration in Craniofacial Reconstruction*, Vol 1 (ed 1). Chicago, Quintessence, 1998, pp 87–88.

3. Arridge SR, Moss JP, Linney AD, et al: Three-dimensional digitization of the face and skull. *J Maxillofac Surg* 1985;13:136–143.

4. Posnick JC, Farkas LG: The application of anthropometric surface measurements in craniomaxillofacial surgery. In Farkas LG (ed): *Anthropometry of the Head and Face* (ed 1). New York, Raven Press, 1994; pp 125–138.

5. Weinberg SM, Scott NM, Neiswanger K, et al: Digital three-dimensional photogrammetry: evaluation of anthropometric precision and accuracy using a Genex 3D camera system. *Cleft Palate Craniofac J* 2004;41:507–518.

6. Davis BK: The role of technology in facial prosthetics. *Curr Opin Otolaryngol Head Neck Surg* 2010;18:332–340.

7. Fourie Z, Damstra J, Gerrits PO, et al: Accuracy and repeatability of anthropometric facial measurements using cone beam computed tomography. *Cleft Palate Craniofac J* 2011;48:623–630.

8. Souccar NM, Kau CH: Methods of measuring the three-dimensional face. *Sem Orthod* 2012;18:187–192.

9. Wong JY, Oh AK, Ohta E, et al: Validity and reliability of 3D craniofacial anthropometric measurements. *Cleft Palate Craniofac J* 2008;45:232–239.

10. Alexander C: Faces of war: amid the horrors of World War I, a corps of artists brought hope to soldiers disfigured in the trenches. *Smithsonian Magazine* 2007;37:72.

11. Beumer J, Wolfaardt J, Lee M: *Maxillofacial Rehabilitation (ed 3)*. Hanover Park, IL, Quintessence, 2011, pp. 282–3, 361-3, 391–394.

12. Germec-Cakan D, Canter HI, Nur B, et al: Comparison of facial soft tissue measurements on three-dimensional images and models obtained with different methods. *J Craniofacial Surg* 2010;21:1393–1399.

13. Scarfe WC, Farman AG, Sukovic P: Clinical applications of cone-beam computed tomography in dental practice. *J Can Dent Assoc* 2006;72:75–80.

14. Kau CH, Olim S, Nguyen JT: The future of orthodontic diagnostic records. *Seminar in Orthodontics* 2011;17:39–45.

15. DeVos W, Casselman J, Swennen GR: Cone-beam computerized tomography (CBCT) imaging of the oral and maxillofacial region: a systemic review of the literature. *Int J Oral Maxillofac Sur* 2009;38:609–625.

16. Heike CL, Cunnigham ML, Hing AV, et al: Picture perfect? Reliability of craniofacial anthropometry using three-dimensional digital stereophotogrammetry. *Plast Reconstr Surg* 2009;124:1261–1272.

17. Plooji JM, Swennen GR, Rangel FA, et al: Evaluation of reproducibility and reliability of 3D soft tissue analysis using 3D stereophotogrammetry. *Int J Oral Maxillofac Surg* 2009;38:267–273.

18. Sabol JV, Grant GT, Liacouras P, et al: Digital image capture and rapid prototyping of the maxillofacial defect. *J Prosthodont* 2011;20:310–314.

19. Aldridge K, Boyadjiev SA, Capone GT, et al: Precision and error of three-dimensional phenotypic measures acquired from 3dMD photographic images. *Am J Med Genet A* 2005;138A:247–253.

20. Wade AL, Dye JL, Mohrle CR, et al: Head, face, and, neck injuries during Operation Iraqi Freedom II: results from the US Navy-Marine Corps combat trauma registry. *J Trauma* 2007;63:836–840.

21. Chan RK, Siller-Jackson A, Verrett AJ, et al: Ten years of war: a characterization of craniomaxillofacial injuries incurred during operations Enduring Freedom and Iraqi Freedom. *J Trauma* 2012;73:453–458.

22. Cohen A, Laviv A, Berman P, et al: Mandibular reconstruction using stereolithograpic 3-dimensional printing modeling technology. *Oral Surg Oral Med Oral Path Oral Rad Endo Nov* 2009;105:661–666.

23. Fruhwald J, Schicho K, Figl M, et al: Accuracy of craniofacial measurements: computed tomography and three-dimensional computed tomography compared with stereolithographic models. *J Cranio Surg* 2008;19:22–26.

24. Taylor JS: Influence of computerized tomography parameters on the quality of stereolithographic models. Biomedical Science [thesis]. San Antonio (TX): University of Texas; 1999.

25. Bouma L: The accuracy of non-contact three-dimensional laser surface scanning in the fabrication of facial moulage. Biomedical Science [thesis]. San Antonio (TX): University of Texas; 2003.

26. Jacobson A: *Radiographic Cephalometry; Basics of Videoimaging*. Chicago, Quintessence, 1995.

27. Williams PL, Warwick R, Dyson M, et al: *Gray's Anatomy* (ed 37). New York, Churchill Livingstone, 1989.

28. Shen, C: Impression materials. In Anusavice KJ (ed): *Phillip's Science of Dental Materials* (edn 11). St. Louis, Saunders, 2003, pp 231–248.

29. Clarke CD: *Prosthetics*. Butler, MD, Standard Arts Press, 1965, Ch 3.

30. Khambay B, Naim N, Bell A, et al: Validation and reproducibility of a high resolution three-dimensional facial imaging system. *Br J Oral Maxillofac Surg* 2008;40:27–32.

31. Weinberg SM, Naidoo S, Govier DP, et al: Anthropometric precision and accuracy of digital three-dimensional photogrammetry: comparing the genex and 3dMD imaging systems with one another and with direct anthropometry. *J Craniofac* 2006;17:477–483.

32. Holberg C, Schwenzer K, Mahaini L, et al: Accuracy of facial plaster casts. *Angle Orthod* 2006;76:605–611.

33. Damstra J, Fourie Z, Huddleston Slater JJR, et al: Accuracy of linear measurements from cone beam computed tomography derived surface models of different voxel sizes. *Am J Orthod Dentofacial Orthop* 2010;137:16.el–16.e6.

34. Stratemann SA, Huang JC, Maki K, et al: Comparison of cone beam computed tomography imaging with physical measures. *Dentomaxillofac Radiol* 2008;37:80–93.

35. Mischkowski R, Reinhard P, Lutz R, et al: Geometric accuracy of a newly developed cone beam device for maxillofacial imaging. *Oral Surg Oral Med Oral Path Oral Rad Endo* 2007;104:551–559.

36. Ghoddousi H, Edler R, Haers P, et al: Comparison of three methods of facial measurement. *Int J Oral Maxillofac Surg* 2007;36:250–258.

37. Lubbers HT, Medinger L, Kruse A, et al: Precision and accuracy of the 3dMD photogrammetric system in craniomaxillofacial application. *J Craniofac Surg* 2010;21:763–767.

38. Jamali AA, Deuel C, Perreira A, et al: Linear and angular measurements of computer generated models: are the accurate, valid, and reliable? *Comput Aided Surg* 2007;12:278–285.

39. Taft RM, Kondor S, Grant GT: Accuracy of Rapid Prototype models for head and neck reconstruction. *J Prosthet Dent* 2011;106:399–408.

40. Esses SJ, Berman P, Bloom A, et al: Clinical applications of physical 3D models derived from MDCT data and created by rapid prototyping. *AJR Am J Roentgenol* 2011;196:683–688.

41. Karayazgan-Saracoglu B, Gunay Y, Atay A: Fabrication of an auricular prosthesis using computed tomography and rapid prototyping technique. *J Craniofac Surg* 2009;20:1169–1172.

42. Turgut G, Sacak, KK, et al: Use of rapid prototyping in prosthetic auricular restoration. *J Craniofac Surg* 2009;20:321–325.

43. Marafon PG, Mattos BS, Saboia AC, et al: Dimensional accuracy of computer-aided design/computer-assisted manufactured orbital prostheses. *Int J Prosthodont* 2010;23:271–276.

44. Maal TJ, Plooji JM, Rangel FA, et al: The accuracy of matching three-dimensional photographs with skin surfaces derived from cone-beam computed tomography. *Int J Oral Maxillofac Surg* 2008;37:641–646.

2

INNOVATIVE APPROACH FOR INTERIM FACIAL PROSTHESIS USING DIGITAL TECHNOLOGY

FUMI YOSHIOKA, DDS, PHD,[1] SHOGO OZAWA, DDS, PHD,[1] IKUO HYODO, MD,[2] AND
YOSHINOBU TANAKA, DDS, PHD[1]

[1]*Department of Removable Prosthodontics, School of Dentistry, Aichi Gakuin University, Nagoya, Japan*
[2]*Department of Plastic and Reconstructive Surgery, Aichi Cancer Center, Nagoya, Japan*

Keywords
Facial prosthesis; interim prosthesis; rapid prototyping; magnetic attachment; surgical prosthesis.

Correspondence
Fumi Yoshioka, 2-11 Suemoridori, Chikusa-ku, Nagoya, Aichi, 4648651, Japan. E-mail: fumi@dpc.agu.ac.jp

Supported by the Hori Sciences and Arts Foundation.

Presented at the Advanced Digital Technology in Head and Neck Reconstruction, 4th International Conference, May 2012; Freiburg, Germany.

The authors deny any conflicts of interest.

Accepted February 20, 2015

Published in *Journal of Prosthodontics* August 2015

doi: 10.1111/jopr.12338

ABSTRACT

Despite the important role of facial prosthetic treatment in the rehabilitation of head and neck cancer patients, delay in its implementation can be unavoidable, preventing patients from receiving a prompt facial prosthesis and resuming a normal social life. Here, we introduce an innovative method for the fabrication of an interim facial prosthesis. Using a 3D modeling system, we simplified the fabrication method and used a titanium reconstruction plate for facial prosthesis retention. The patient received the facial prosthesis immediately after surgery and resumed a normal social life earlier than is typically observed with conventional facial prosthetic treatment.

A facial prosthesis is a treatment option for repairing facial defects in head and neck cancer patients. Following surgery, facial prosthesis fabrication is often delayed due to a number

of factors. For one, patients are not referred to a prosthodontist until the surgeon has confirmed that the surgical site has completely healed with no tumor recurrence. In addition, prosthodontists do not initiate treatment until the wound has completely healed, as modification of silicone material is difficult once it has cured; however, physicians should carefully consider the psychological impact following loss of part of the face, even in the wound-healing period.[1]

Facial prosthesis fabrication via the conventional method consists of many steps, as follows: making an impression, building a wax sculpture for the missing structure, converting it into silicone material, and matching intrinsic and extrinsic coloration with the skin. To reduce the time required to construct a prosthesis, a rapid prototyping (RP) system has been applied to prosthodontic treatment[2] and facial prosthesis fabrication.[3–7] We applied a 3D digitizer and RP system to the fabrication of orbital prostheses[7] and found that treatment time was markedly reduced.

This new, rapid system has since been used for the simple fabrication of facial prostheses,[8] supporting the potential to deliver facial prostheses immediately after surgery to repair the facial defect and decrease the psychological depression of patients. Here, we introduce an innovative method for the immediate fabrication of facial prostheses using a 3D RP system.

CLINICAL REPORT

A 44-year-old woman with nasal cancer was scheduled to undergo a rhinectomy. The histopathologic nature was squamous cell carcinoma. Induction or adjuvant chemotherapy or radiotherapy was not planned. On surgical planning, however, nasal reconstructive surgery was deemed insufficient by the plastic surgeon. The patient was therefore referred to a maxillofacial prosthodontist as a candidate for prosthodontic

treatment in combination with lip reconstruction surgery. The patient was informed that the resected area would be extended to the external nose, upper lip, and bilateral maxilla on presurgical planning. A combination of myocutaneous forearm free-flap reconstruction and facial prosthesis of the upper lip and nose was planned for the midfacial defect. A titanium reconstruction plate (UCMF primary reconstruction plate; Stryker Corp., Kalamazoo, MI) was designed for the retention of an interim nasal prosthesis.

Presurgical Consult and Data Acquisition

Before surgery, a digital image was acquired using a 3D digitizer (Rexcan 3; Solutionix Co., Seoul, South Korea). This 3D digitizer consisted of an industrial 3D scanner using phase-shifting optical triangulation and CCD twin-camera technology, and enabled 3D data to be acquired within a short duration (2 seconds) and purported excellent accuracy (± 0.001 mm). Computed tomography (CT) data for the diagnosis were used for data establishment. Both sets of digital data were converted into STL format and aligned using 3D transforming software (Geomagic Studio; Geomagic, Morrisville, NC; Fig 2.1). The surgeon then estimated the ablation site by referencing CT data, prosthodontists designed a virtual prosthesis with reference to scanned data, and CT data were aligned using CAD software (Free-Form Modeling; Sensable, Wilmington, MA; Fig 2.2). A facial model combined with the designed prosthesis was manufactured with dental stone (New Plastone 2; GC Corp., Tokyo, Japan) using a 3D milling machine (MDX-40; Roland DG, Shizuoka-ken, Japan). A surgical template made from a formed thermoplastic polyethylene terephthalate glycol plate (Erkodur; Erkodent, Pfalzgrafenweiler,

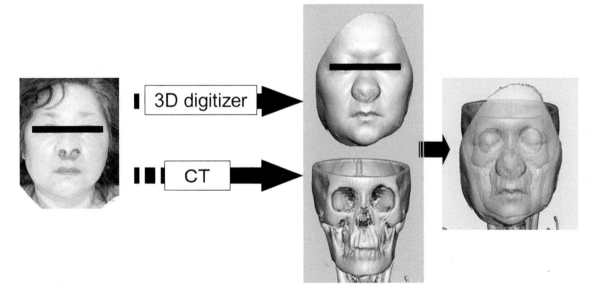

FIGURE 2.1   Schema of 3D image establishment. Scanned surface data and CT data were aligned.

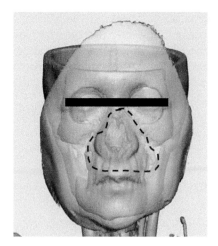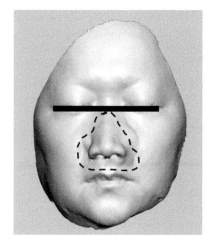

FIGURE 2.2   Estimated resected site and designed virtual facial prosthesis in place (perforated line).

Germany) was fabricated using a vacuum-forming machine (Erkopress; Erkodent; Fig 2.3).

During surgical reconstruction, the titanium reconstruction plate was bent and inserted at an appropriate position, where the retentive force of the prosthesis is most effective, and the plate would not disturb the morphology of the prosthesis. The surgical template was used to determine the position by referring to presurgical planning (Fig 2.4), and the plate was fixed on the anterior wall of the maxilla. The template was also used as reference to position the forearm flap.

Postsurgical Data Acquisition and Fabrication of Facial Prosthesis

Following surgery, another digital image was acquired using the 3D digitizer, and a postoperative facial mold was manufactured using the 3D milling machine (Fig 2.5). A postoperative template made of formed thermoplastic polymethylmethacrylate (PMMA) plate was fabricated using the vacuum-forming machine. Pre- and postsurgical templates were combined to make the substructure of the prosthesis. The outer side of the substructure was then covered

with a thin layer of wax to represent skin color and texture (Fig 2.6). Skin-colored wax was used for sculpting, which is better and easier for us and the patient to capture the form of the prosthesis during sculpting when tried in.

The prototype was invested, and a silicone adhesive was applied to the surface of the substructure. The wax surface was converted into intrinsically colored silicone material (A2186F; Factor II, Lakeside, AZ). Following polymerization, the facial prosthesis was removed from the mold and tried on the patient. Magnetic keepers (Gigauss D800; GC Corp.) were attached to the titanium reconstruction plate (Fig 2.7), and magnetic assemblies were fixed onto the inner side of the prosthesis using self-cured resin. In this case, it took a week for initial wound healing when the resected area had been covered with the gauze. One week after surgery, an interim facial prosthesis was delivered to the patient, and the fit and orientation to the adjacent tissue as well as the retention were assessed (Fig 2.8). The side of the prosthesis facing the tissue was made of a thin plastic plate to enable modification using self-curing resin to adapt to wound healing. The outer side of the prosthesis was constructed from silicone material to represent skin color and texture. The patient was instructed to clean the plate with swabs,

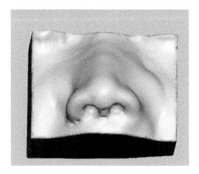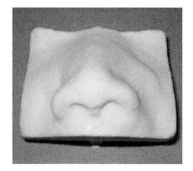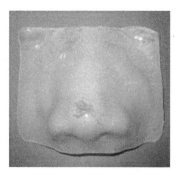

FIGURE 2.3   Planned and manufactured models (left and center) and fabricated surgical template.

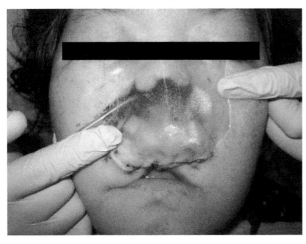

FIGURE 2.4   The surgical template in place during surgery.

particularly in the area between skin and plate, and no inflammation was shown. She left the hospital 3 weeks after surgery with the prosthesis. It was used for about 6 months, until the surgical site was completely healed and ready for the final prosthesis.

DISCUSSION

Our newly developed system used an industrial noncontact 3D scanner consisting of phase-shifting optical triangulation and CCD twin-camera technology enabling us to easily acquire precise 3D curvature via the computer. In this case, optical facial impression of the nasal area was made with the 3D scanner, though it could be sensitive before and after surgery. In combination with CT data, the surgeon and

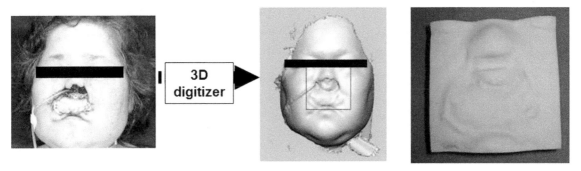

FIGURE 2.5   Postsurgical scanned data and postsurgical template.

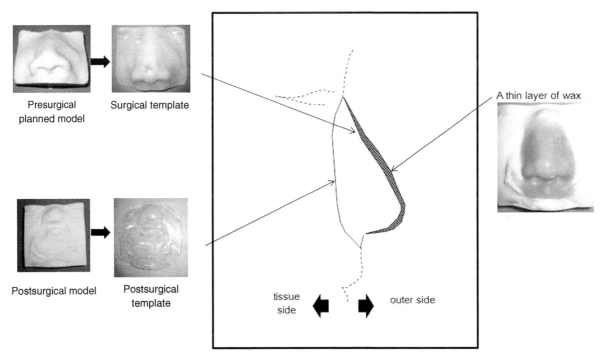

FIGURE 2.6   Schema of the substructure of the wax prototype for the interim facial prosthesis. Two templates were combined, and outer side was covered with a thin layer of wax.

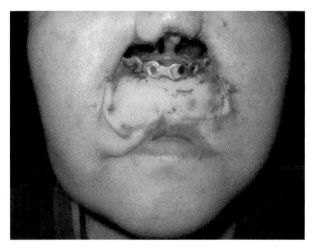

FIGURE 2.7 Magnetic attachments attached to the titanium plate.

prosthodontists were able to acquire the defected facial image and discuss postsurgical rehabilitation, including postsurgical appearance.

Presurgical planning using computer technology has become increasingly common in the dental and medical fields and may prove useful in a team approach. In this case, the surgeon and prosthodontists had the opportunity to consult each other concerning surgical planning and postsurgical rehabilitation using 3D facial and CT data. The surgeon was able to obtain the final image for rehabilitation during surgery, and the prosthodontist was able to convey the necessity for the construction of a retaining structure for the interim facial prosthesis.

The facial prosthesis was easily designed using CAD software referring to the presurgical data. It saved time as compared to the conventional way to fabricate facial prostheses using CAD software. In this case, the prosthesis framework was fabricated with PMMA plate, so the modification using self-curing resin could be achieved during wound healing, and the weight of the prosthesis became light. An outer-side layer of silicone represented skin color and texture.

Facial prosthesis retention is commonly achieved via adhesives, mechanical retention, anatomical retention, or implants.[9] However, during the wound-healing period of an interim facial prosthesis, the skin surrounding the defected area should not be irritated by adhesives or mechanical stimulus. Furthermore, the craniofacial implant should be inserted simultaneously or delayed until after tumor resection.[10] In both cases, a period of rest until secondary surgery has historically been necessary for osseointegration, and implant retention should not be applied to interim facial prostheses. In this study, a titanium reconstruction plate and magnetic attachment were used to achieve facial prosthesis retention. The Ti reconstruction plate was screwed to the anterior wall of the maxilla, and magnetic attachments were fixed using self-curing resin.

CONCLUSION

In this study, the patient received the interim facial prosthesis immediately after surgery using digital technology and resumed her social life earlier than is typically observed with conventional treatment.

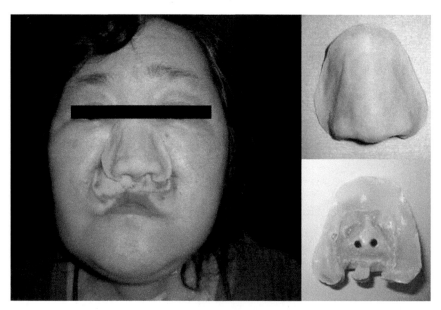

FIGURE 2.8 Delivery of interim facial prosthesis to the patient.

REFERENCES

1. Kapp-Simon KA: Psychological approaches to patient management. In McKinstry RE (ed): *Fundamentals of Facial Prosthetics*, Vol. 1 (ed 2). Arlington, VA, ABI Professional, 1995, pp. 1–3.

2. Strub JR, Rekow ED, Witkowski S: Computer-aided design and fabrication of dental restorations: current systems and future possibilities. *J Am Dent Assoc* 2006;137:1289–1296.

3. Ciocca L, Mingucci R, Gassino G, et al: CAD/CAM ear model and virtual construction of the mold. *J Prosthet Dent* 2007;98:339–343.

4. Westermark A, Zachow S, Eppley BL: Three-dimensional osteotomy planning in maxillofacial surgery including soft tissue prediction. *J Craniofac Surg* 2005;16:100–104.

5. Jiao T, Zhang F, Huang X, et al: Design and fabrication of auricular prostheses by CAD/CAM system. *Int J Prosthodont* 2004;17:460–463.

6. Coward TJ, Scott BJ, Watson RM, et al: Comparison between computerized tomography, magnetic resonance imaging, and laser scanning for capturing 3-dimensional data from an object of standard form. *Int J Prosthodont* 2005;18:405–413.

7. Yoshioka F, Ozawa S, Okazaki S, et al: Fabrication of an orbital prosthesis using a noncontact three-dimensional digitizer and rapid-prototyping system. *J Prosthodont* 2010;19:598–600.

8. Ariani S, Visser A, vanOort RP, et al: Current state of craniofacial prosthetic rehabilitation. *Int J Prosthodont* 2013;26:57–67.

9. McKinstry RE: Retention and facial prostheses. In McKinstry RE (ed): *Fundamentals of Facial Prosthetics*, Vol 1 (ed 2). Arlington, VA, ABI Professional Publications, 1995, pp. 19–30.

10. Karakoca S, Aydin C, Yilmaz H, et al: Retrospective study of treatment outcomes with implant-retained extraoral prostheses: survival rates and prosthetic complications. *J Prosthet Dent* 2010;103:118–126.

3

UPDATES ON THE CONSTRUCTION OF AN EYEGLASS-SUPPORTED NASAL PROSTHESIS USING COMPUTER-AIDED DESIGN AND RAPID PROTOTYPING TECHNOLOGY

Leonardo Ciocca, dds, phd,[1] Achille Tarsitano, md,[2] Claudio Marchetti, dmd, dds,[3] and Roberto Scotti, dmd, dds[4]

[1]Section of Prosthodontics, Department of Biomedical and Neuromotor Science, Alma Mater Studiorum University of Bologna, Bologna, Italy
[2]Maxillofacial Surgery Unit, S. Orsola-Malpighi Hospital, Department of Biomedical and Neuromotor Science, Alma Mater Studiorum University of Bologna, Bologna, Italy
[3]Alma Mater Studiorum University of Bologna, Bologna, Italy
[4]Department of Biomedical and Neuromotor Science, Alma Mater Studiorum University of Bologna, Bologna, Italy

Keywords
Maxillofacial prosthodontics.

Correspondence
Leonardo Ciocca, Via S. Vitale 59, 40125 Bologna, Italy.
E-mail: leonardo.ciocca@unibo.it

The authors deny any conflicts of interest.

Accepted April 11, 2015

Published in *Journal of Prosthodontics* August 2015

doi: 10.1111/jopr.12332

ABSTRACT

This study was undertaken to design an updated connection system for an eyeglass-supported nasal prosthesis using rapid prototyping techniques. The substructure was developed with two main endpoints in mind: the connection to the silicone and the connection to the eyeglasses. The mold design was also updated; the mold was composed of various parts, each carefully designed to allow for easy release after silicone processing and to facilitate extraction of the prosthesis without any strain. The approach used in this study enabled perfect transfer of the reciprocal position of the prosthesis with respect to the eyeglasses, from the virtual to the clinical environment. Moreover, the reduction in thickness improved the flexibility of the prosthesis and promoted adaptation to the contours of the skin, even during functional movements. The method described here is a simplified and viable alternative to standard construction techniques for nasal prostheses and offers improved esthetic and functional results when no bone is available for implant-supported prostheses.

Nasal prostheses represent a viable option for patients after rhinectomy when surgical reconstruction cannot be performed due to the size of the residual defect. Two alternatives to support a nasal prosthesis exist: a craniofacial implant and eyeglasses.[1–4] In the past, adhesive prostheses were widely used for small nasal defects; however, at this time, an adhesive prosthesis may not be considered a suitable solution for patients, given the risk of skin reactions and decay of the adhesion during use. Implant- and eyeglass-supported prostheses have specific indications related to the available quality and quantity of bone for inserting a craniofacial implant (i.e., tumor recurrence potential and esthetic demands). If bone is present in the glabella and the premaxilla, implants should be used to secure the nasal prosthesis to the face without any other mechanical support, giving the patient a good restorative result in terms of esthetic and social demands.[5] However, if no anchoring implant can be inserted, an eyeglass-supported prosthesis is indicated to restore the contour of the face (Fig 3.1). Many approaches have been presented over the last two decades for creating a convenient and secure connection between eyeglasses and a nasal prosthesis.[6–10] Modern computer-aided design and computer-aided manufacturing (CAD/CAM) technology has facilitated customized clinical solutions, including a simplified connection between the substructure and eyeglasses. Recently, Ciocca and Scotti[11] proposed that an oculo-facial prosthesis be secured to eyeglasses using CAD/CAM and rapid prototyped (RP) scaffold construction. The prosthesis was anchored to eyeglasses by means of strategic arms that enveloped the frame, thus connecting the volume of the oculo-facial prosthesis to the right lens frame and lateral shaft of the eyeglasses. The method also used the substructure to support the ocular bulb of the facial prosthesis.

The aim of this study was to use CAD/CAM technology to improve and simplify the protocol for constructing the connection system of an eyeglass-mounted nasal prosthesis. A sample case was used to document the procedure used for all patients scheduled for a nasal prosthesis when no surgical nasal reconstruction is possible and no craniofacial implant can be inserted.

UPDATED CONSTRUCTION TECHNIQUE

The technique used to design and produce the prototype of the eyeglass-supported nasal prosthesis had steps similar to a previous study.[8] Briefly, a digital impression of the entire face was made using a 3D laser scanner (3dMDface System; 3dMD Ltd., London, UK) to analyze the complete defect with all undercuts and the upper anterior part of the auricular region, where the eyeglasses rest on the ears. The use of this scanner was the first update: this scanner uses a noninvasive

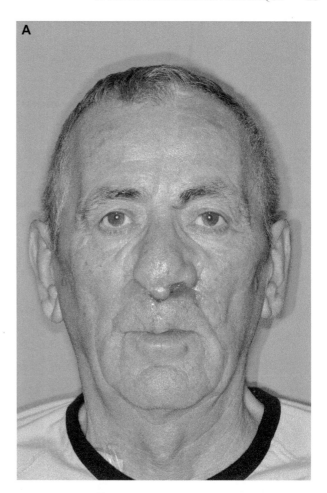

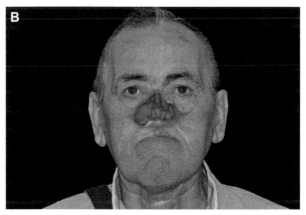

FIGURE 3.1 Before (A) and after (B) rhinectomy appearance of the patient.

imaging technique and allows a 180° image to be captured (ear to ear) with a capture speed of about 1.5 ms at high resolution; thus, the patient has no difficulty maintaining a single facial expression during scanning. The scanning system generated a geometry of one continuous point cloud from the two stereo camera viewpoints, thereby eliminating the

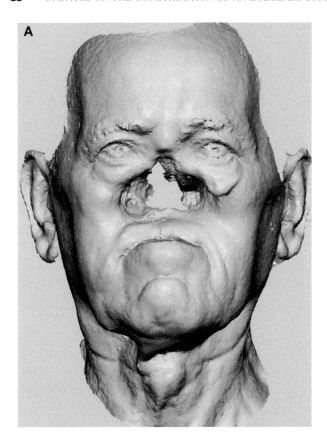

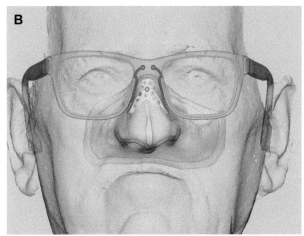

FIGURE 3.2   CAD projection.

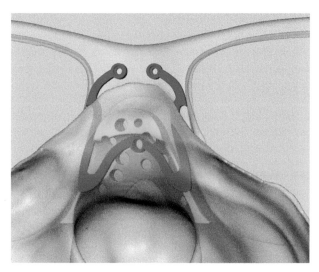

FIGURE 3.3   Design of the substructure and retentive system.

solution was achieved virtually, the digitized eyeglasses were superimposed using the ClayTools system (Freeform Modeling Plus software and Phantom Desktop Haptic device; Sensable, Wilmington, MA) (Fig 3.3). For optimal virtual eyeglass positioning, it was necessary to print a resin model of the final nasal prosthesis for trying on the patient. The position was recorded using impression material (Occlu-fast CAD-CAM; Zhermack, Badia Polesine, Italy); after positioning the resin model in the facial defect, the eyeglasses were leaned in place on the resin try-in prosthesis. The reciprocal position of eyeglasses and prosthesis was registered in the glabella using the silicone impression material. The silicone position check was scanned to generate an STL file so that the informatics technician could superimpose the eyeglasses onto the nasal prosthesis in the correct clinical position.[8]

Framework and Substructure Design

The main update regarded the procedure used to design the substructure. It was developed with two main endpoints in mind: (1) the connection to the silicone and (2) the connection to the eyeglasses. The first endpoint was obtained by means of a framework of polyamide resin that allowed for mechanical engagement of the silicone prosthesis to the inner holes of the framework. The design of the resin framework presented 1.2 to 2.0 mm diameter holes and a precise slot for the metal framework. The second endpoint was achieved using a laser-melted cobalt-chrome framework to engage both the eyeglasses and the polyamide substructure. This metal framework was designed to screw into the back of the interocular eyeglass frame so as to be invisible from the front. It was conceived for sustaining the main supportive forces and for this reason was prototyped

errors associated with merging/stitching datasets together (Fig 3.2). After the eyeglasses were scanned too, two standard triangulation language (STL) files (face and eyeglasses) were generated. To better reconstruct the nose of the patient, the digital ear and nose library may not be used if a preoperative face scan exists, or if a model (e.g., the patient's son) is available. The nasal anatomy may be copied from one of these sources to duplicate the missing facial volume and integrate it onto the patient's face. Once the STL files of the patient and model were integrated, and a good esthetic

in metal. Both components were produced using an RP machine (Eosint P100 Formiga; Electro Optical Systems GmbH, Munich, Germany).

Mold Design

The mold design represents an updated version of a protocol described previously.[8] This update consists of the diverse parts that composed the mold, each of which was carefully

designed to allow for easy release after silicone processing and to facilitate extraction of the prosthesis without any strain. The main body (Fig 3.4A) of the mold was designed in two parts: the front and the back. The front was composed of two pieces (Fig 3.4E), the minor one for the nostrils in order to create open breathing channels (Fig 3.4F). The component visible in Figure 3.4E had to be removed first, so that the rear part of the nostrils could be disengaged during removal of the prosthesis. The back of the mold was

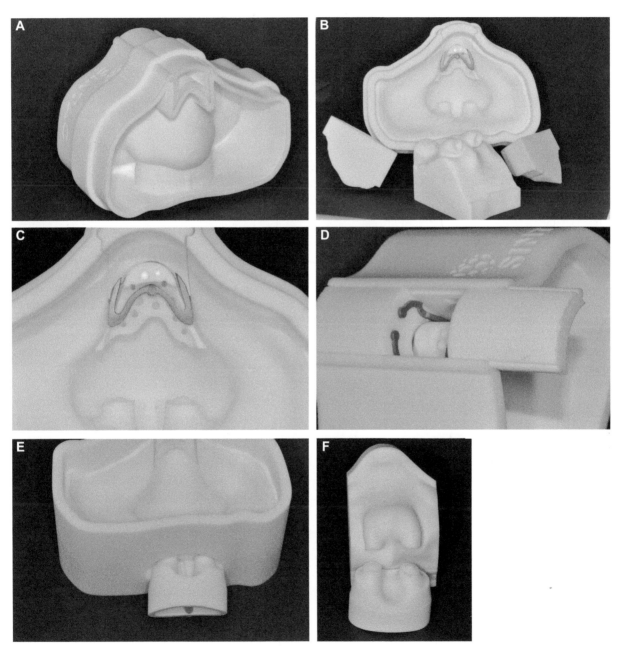

FIGURE 3.4   RP of the mold: (A) the assembled mold; (B) the three parts of the back portion; (C) the resin and the metal framework in position; (D) the two-piece securing system; (E) anterior mold component for nostrils; and (F) the two components for the nostril holes.

composed of three parts (Fig 3.4B) in such a way that the lateral parts could be extracted first, allowing for removal of the residual central component with little force. Thus, the central part was easily removed.

Also, the retaining system was an update of previous techniques. It was designed to stabilize the substructure and metal framework at the inner mold during silicone processing. It was necessary to secure the metal framework in exactly the virtually planned position with respect to the substructure and the prosthesis. Thus, two sliding slot slices (Figs 3.4C and 3.4D) were created to secure the framework and substructure during molding. This is a fundamental innovative point because during silicone processing, high hydrostatic pressure is developed when the mold is pressed in the vise, and the substructure and metal framework can be consequently dislodged in the wrong position. This would, in turn, result in incongruent eyeglass-prosthesis malposition.

DISCUSSION

The main outcome of this updated procedure for connecting a nasal prosthesis to eyeglasses was the perfect transfer of the position in the virtual environment to the actual prosthesis after molding. This connection system will simplify previous technological solutions, making it possible to position two securing screws straight in the eyeglass interocular frame without the use of other components.[10]

A secondary result was the reduction in prosthesis weight, which was obtained by reducing the thickness by 1.7 mm in the facial part of the prosthesis. This made the facial portion of the prosthesis surface extremely flexible and similar to the consistency of natural skin when touched. This flexible portion will make it possible for the prosthesis to follow facial movements during mastication, speaking, and smiling.

New CAD/CAM technologies have led to improved approaches for the construction of nasal prostheses. In the last decade,[6–10] scientists have reported the automation of impression making for nasal prostheses and diagnostic wax-up, substructure design by CAD and printing by means of RP machines, try-in automation and the elimination of stone molds, and optimized surface roughness due to changes in the surface of the prototyped mold. When a nasal prosthesis has to be stabilized in place through mechanical support (e.g., eyeglasses) rather than implants, long-term follow-up of the connection system is very important. The main features of this connection should be esthetic invisibility and sufficient mechanical support for the prosthesis during function. In this protocol, a novel substructure design for a metal framework and the connection for a nasal prosthesis were created for patients in whom no craniofacial implant could be used.

To obtain good esthetic results, two challenges had to be overcome: the design of the connection system itself and its positioning in the mold prototype. The connection was designed in two parts, one for engaging the silicone (polyamide resin framework) and one for securing the prosthesis to the eyeglasses and the resin framework (laser-melted metal structure). The polyamide resin structure was designed as a 1.5- to 2.0-mm network for mechanical retention of the silicone and engagement to the metal framework to ensure optimal distribution of the loading force between the prosthesis and eyeglasses. To ensure sufficient mechanical support, the metal framework possesses two screw holes for retention on the eyeglass frame. In the mold, it is positioned by means of a female slot to guarantee the correct location; in the eyeglasses, it is positioned using the precise engagement with the frame. The effect of the screws on stabilization is augmented by their duplicity (two screws), making rotation impossible.

A novel system for molding is hereby proposed. As shown in Figures 3.4C and 3.4D, a special system for recombining the sliding parts of the mold was constructed not only to ensure the correct position but also to secure the resin/metal connection during silicone processing. Indeed, without constructing a two-piece securing system (Fig 3.4D), the resin/metal connection system may shift during compression when the silicone is poured into the mold. These two sliding pistons guarantee secure engagement of the connection system in the required position due to their precise dimensions with respect to the external margin of the mold. In this way, when the mold is compressed between the two parallel planes of the vise (top and bottom), the sliding components cannot shift and remain in position.

A minor feature of this updated method is the reduction in thickness of the prosthesis. This influences the weight and peripheral margin flexibility of the silicone, allowing for optimal adaptation to the skin during physiologic functions (e.g., swallowing, speaking, and smiling). This adaptive effect is a side product of the mold design. As described by Ciocca et al,[12] the 1.5-cm marginal area of the prosthesis is CAD-modeled with a light depression (5–8 mm) toward the virtual face volume along the contact prosthesis profile with the skin. The thinness of the silicone at the periphery and the artificial depression allow for the adaptive effect during physiological function, due to the creation of flexible and compressive margins. Moreover, the reduced thickness of the entire prosthesis (apart from the nasal pyramid) confers a natural consistency to the prosthesis that mimics natural skin, and which patients usually enjoy (Fig 3.5). The cost of this procedure was €1200 and the working hours for the CAD technician were 34.

Limitations of this technique may be the final esthetic result, due to the use of eyeglasses and to the difficulty obtaining a correct profile when a large part of the premaxilla was ablated during cancer surgery. The upper lip, as presented here, may be withdrawn, resulting in a nose in disharmony with the lower portion of the face; however, even if only a partial restoration of the esthetics may be

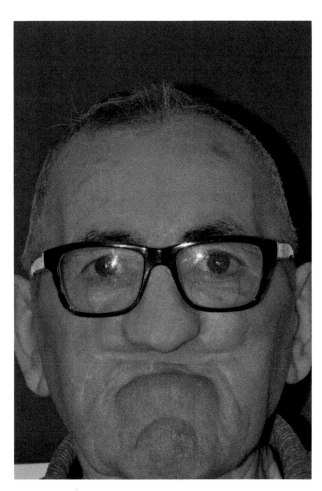

FIGURE 3.5 Extrinsic coloring and delivery.

obtained, the patient is no longer obliged to wear a bandage to cover the defect and can wear his therapeutic eyeglasses.

CONCLUSIONS

The updated CAD/CAM technique used in this study to construct a novel engagement system for eyeglass-mounted nasal prostheses allows for simplification of the design and esthetic improvement with respect to previous techniques, and it may represent a viable protocol for patients in whom no bone is available for craniofacial implants to support a nasal prosthesis.

ACKNOWLEDGMENT

The authors thank Dr. Andrea Sandi (Sintac srl, Trento, Italy) for his valuable work in the CAD design and in the rapid prototyping of the mold and substructure.

REFERENCES

1. Ugadama A, King GE: Mechanically retained facial prostheses: helpful or harmful? *J Prosthet Dent* 1983;49:85–86.
2. Parel SM, Branemark P, Tjellstrom A, et al: Osseointegration in maxillofacial prosthetics. Part II: extraoral applications. *J Prosthet Dent* 1986;55:600–606.
3. Dumbrigue HB, Flyer A: Minimizing prosthesis movement in a midfacial defect: a clinical report. *J Prosthet Dent* 1997;78:341–345.
4. Flood TR, Russell K: Reconstruction of nasal defects with implant-retained nasal prosthesis. *Br J Oral Maxillofac Surg* 1998;36:341–345.
5. Goiato MC, Delben JA, Monteiro DR, et al: Retention systems to implant-supported craniofacial prostheses. *J Craniofac Surg* 2009;20:889–891.
6. Karakoca S, Ersu B: Attaching a midfacial prosthesis to eyeglass frames using a precision attachment. *J Prosthet Dent* 2009;102:264–265.
7. Ciocca L, Fantini M, De Crescenzio F, et al: New protocol for construction of eyeglasses-supported provisional nasal prosthesis using CAD/CAM techniques. *J Rehabil Res Dev* 2010;47:595–604.
8. Ciocca L, Fantini M, Marchetti C, et al: Immediate facial rehabilitation in cancer patients using CAD-CAM and rapid prototyping technology: a pilot study. *Support Care Cancer* 2010;18:723–728.
9. Ciocca L, Bacci G, Mingucci R, et al: CAD-CAM construction of a provisional nasal prosthesis after ablative tumour surgery of the nose: a pilot case report. *Eur J Cancer Care (Engl)* 2009;18:97–101.
10. Ciocca L, Maremonti P, Bianchi B, et al: Maxillofacial rehabilitation after rhinectomy using two different treatment options: clinical reports. *J Oral Rehabil* 2007;34:311–315.
11. Ciocca L, Scotti R: Oculo-facial rehabilitation after facial cancer removal: updated CAD/CAM procedures. A pilot study. *Prosthet Orthot Int* 2014;38:505–509.
12. Ciocca L, De Crescenzio F, Fantini M, et al: CAD/CAM bilateral ear prostheses construction for Treacher Collins syndrome patients using laser scanning and rapid prototyping. *Comput Methods Biomech Biomed Engin* 2010;13:379–386.

4

OCULAR DEFECT REHABILITATION USING PHOTOGRAPHY AND DIGITAL IMAGING: A CLINICAL REPORT

Muaiyed M. Buzayan, bds, mclindent,[1] Yusnidar T. Ariffin, bds, msc,[2] Norsiah Yunus, bds, msc,[2] and Wan Adida Azina Binti Mahmood, bds, mdsc[2]

[1]Department of Prosthodontics, Faculty of Dentistry, University of Tripoli, Tripoli, Libya
[2]Department of Prosthetic Dentistry, Faculty of Dentistry, University of Malaya, Kuala Lumpur, Malaysia

Keywords
Custom-made ocular prosthesis; photographic iris; digital imaging; digital photography.

Correspondence
Muaiyed M. Buzayan, Department of Prosthodontics, Faculty of Dentistry, University of Tripoli, Tripoli, Libya.
E-mail: Muaiyed_zyan@hotmail.com

The authors deny any conflicts of interest.

Accepted May 25, 2014

Published in *Journal of Prosthodontics* August 2015; Vol. 24, Issue 6

doi: 10.1111/jopr.12235

ABSTRACT

Ocular disorders occasionally necessitate surgical intervention that may lead to eye defects. The primary objective in restoring and rehabilitating such defects with an ocular prosthesis is to enable patients to cope better with associated psychological stress and to return to their accustomed lifestyle. A series of detailed steps for custom-made ocular prosthesis fabrication using the advantages of digital photography to replace the conventional oil paint and monopoly iris painting technique are presented in this article. In the present case, a digital photograph of the patient's iris was captured using a digital camera and manipulated on a computer using graphic software to produce a replica of the natural iris. The described technique reduces treatment time, increases simplicity, and permits the patient's natural iris to be replicated without the need for iris painting and special artistic skills.

Loss of an eye can be caused by a congenital anomaly, trauma, tumor, or even the need for histological confirmation of a suspected diagnosis.[1] The resultant facial disfigurement can cause significant physical, emotional, and psychological consequences. The rehabilitation of a patient suffering such loss requires an ocular prosthesis. The primary purpose of any ocular prosthetic rehabilitation is to regain eye socket volume and produce the illusion of a normal healthy eye and surrounding tissues.[2]

Artificial eyes consist of two components.[2] The first is the orbital implant, which should be placed at the time of the enucleation or evisceration and fills the eye socket. Orbital implants can be fabricated from silicone, hydroxyapatite, and porous polyethylene.[3] The second component of the artificial eye is the ocular prosthesis. It is placed between the eyelids and the orbital implant. This component makes the artificial eye appear lifelike, is inserted 6 to 8 weeks postenucleation/evisceration, and can be either a stock or custom-made prostheses made from either methyl methacrylate (MMA) or glass.[4–8] The fabrication of a custom-made acrylic resin eye provides more esthetic and precise results than a stock eye. In the custom-made eye technique, the prosthesis is advantageous, as the adaptation to underlying tissues is improved, mobility of the prosthesis increased, and esthetics enhanced. On the other hand, a custom-made ocular prosthesis is more expensive than a stock prosthesis, and several steps are essential for its fabrication.[9] In general, MMA is preferred as the material of choice for the orbital prosthesis fabrication compared to glass.[5] It has a longer life expectancy and is more durable than glass.[5]

The ocular prosthesis should be as similar as possible to the natural eye, particularly the iris, which determines eye color. Reproduction of the prosthetic iris is a crucial step during the fabrication of the ocular prosthesis.[10,11] Several articles have described reproduction of the iris using materials like paints, pigments, and papers, such as white and black cardboard with watercolor paint and oil paint.[10,12,13] However, these techniques consume time and require artistic skills. One of the recent iris reproduction techniques reported in the literature is the digital imaging technique.[10,14] In both techniques, a digital photograph of the patient's natural iris is made using a digital camera and manipulated using graphic software to get a replica of the natural iris. The use of such technique for iris replication has the advantage of acceptable esthetics with reduced treatment time compared to the conventional oil paint and monopoly iris painting technique.[14]

This article attempts to simplify the painting process of the iris disc and ocular prosthesis fabrication by means of digital photography while providing natural esthetics, saving time, and precluding the need for artistic skill.

CLINICAL REPORT

A 28-year-old man presented to the Department of Prosthetic Dentistry Dental Faculty Practice, University of Malaya (Kuala Lumpur, Malaysia) for a new orbital prosthesis to restore his missing right eye (Fig 4.1). History revealed surgical removal (enucleation) of the eyeball after a traumatic injury in a car accident. Examination of the eye socket showed healthy conjunctival lining. The treatment plan included fabrication of a custom-made ocular prosthesis. The rehabilitation team included a prosthodontist and an ophthalmologist. The fabrication procedure, maintenance, and limitations were explained to the patient.

Procedure

An impression of the ocular defect was made with an ocular-shaped acrylic impression tray. Using another patient's eye prosthesis mold, a suitable ocular impression tray was made with light-curing acrylic resin (Kemdent; Swindon, UK). The tray was designed with retention holes and a hollow handle extension, to accommodate the impression syringe tip (Fig 4.2). The tray was adjusted to fit in the enucleated socket, and various eye movements were performed to ensure passivity (Fig 4.3). Medium body polyvinyl siloxane (PVS) (GC Exaflex regular; GC America, Alsip, IL) was injected into the socket through the hollow tray handle (Fig 4.4), and the patient was instructed to perform different eye movements to mold the impression during setting.

The ocular impression was retrieved, and type IV dental stone (Elite Stone; Zhermack, Badia Polesine, Italy) was mixed and poured to fill the inner concave tissue surface of the impression. The impression was then inverted into the plastic cup, which had already been partially filled with stone mixture. Once set, several keyholes were prepared on the periphery of the master cast. For easy retrieval, a second layer was poured on two steps to obtain a three-piece cast. That was accomplished by separating the upper two halves with a wax barrier (Fig 4.5).

The impression was removed, and the sclera wax pattern was prepared by pouring molten wax into the resultant mold. The sclera wax pattern was smoothed, polished, and tried in for eye socket contour and lid movements. The fit was also confirmed by gently lifting the eyelids and observing the pattern extensions into the fornices. The eyelids should be able to completely close over the wax pattern to reduce potential irritation of the adjacent tissues.[2] The height of convexity of the sclera pattern was verified to be centered over the pupil area, then it was marked and accentuated with a droplet of wax. The wax pattern was invested in a small metal flask and processed in white shade heat-cured acrylic resin (color grade 1; AD Stellon C, London, UK).

The finished acrylic sclera was tried in the eye socket to check for fit and contour (Fig 4.6). The patient was instructed to look straight ahead at a distant point. The pupil position was confirmed with the help of the other natural eye and anatomical landmarks. The diameter of the patient's natural iris was measured with a millimeter ruler. In this case, it was

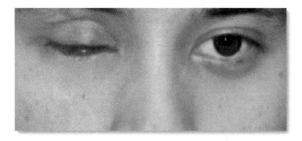

FIGURE 4.1   Frontal view.

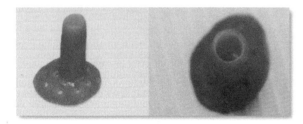

FIGURE 4.2   Ocular-shaped impression tray with hollow handle.

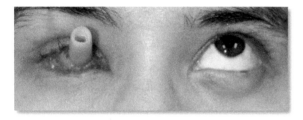

FIGURE 4.3   Ocular tray being verified for passive fit within the eye defect.

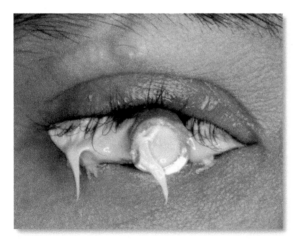

FIGURE 4.4   PVS impression material was injected through the tray's hollow handle.

around 11.5 mm. To preserve the shape of the acrylic scleral blank, a mold was prepared using silicon putty impression material.

A digital photograph of the patient's iris was captured using a digital camera (Canon EOS Digital Rebel; Canon Inc, Tokyo, Japan; Fig 4.7), and it was compared with the patient's natural iris. The color, brightness, contrast, and hue of the image was adjusted and formatted on a computer using graphic software (Paint Shop Pro X4 version 14.0.0.322; Corel®, Ottawa, Canada). The adjusted iris image was printed on photo paper (Prinzet Inkjet photo paper 265gm 4r professional glossy) and then checked chairside for the correct color (Fig 4.7). The diameter of the printed iris should be 1 mm less than that of the natural iris measured earlier to compensate for the magnification caused by the clear corneal prominence.

The acrylic anterior sclera curvature was reduced to about 2 mm thick in the iris region (corneal area), for better adaptation of the printed iris disc on to the acrylic sclera. The printed iris was cut and temporarily adapted within the space using a wax droplet. The assembly was then tried in the patient's eye to confirm the shape, size, and color of the artificial eye (Fig 4.8). The patient fixed his gaze on a predetermined object kept at least 3 feet in front and at natural eye level. Once verified, the iris disc was fixed to the scleral blank using cyanoacrylate adhesive, and using the previously prepared sclera putty mold, the sclera form and contour were reestablished in wax (Fig 4.9). It was invested and processed with a layer of clear heat-cured acrylic resin (Impact; DEL, London, UK) to give a glossy, realistic appearance. For scleral vein characterization, red silk fibers were added at the time of trial packing before final processing (Fig 4.10). At the insertion visit, the prosthesis was evaluated for fit, and the patient was advised on hygiene and how to wear and remove the prosthesis (Fig 4.11).

DISCUSSION

Several techniques and materials have been introduced throughout the years to fabricate ocular prostheses, including custom-made and modified stock ocular prostheses, made from glass or MMA.[2,14] Similarly, various techniques of iris painting have been introduced: paper iris disc technique, black iris disc technique, and monopoly with dry earth pigment. Recently, digital imaging has been used to replicate irises.[10,14] The use of digital imaging for iris replication in the construction of ocular prostheses has the advantage of acceptable esthetics with reduced treatment time compared to the conventional oil paint and monopoly iris painting technique.[14]

The ocular prosthesis fabrication technique described in this article is uncomplicated, reduces treatment time, and requires less artistic skill, unlike the iris painting technique,

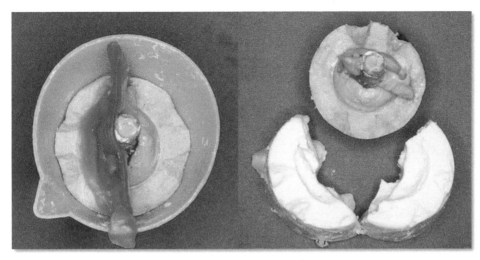

FIGURE 4.5   Three-piece cast was made.

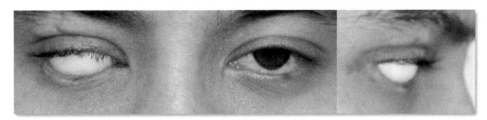

FIGURE 4.6   Acrylic sclera at try-in.

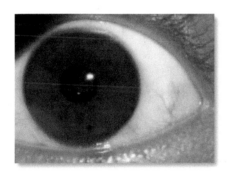
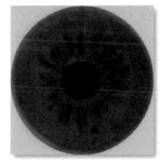

FIGURE 4.7   Digital photograph of the patient's iris (left) and the adjusted iris image (right).

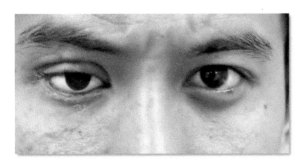

FIGURE 4.8   Acrylic sclera with attached printed iris disc for verification of iris color, size, and position.

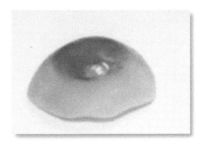

FIGURE 4.9   The sclera anterior curvature was restored with wax before processing.

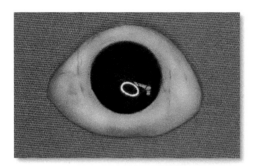

FIGURE 4.10   Processed ocular prosthesis.

in which artistic skill is a must.[8] On the other hand, special digital photography equipment and settings, as well as computer software that allows for image adjustments, are required.[10,14]

In the digital photography technique, three stages are needed: first, impression taking and natural iris photograph capturing; second, try-in stage for both the acrylic sclera and the printed iris with different contrast and brightness; third, ocular prosthesis delivery. The conventional iris painting procedure needs more time, which varies according to the ocularist's skill. The painting stage itself may need half an hour to 1 hour. On the other hand, the painting stage would not be needed in case of digital photography; however, the iris image would need digital adjustment with an average time of 10 to 20 minutes or less. This amount of time could be further reduced if an iris digital photograph gallery was made available.

The digital imaging technique described in this article was similar to that described by Artopoulou et al.[14] However, in the present report, the printed iris disc was directly pasted to the acrylic scleral blank. This eliminated the need for additional armamentarium such as the ocular button to carry the iris disc. Moreover, in patients whose scleral thickness is limited in the anteroposterior dimension, the additional thickness of the ocular button could limit its use.

At the iris disc try-in procedure, unlike Artopoulou et al,[14] who tried the iris disc on waxed sclera, in the present case, a processed acrylic sclera was used. Therefore, tendency for error in iris disc positioning relative to the eyelids was less, as the fit and contour of the sclera were already established earlier. Unlike previously described techniques,[10,14] the anterior curvature of the scleral blank was preserved before the cut-back and iris disc try-in procedure that reduced the needed prosthesis adjustments at the insertion visit.

The final position of the iris in the present method only required commonly available adhesive and a conventional denture process to restore the anterior curvature in the corneal region with a layer of clear heat-cured acrylic resin; however, the color replication of the iris depends on several factors: the quality of the printer ink and the printer paper type and quality. These factors may lead to unstable results and affect the iris color replication. Therefore, it is essential to use waterproof and glossy photo paper to achieve an acceptable iris replication as opposed to the use of an ocular button.

In the digital photography technique, special digital photography equipment, computer software that allows for image adjustments, and the skills needed to use such software are required. All of these could be considered as drawbacks to this technique. Another question to be answered is how long the color of these printed iris discs will last. Furthermore, there is as yet no definitive protocol to follow in ocular prosthesis construction. Improving digital photography technique and using it as a starting point to potentially fabricate a CAD/CAM ocular prosthesis that could be constructed in one visit, a technique that would require no special skill, should be the goal for future ocular prosthesis construction.

SUMMARY

In the technique described, digital imaging was used to replicate the patient's remaining natural iris. The treatment time reduction and simplicity of the followed technique make this method a viable alternative for ocular prosthesis fabrication; however, further research is essential to evaluate the long-term color stability and aging of the ocular prostheses produced by this technique.

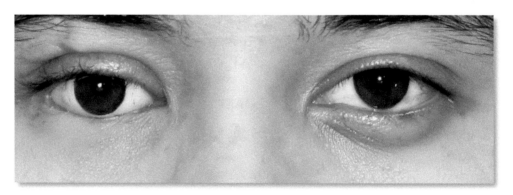

FIGURE 4.11   The ocular prosthesis in place.

REFERENCES

1. Raflo GT: Enucleation and evisceration. In Tasmun W, Jaeger E (eds): *Duane's Clinical Ophthalmology*, Vol 5. Philadelphia, Lippincott-Raven, 1995, pp. 1–25.

2. Jain DC, Hegde V, Aparna IN, et al: Ocular prosthesis: an esthetic vision. *J Nepal Dent Assoc* 2010;11:101–106.

3. Custer PL, Kennedy RH, Woog JJ, et al: Orbital implants in enucleation surgery: a report by the American Academy of Ophthalmology. *Ophthalmology* 2003;110:2054–2061.

4. Nunnery WR, Ng JD: Enucleation and evisceration. In Spaeth G (ed): *Ophthalmic Surgery: Principles and Practice* (ed 3) Philadelphia, Elsevier, 2003, pp. 485–507.

5. Patil SB, Meshramkar R, Naveen BH, et al: Ocular prosthesis: a brief review and fabrication of an ocular prosthesis for a geriatric patient. *Gerodontology* 2008;25:57–62.

6. Taicher S, Steinberg HM, Tubiana I, et al: Modified stock-eye ocular prosthesis. *J Prosthet Dent* 1985;54:95–98.

7. Benson P: The fitting and fabrication of a custom resin artificial eye. *J Prosthet Dent* 1977;38:532–538.

8. Beumer J, Curtis TA, Marunick MT: *Maxillofacial Rehabilitation: Prosthodontic and Surgical Considerations*. St. Louis, MO, Ishiyaku EuroAmerica, Inc., 1996, pp. 425–431.

9. Matthews MF, Smith RM, Sutton AJ, et al: The ocular impression: a review of the literature and presentation of an alternate technique. *J Prosthodont* 2000;9:210–216.

10. Jain S, Makkar S, Gupta S, et al: Prosthetic rehabilitation of ocular defect using digital photography: a case report. *J Indian Prosthodont Soc* 2010;10:190–193.

11. Murphey PJ, Pitton RD, Schlossberg L, et al: The development of acrylic eye prosthesis at the National Naval Medical Center. *J Am Dent Assoc* 1945;32:1227–1244.

12. Raizada K, Rani D: Ocular prosthesis. *Contact Lens Anter Eye* 2007;30:152–162.

13. Brown KE: Fabrication of an ocular prosthesis. *J Prosthet Dent* 1970;24:223–225.

14. Artopoulou II, Montgomery PC, Wesley PJ, et al: Digital imaging in the fabrication of ocular prostheses. *J Prosthet Dent* 2006;95:327–330.

PART II

MANAGEMENT OF TOOTH WEAR

5

FULL-MOUTH REHABILITATION OF A PATIENT WITH GASTROESOPHAGEAL REFLUX DISEASE: A CLINICAL REPORT

JUANLI GUO, DMD, MS, PHD, FACP,[1] GLENN RESIDE, DMD,[2] AND LYNDON F. COOPER, DDS, PHD, FACP[3]

[1]Private Practice, Vienna, VA
[2]Department of Oral and Maxillofacial Surgery, School of Dentistry, , University of North Carolina, Chapel Hill, NC
[3]Department of Prosthodontics, School of Dentistry, , University of North Carolina, Chapel Hill, NC

Keywords
GERD; full-mouth rehabilitation; dental erosion; caries.

Correspondence
Juanli Guo, 8321 Old Courthouse Rd, Suite 120, Vienna, VA 22182. E-mail: ImplantDentalArt@gmail.com

Accepted August 18, 2011

Published in *Journal of Prosthodontics* October 2011; Vol. 20, Suppl 2

doi: 10.1111/j.1532-849X.2011.00785.x

ABSTRACT

Gastroesophageal reflux disease (GERD)is a chronic condition caused by stomach acid regurgitating into the esophagus or oral cavity, often causing heartburn. Tooth erosion and wear are common oral manifestations of GERD. This clinical report describes the full-mouth rehabilitation of a patient with over 30 years of GERD, causing wear of maxillary and mandibular anterior teeth, along with complications associated with past restorations. Full-mouth rehabilitation of natural teeth in conjunction with dental implants was selected as the treatment option. Ideal occlusal design and optimal esthetics, along with reinforcement of oral hygiene, ensure a favorable prognosis.

Patients with severely worn dentition frequently require full-mouth rehabilitation due to the associated occlusal discrepancy. It is critical to identify the etiology of the worn dentition before a proper treatment is initiated. The pathological loss of tooth structure can be caused by different processes: (1) abnormal attrition, loss of tooth structure, or restorative material due to tooth-tooth contact, such as bruxism; (2) abrasion, loss of tooth structure due to factors other than tooth contacts (brushing, tobacco chewing, etc.); and (3) erosion, chemical loss of tooth structure without bacteria involvement, usually demineralization of enamel or dentin by acid.[1] Based on the source of the acid, dental erosion can be differentiated into extrinsic erosion, where the acid is mainly from dietary consumption, or intrinsic erosion, where acid is mainly from gastric fluid, such as, in patients with bulimia or gastroesophageal reflux disease (GERD). The critical pH value of enamel (when it begins to dissolve) is around 5.2. The pH value of most acidic beverages and gastric fluid is below 2.0.[2] The cause of erosion sometimes can be differentiated based on the wear pattern. Intrinsic erosion generally occurs on the palatal surfaces of the maxillary anterior teeth and the mandibular posterior teeth.[3] The prevalence of dental erosion in adult GERD patients has been documented to be around 25%.[4] However, the correlation between GERD and the prevalence of dental caries appears to be negative or even a reverse relationship.[5]

This report focuses on a patient with a long history of GERD, and a presentation of tooth wear on the maxillary and the mandibular anterior teeth, along with heavily restored dentition and a failing five-unit fixed dental prosthesis (FDP).

CLINICAL REPORT

Preoperative Information, Diagnosis, and Treatment Plan

A 58-year-old woman presented with the chief complaint of a loose FDP. She lacked self-confidence due to thin and unaesthetic anterior teeth. A review of the patient's medical history revealed she had GERD for more than 30 years, and was taking an over-the-counter H2 blocker, Prevacid. She had a cholecystectomy and hysterectomy 1 year before her initial prosthodontic office visit, and was taking Progestin for hormonal replacement. She had a history of high blood pressure that was under control with medication (Terazosin). She had no known drug allergy. She did not smoke, and consumed alcohol occasionally. The patient had no medical contraindications to dental treatment.

Over the past 35 years, the patient had extensive dental treatment, including root canal treatment (RCT), fillings, crowns, and FDPs. The upper-left FDP had been loose for more than 6 months. Clinical exam revealed that a five-unit FDP on teeth #11 to 15 was loose. After removal of the FDP, abutment tooth #11 was noted to have deep caries below the gingival level and was determined nonrestorable. The patient also presented with moderately worn dentition and restorations. Defective composite restorations were present on most of the anterior teeth. Multiple fixed restorations were in place, including porcelain-fused-to-metal (PFM) crowns on teeth #4, 5, 7, 21, 22, 27, and 28, full-gold crowns on teeth #2 and #17, a 7/8 gold crown on tooth #3, a PFM-FDP on teeth #18 to 20, and a gold FDP with mesial retainer facial porcelain veneer on #29 to 31. Secondary caries was noticed on teeth #2, 6, 8, 9, 10, 11, 17, 18, 20, and 29. The patient had an Angle's Class I canine relationship and an Angle's Class III

molar relationship. The mandibular midline was coincident with the facial midline, whereas the maxillary midline was 2 mm to the left. The occlusal vertical dimension (OVD) was deemed reduced after evaluation of esthetics and phonetics. The patient's centric occlusion and maximal intercuspal position (MIP) were coincident. Radiographic findings revealed generalized mild to moderate bone loss (Fig 5.1). Using the American College of Prosthodontists' Prosthodontic Diagnostic Index (PDI) for partial edentulism, the patient was classified as Class IV.[6]

The options of single implant versus 3-unit FDPs in the edentulous areas of #19 and #30 were discussed with the patient. She decided to have FDPs due to financial concerns. Maxillary anterior crown lengthening and orthodontic treatment to correct malocclusion before definitive prosthodontic treatment were also proposed to the patient, but were rejected.

Treatment Procedures

A caries management program, including dietary assessment and reinforcement of oral hygiene measures, was initiated before the treatment was started. Periodontal treatment was completed before starting other treatment procedures. A lateral window approach sinus floor augmentation was performed, and the grafted area was allowed to heal for 6 months before implant placement. Three months after sinus floor augmentation, the existing FDP #11 to 15 was sectioned at the mesial of abutment tooth #15. The nonrestorable tooth #11 was extracted, and ridge augmentation was completed. An interim PRDP was inserted during healing. After healing of the sinus floor augmentation and the ridge augmentation, three dental implants were placed at #11, 13, and 14 with the aid of a surgical guide (Fig 5.2).

A set of diagnostic casts was made and articulated on a Hanau Wide-Vue articulator (Waterpik Technologies, Fort Collins, CO) using a Hanau Springbow and a centric relation record. Diagnostic wax-up was done to plan the anticipated occlusion and to foresee any potential problems (Fig 5.3). OVD was restored by opening about 1.5 mm on the incisal guide pin to compensate the lost OVD.

During the healing of bone grafting and implant surgery, all defective restorations on teeth #6 to 10 and #23 to 26 were removed, and secondary caries excavated. The cavities were restored with composite resin. All existing crowns and FDPs were sectioned and removed. All abutment teeth were thoroughly examined, and secondary caries excavated. Tooth #17 had lost extensive tooth structure and was extracted due to nonpredictable RCT. Teeth #2 and 20 had lost extensive tooth structure, and were recommended to have selective RCT and dowel-core buildup before new crowns were fabricated. Teeth #3, 4, 18, 20, 21, and 31 did not have enough remaining coronal tooth structure for adequate ferrule effect. Therefore, crown-lengthening surgery was

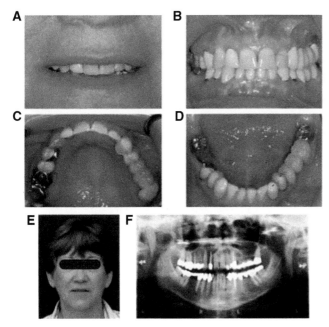

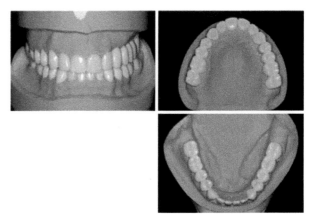

FIGURE 5.3   Diagnostic wax-up.

FIGURE 5.1   Preoperative images and panoramic radiograph. (A) Close-up frontal view showing thin maxillary incisors. Intraoral images; (B) Frontal view at maximum-intercuspal position (MIP); (C) Maxillary occlusal; and (D) Mandibular occlusal views. (E) Preoperative smile image. (F) Preoperative panoramic radiograph.

recommended. Teeth #3, 5, 15, 18, and 31 lost some tooth structure, but were determined to be restorable and have a favorable prognosis. They were restored with amalgam, with pins placed on teeth #3 and 31 to assist core retention. A cast dowel-core of tooth #21 became loose and was removed. Teeth #2, 4, 7, 20, 21, and 29 were recommended to have RCT. Dowel spaces were prepared on #2, 4, 7, 20, and 21 using a ParaPost XP System (Coltene Whaledent Inc., Cuyahoga Falls, OH). Prefabricated stainless steel Para-Posts was

bonded with resin cement (MaxCem Resin Cement, Kerr Corporation, Orange, CA), and the teeth were then restored with amalgam. Tooth #29 had adequate tooth structure after RCT and was restored with amalgam. The preparations were refined. Provisional crowns and FDPs were fabricated using autopolymerized acrylic resin.

The implants were uncovered during second stage surgery after 3 months healing, and a screw-retained provisional FDP was fabricated at #11 to 13–14 area. Teeth #6 to 10 were prepared for zirconium-based all-ceramic crowns. Teeth #23 to 26 were prepared for Empress all-ceramic crowns (Ivoclar Vivadent, Amherst, NY). A set of new provisional crowns and FDPs was fabricated and delivered at the increased OVD (Fig 5.4). After the patient felt comfortable with the new interim prostheses for a month, impressions of the interim prostheses were made, and casts were poured (Fig 5.5). Casts were mounted on a Hanau Wide-Vue semi-adjustable articulator. A custom incisal guide table was fabricated. Final impressions were made of all prepared natural teeth and

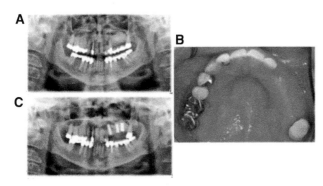

FIGURE 5.2   (A) Panoramic radiograph after the lateral window sinus augmentation. (B) Intraoral maxillary view after the sinus augmentation and the ridge augmentation. (C) Panoramic radiograph after implant placement.

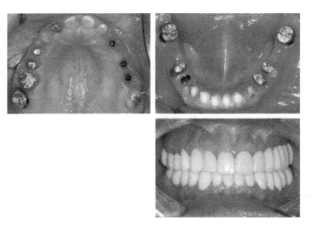

FIGURE 5.4   Tooth preparations and interim prostheses.

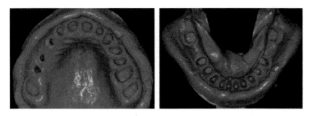

FIGURE 5.5 Final impressions.

implant fixtures with vinylpolysiloxane (VPS) impression material. Centric relation interocclusal records, including preparation against preparation, and preparation against interim prostheses, were made with VPS material and the aid of a Lucia Jig, which was fabricated at the same OVD as the interim prostheses. Master casts were cross mounted against the casts of the interim prostheses. The interim prostheses were used to guide the fabrication of the final prostheses. In this case, computer-aided design/computer-aided manufacture (CAD/CAM) abutments were used for the implant-supported, cement-retained FDPs. The final prostheses were designed as follows: full-gold crowns on teeth #2

and #15; PFM crowns on teeth #3, 4, 5, 14, 21, and 28; PFM-FDPs on teeth/implants #11 to 13, 18 to 20 (#18 as full gold retainer), and 29 to 31 (#31 as full gold retainer); zirconium-based all-ceramic crowns (Lava, 3M ESPE, St. Paul, MN) on teeth #6 to 10, 22, and 27; and IPS Empress Esthetics (Ivoclar Vivadent, Amherst, NY) all-ceramic crowns on teeth #23 to 26. The occlusion was constructed as mutually protected occlusion with anterior guidance at protrusion and lateral excursion (Fig 5.6). The IPS Empress all-ceramic crowns were etched with hydrofluoric acid, conditioned with saline coupling agent, and bonded to the abutment teeth using light-polymerized resin cement (Variolink, Ivoclar Vivadent, Amherst, NY). The remaining crowns and FDPs were cemented using resin-modified glass ionomer (GC FujiCEM, GC America, Alsip, IL).

Posttreatment Therapy and Prognosis

One week after the final prostheses were delivered, the patient returned to the clinic for reevaluation. A maxillary occlusal splint was delivered 2 weeks after the treatment. She

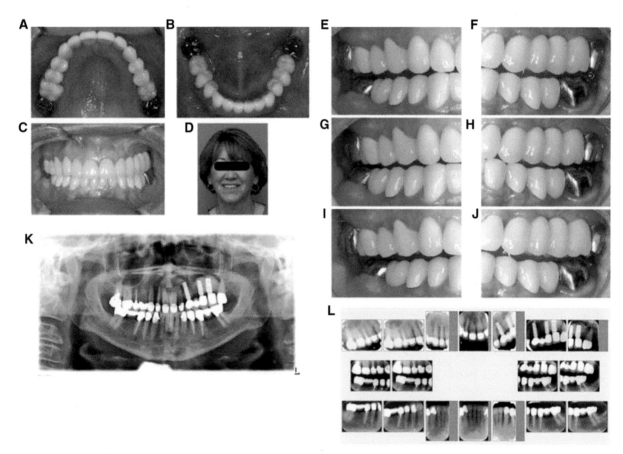

FIGURE 5.6 Postoperative images and radiographs. (A) Maxillary occlusal view. (B) Mandibular occlusal view. (C) Frontal view at MIP. (D) Patient's facial frontal smile view. (E, F) Lateral view at protrusion. (G, H) Lateral view at laterotrusion. (I, J) Lateral view at mediotrusion. (K) Postoperative panoramic radiograph. (L) Postoperative full-mouth series radiograph.

was satisfied with the treatment and was very motivated to maintain the final prostheses with excellent oral hygiene practices. Oral hygiene instruction was reinforced throughout the treatment and after the treatment. The patient was placed on a 6-month recall schedule. The restoration of the patient's dentition, coupled with the development of an ideal occlusal scheme, excellent oral hygiene practices, and a positive attitude assures a favorable long-term prognosis.

DISCUSSION

Multiple factors, including attrition, abrasion, and erosion, contribute to tooth wear. It has been well documented that GERD can cause dental erosion; however, whether there is a correlation between GERD and dental caries is not well known. It has been proposed that due to the strong acidity of gastric acid, GERD patients typically are less prone to dental caries, partly because of the inhibition effect of strong gastric acid on bacteria.[5] However, dental caries is a multi-factorial disease. The patient's dietary habits, intake of medicine, oral hygiene, history of dental treatment, and the predisposed tooth structure could also contribute to caries formation. In this patient, previous extensive dental treatment including tooth-colored (composite resin) restorations, crowns, and FDPs, instead of GERD itself, may have caused higher caries risk. In addition, the daily intake of multiple medicines and limited oral hygiene measures also increased the dental caries risk. It is not surprising for the patient to present with both secondary caries and dental erosion. Management of dental erosion is mainly focused on preventive strategies; therefore, identifying the source of erosion is very important. These strategies include: (1) to identify the source of erosive tooth wear; (2) to refer to a physician if it is intrinsic erosion; (3) to reduce acid intake; (4) to reduce the level of oral acidity; (5) to increase salivary flow; (6) to remineralize the eroded areas; (7) to reduce abrasion; (8) to protect the exposed dentin with resin restorations or lingual veneers; (9) to fabricate an occlusal night guard.[7] When restoration is necessary, it is recommended to be conservative when the erosion is not accompanied with occlusal discrepancy or reduced OVD.[8] Based on the severity of erosion, choices of restoration could range from sealants to composite restorations to indirect restorations, such as inlays, onlays, and crowns. In severe cases, when there is occlusal discrepancy and reduced OVD, full-mouth rehabilitation is often indicated.

In this case, the patient had previous restorations with an occlusal plane discrepancy and occlusal interference. Full-mouth rehabilitation was indicated. The moderately worn palatal surfaces of the maxillary anterior teeth and the worn and lingually inclined mandibular anterior teeth make it challenging to restore the dentition at the preoperative OVD. Due to the loss of palatal tooth structure on maxillary anterior teeth and lingual inclination of mandibular anterior teeth, minimal preparation on the palatal surfaces of maxillary anterior teeth and facial surfaces of mandibular anterior teeth was indicated. Subgingival margins were indicated in this case to prevent future erosion of tooth structures due to GERD. When considering cement selection, there are no guidelines available to compare the solubility and bio-mechanical behaviors of different cements in an acidic environment; however, it has been reported when cement materials, such as glass ionomer, resin-modified glass ionomer, and composite resin, are used as restorative materials, they are more resistant to erosive wear when compared to enamel. Differences have been reported among restorative materials, with glass ionomer most susceptible to acid, resulting in lower erosive wear resistance and microhardness, and composite resin the most resistant to acid.[9,10] For this patient, composite resin was used to bond the anterior restorations due to its higher acidic resistance and stronger bonding strength. Resin-modified glass ionomer was used to cement the other restorations due to its lower technique sensitivity and reasonable acidic resistance.

REFERENCES

1. Eccles JD: Tooth surface loss from abrasion, attrition, and erosion. *Dent Update* 1982;9:373–381.
2. Larsen MJ: Chemical events during tooth dissolution. *J Dent Res* 1990;69(spec Issue): 575–580.
3. Bartlett DW, Evans DF, Anggiansah A, et al: A study of the association between gastro-oesophageal reflux and palatal dental erosion. *Br Dent J* 1996;181:125–131.
4. Pace F, Pallotta S, Tonini M, et al: Systematic review: gastro-oesophageal reflux disease and dental lesions. *Aliment Pharmacol Ther* 2008;27:1179–1186.
5. Munoz JV, Herreros B, Sanchiz V, et al: Dental and periodontal lesions in patients with gastro-oesophageal reflux disease. *Dig Liver Dis* 2003;35:461–467.
6. McGarry TJ, Nimmo A, Skiba JF, et al: Classification system for partial edentulism. *J Prosthodont* 2002;11:181–193.
7. Donovan T: Dental erosion. *J Esthet Restor Dent* 2009;21:359–364.
8. Reis A, Higashi C, Loguercio AD: Reanatomization of anterior eroded teeth by stratification with direct composite resin. *J Esthet Restor Dent* 2009;21:304–316.
9. Shabanian M, Richards LC: In vitro wear rates of materials under different loads and varying pH. *J Prosthet Dent* 2002;87:650–656.
10. Honorio HM, Rios D, Francisconi LF, et al: Effect of prolonged erosive pH cycling on different restorative materials. *J Oral Rehabil* 2008;35:947–953.

6

REHABILITATION OF A BULIMIC PATIENT USING ENDOSTEAL IMPLANTS

ALBERTO AMBARD, DDS, MS[1] AND LEONARD MUENINGHOFF, DDS[2]

[1] Fellow, Maxillofacial Prosthetics Clinic, Department of Surgery, University of Chicago, Chicago, IL

[2] Professor, Department of Prosthodontics and Biomaterials, Director of Graduate Prosthodontics and Continuing Dental Education, The University of Alabama at Birmingham, Birmingham, AL,

Keywords
Bulimia; dental treatment; eating disorder; prosthodontics.

Correspondence
Dr. Alberto J. Ambard, 30 South Ellsworth St., Naperville, IL 60540. E-mail: aambard@mac.com

This article was presented as a poster at the American Prosthodontic Society annual meeting in Chicago, February 2002.

Accepted June 18, 2002

Published in *Journal of Prosthodontics* September 2002; Vol. 11, Issue 3

doi:10.1053/jpro.2002.127593

ABSTRACT

This article describes the dental rehabilitation of a bulimic patient using endosteal implants. Although the patient, a 31-year-old woman with a long history of bulimia nervosa, had been receiving medical and psychological treatment, the condition was not completely controlled. Clinical examination revealed multiple crowns with extensive cervical caries. The prognosis for all remaining teeth was poor. After extractions, implant therapy was implemented to provide support for fixed prostheses. After the implants were uncovered and during provisional therapy, the peri-implant tissue exhibited inflammation and lack of keratinized tissue requiring additional periodontal procedures before definitive restorations could be placed. Because of the difficulty in managing the peri-implant tissue during the many phases of implant therapy, treatment was challenging. One year after treatment, the patient's low self-esteem had improved substantially and her restorations provided satisfactory esthetics and function.

BULIMIA NERVOSA, a psychological disorder characterized by a pattern of binge eating followed by fasting, over-exercise, and/or various methods of purging, including self-induced vomiting and abuse of laxatives or diuretics, affects 7.5 million people in the United States.[1] Binges of 500 to 20,000 calories usually consist of sweets or salty carbohydrates.[2] About 90% of the affected population are white females of middle to upper socioeconomic strata.[3] Between 5 and 20% of college women in the United States are affected.[4,5] The prognosis for the disease is relatively poor; only 37% of patients experience complete recovery.[6]

Clinical signs and symptoms of bulima include dehydration, edema, electrolyte imbalances, and blisters on the dorsum of the hand (Russell's sign). Complications may occur, such as gastric ruptures and potassium depletion, leading to cardiac irregularities.[3] These patients exhibit low self-esteem, guilt, depression, excessive concern with body shape and esthetics, a need for constant approval, and a fear of rejection.[2,3,7] Oral signs and symptoms include hypersensitivity, generalized erythema, erosion of the lingual surface of maxillary teeth, anterior open bite, xerostomia, enlarged parotid glands (hamster-like appearance), enamel loss, sore throat, gingival bleeding, and caries.[2,7] The prosthodontist caring of such patients should be encouraging and supportive. A confrontational approach at any phase of treatment may produce resistance, denial, hostility, and fear in the patient.[8]

Endosteal dental implants have been used successfully over the past 20 years.[9–11] Although several reports have described oral rehabilitations in bulimic patients,[12–15] the prognosis for endosteal implants and peri-implant tissue in active bulimic patients has not been reported. Concerns relate to the possibility of continuous exposure to a strongly acidic environment. This article describes the management of an active bulimic patient treated with endosteal implants.

CLINICAL REPORT

Patient History

The patient, a 31-year-old professional woman who had suffered from bulimia nervosa for almost 10 years, sought medical help because of frequent hematemesis, resulting from 3 to 4 daily binge-eating episodes followed by self-induced vomiting. The treatment team included a psychologist, a primary physician, and a dietician. Treatment consisted of psychological therapy, education, diet control, and group support. Pharmacologic therapy was not used. At the time of the prosthodontic consultation, the patient, who remained under medical and psychological supervision, experienced approximately 1 bulimic episode a week. She had no other medical problems and did not smoke. When explaining the detailed history of her disease, she expressed willingness to cooperate with treatment. Psychologically, she exhibited low self-esteem, a need for approval, and a concern with treatment outcome, a profile that persisted throughout treatment. Clinical and radiographic examinations revealed crowns on all remaining teeth. Lingual surfaces and the margins of all crowns exhibited extensive erosion and caries. Crown/root ratios were compromised. Most of the remaining teeth had been endodontically treated with what appeared

radiographically to be prefabricated dowels (Fig 6.1). The periodontal tissue was generally erythematous, periodontal charting revealed probing depths of 4 mm or less, and mild bleeding was observed on probing.

Treatment Plan

The treatment plan included extraction of all remaining teeth followed by implant placement and fixed restorations. Other prosthetic options presented were conventional complete denture therapy, implant-retained overdentures, and fixed detachable prostheses. The retention of remaining teeth represented an unfavorable option because of the extent of the caries and the compromised crown/root ratios.

The goal of the prosthodontic plan was to provide the patient with first molar occlusion using eight implants in the maxilla and six in the mandible (Steri-Oss; Nobel Biocare USA, Yorba Linda, CA) to provide prosthesis retention.

Initial Surgical and Prosthodontic Treatment. Preliminary diagnostic treatment followed conventional prosthodontic protocols. The teeth were extracted in stages to reduce psychological trauma, to enhance implant placement and, to facilitate provisional treatment. Surgical treatment was performed as follows: extraction of all posterior teeth, posterior implant placement, extraction of anterior teeth and anterior implant placement with time allowed between procedures for adequate healing. Interim complete dentures provided provisional occlusion and esthetics.

Late Surgical and Prosthodontic Treatment. Six months after maxillary implant placement, the patient returned for implant uncovering. Three weeks later, the status of the implants was assessed. The peri-implant tissue was moderately inflamed, although no calculus or plaque was found. The condition of the tissue suggested that the patient had experienced bulimic episodes after the implants had been uncovered. The implants exhibited neither mobility nor pain on percussion, and radiographic examination revealed adequate relation between bone and implants. No periodontal probing was performed. Three weeks later, fixed provisional restorations were placed in the maxilla. Because the area of the maxillary right canine implant completely lacked keratinized tissue, a split-thickness flap was elevated from the palate and placed buccal to the implant. Although the area showed improvement after 10 weeks, the peri-implant tissue near most implants remained mildly inflamed and exhibited some nonkeratinized areas. In addition, the gingiva generally remained erythematous. No improvement in this condition had occurred after 8 more weeks. Moreover, some implant collars were slightly exposed and, although the smile line of the patient was low (Fig 6.2), she was self-conscious about the esthetics of her

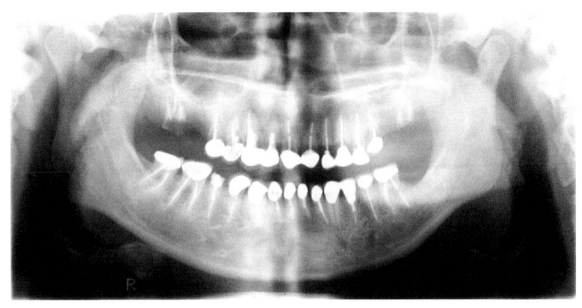

FIGURE 6.1 Initial panoramic radiograph.

appearance. For these reasons, 1 day after delivery of the mandibular fixed provisional restorations, a maxillary allo-derm graft was performed from first premolar to first premolar. Although the esthetic limitations of this

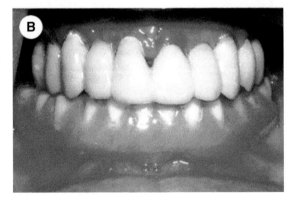

FIGURE 6.2 Patient with maxillary fixed provisional restorations and mandibular interim dentures. (A) Facial view; (B) Intra-oral view.

procedure were considered, the attempt was deemed justi-fied by the need for more keratinized peri-implant tissue (Fig 6.3).

Three months after this procedure, the condition and appearance of the gingival tissue was satisfactory. Fabrica-tion of the final restorations was then scheduled.

Definitive Prosthetic Treatment. Metal ceramic restora-tions were fabricated as originally planned. Although the peri-implant tissue remained mildly erythematous at the time of delivery, the patient expressed pleasure with the results. Oral hygiene instructions included the conventional protocol for implant patients with fixed prostheses. Instructions relat-ing to the bulimia included rinses with water or a basic solution immediately after purging.

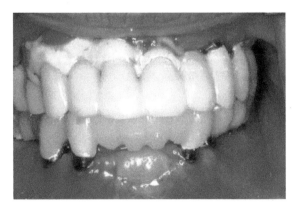

FIGURE 6.3 Patient 2 weeks postperiodontal surgery to gain keratinized peri-implant tissue and improve esthetics.

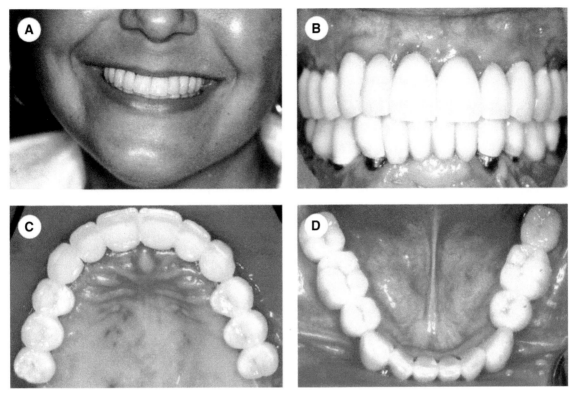

FIGURE 6.4   Patient at 1-year follow-up. (A) Facial view (B) intra-oral facial view (C) intra-oral occlusal view of maxillary arch, and (D) intra-oral occlusal view of mandibular arch

Follow-Up

When the patient returned for evaluation 1 year after delivery, both her self-esteem and the bulimic condition showed improvement. The patient reported experiencing only 1 bulimic episode every 1 to 2 months and was no longer participating in group therapy. She saw her primary physician every 6 months. Examination of her oral cavity showed that erythema and inflammation were no longer present. Peri-implant tissue appeared healthy, and exposure of metal implant components was less evident. The restorations were judged successful in improving esthetics and function (Fig 6.4).

DISCUSSION

Whether or not to proceed with implant therapy in an active bulimic patient is a difficult decision. Hazelton and Faine[7] have proposed limiting dental care in an active bulimic patient to preventive therapy unless the individual acknowledges the problem, receives medical help and counseling, and does not have active caries. Although these authors also suggested that normal treatment could be provided if the bulimia is no longer active, they did not discuss dental implants.[7]

The decision to provide definitive treatment for this patient was supported by the patient's expression of willingness to cooperate with the dental and medical treatment, the actual need for dental care, and evidence of improvement of the disease. Caries control was not a factor, because all remaining teeth were indicated for extraction. The patient's age, the need to maintain alveolar bone, and the patient's concerns regarding esthetics and comfort all suggested implant therapy as an appropriate option.

Slow healing, reduced keratinized peri-implant tissue, and generalized inflammation around the implants, observed after the implants were uncovered, suggested that the patient's bulimic episodes were continuing. Further periodontal procedures were required to achieve acceptable results. Surgical procedures had been performed after acceptable protocols, and the patient was young, healthy, and did not smoke. Moreover, her oral hygiene was optimal. Although she reported only 4 to 5 bulimic episodes during the period after the implants were uncovered, the mild xerostomia and generalized erythema of the oral cavity noted during this phase have been described as typical signs of bulimia.[2,7] Epithelialization of the sulci usually occurs about 2 weeks after implants are uncovered. In this case, moderate inflammation was found in the peri-implant tissue 3 weeks after uncovering and never completely resolved. Normally, clinical healing after a split-thickness flap procedure such as that performed in this patient occurs 6 to 8 weeks after surgery. In this case, the tissue remained inflamed after 10 weeks, and 8 additional weeks were required for clinically healing.

From the beginning of treatment, the patient showed low self-esteem, fear of rejection, and a marked need of approval. These characteristics have been described as common in bulimic patients.[2,3,7] However, the patient was always very cooperative and followed postoperative instructions and oral hygiene effectively. Because of this psychological profile, it was important to express optimism and encouragement to the patient, regardless of the bulimic episodes.

One year after treatment, implants and restorations continue to provide acceptable function and esthetics. Medical and psychological treatments, coupled with the patient's determination, have been effective in nearly eliminating the bulimia. It seems reasonable to conclude that improved oral health and esthetic appearance also contributed to the patient's ability to control the disorder.

REFERENCES

1. Roberts MW, Tylenda CA: Dental aspects of anorexia and bulimia nervosa. *Pediatrician* 1989;16:178–184.

2. Montgomery MT, Ritvo J, Ritvo J, et al: Eating disorders: Phenomenology, identification, and dental intervention. *Gen Dent* 1988;36:485–488.

3. Kreipe RE, Birndorf DO: Eating disorders in adolescents and young adults. *Med Clin North Am* 2000;84:1027–1049.

4. Herzog DB, Copeland PM: Eating disorders. *N Eng J Med* 1985;313:295–303.

5. Pyle RL, Harlvorson P, Neumann P, et al: The increasing prevalence of bulimia in freshman college students. *Int J Eating Dis* 1983;2:75–85.

6. Norring CE, Sohlberg SS: Outcome, recovery, relapse and mortality across 6 years in patients with clinical eating disorders. *Acta Psychiatr Scand* 1993;87:437–444.

7. Hazelton LR, Faine MP: Diagnosis and dental management of eating disorder patients. *Int J Prosthodont* 1996;9:65–73.

8. Schmidt U, Treasure J: Eating disorders and the dental practitioner. *Eur J Prosthodont Restor Dent* 1997;5:161–167.

9. Adell R, Lekholm U, Rockler B, et al: A 15-year study of osseointegrated implants in the treatment of the edentulous jaw. *Int J Oral Surg* 1981;10:387–416.

10. Lindquist LW, Carlsson GE, Jemt T: A prospective 15-year follow-up study of mandibular fixed prostheses supported by osseointegrated implants. Clinical results and marginal bone loss. *Clin Oral Implants Res* 1996;7:329–336.

11. Albrektsson T, Zarb G, Worthington P, et al: The long-term efficacy of currently used dental implants: A review and proposed criteria of success. *Int J Oral Maxillofac Implants* 1986;1:11–25.

12. Bonilla ED, Luna O: Oral rehabilitation of a bulimic patient: A case report. *Quintessence Int* 2001;32:469–475.

13. Hastings JH: Conservative restoration of function and aesthetics in a bulimic patient: A case report. *Pract Periodontics Aesthet Dent* 1996;8:729–736.

14. Milosevic A, Jones C: Use of resin-bonded ceramic crowns in a bulimic patient with severe tooth erosion. *Quintessence Int* 1996;27:123–127.

15. Shaw BM: Orthodontic/prosthetic treatment of enamel erosion resulting from bulimia: A case report. *J Am Dent Assoc* 1994;125:188–190.

7

FIXED PROSTHODONTIC REHABILITATION IN A WEAR PATIENT WITH FABRY'S DISEASE

AVINASH S. BIDRA, BDS, MS, FACP

Department of Reconstructive Sciences, University of Connecticut Health Center, Farmington, CT

Keywords

Fabry's disease; medical management; tooth wear; bruxism; diastema; esthetics; fixed rehabilitation; partial group function.

Correspondence

Avinash S. Bidra, Department of Reconstructive Sciences, University of Connecticut Health Center, 263 Farmington Ave., L6078, Farmington, CT 06030. E-mail: avinashbidra@yahoo.com

Accepted March 28, 2011

Published in *Journal of Prosthodontics* October 2011; Vol. 20, Suppl 2

doi: 10.1111/j.1532-849X.2011.00764.x

ABSTRACT

Fabry's disease is an uncommon X-linked metabolic disorder that leads to abnormal accumulation of glycosphingolipids in the body resulting in a variety of systemic disorders. Few reports have addressed dental findings and management of these patients. This clinical report describes the fixed prosthodontic rehabilitation of an adult male patient with Fabry's disease, who presented with generalized severe wear of the dentition. In addition to numerous systemic morbidities, the patient also presented with intraoral angiokeratomas, telangiactasias, anterior diastemata, bimaxillary prognathism, and other oral findings known to be prominent in these patients. The patient was managed by an interdisciplinary team of dental specialists in close coordination with his nephrologist. The prosthodontic treatment included restorations on all teeth, except mandibular anterior teeth, and the patient was restored with a partial group function scheme of occlusion. At the 3.5-year follow-up appointment, the patient's oral health and integrity of the restorations remained stable. This is the first clinical report describing the prosthodontic management of a patient with Fabry's disease. Unique features related to this patient's fixed prosthodontic treatment include accommodation to complex medical problems, management of maxillary diastemata, and choice of occlusal scheme.

Journal of Prosthodontics on Complex Restorations, First Edition. Edited by Nadim Z. Baba and David L. Guichet.
© 2016 American College of Prosthodontists. Published 2016 by John Wiley & Sons, Inc.

Fabry's disease is a rare X-linked recessive, lysosomal storage metabolic disorder described by Fabry and Anderson in 1898.[1,2] It is caused by a deficiency of lysosymal enzyme α-galactosidase A (AGA).[1] The altered gene is on the mother's X-chromosome, hence her sons have 50% chance of inheriting the disorder and daughters have a 50% chance of being carriers.[3] Hemizygous males usually have more pronounced disease manifestations than heterozygous females.[2] The incidence has been estimated at 1:40,000 to 1:117,000 people worldwide, but absolute numbers are unavailable.[1] A mutation in the gene that controls the AGA enzyme causes insufficient breakdown of lipids that builds up harmful levels of glycosphingolipids in the kidneys, eyes, autonomous nervous system, and cardiovascular system. This results in several clinical signs and symptoms and substantial morbidity and mortality.[1]

Systemic manifestations of this disease include cardiovascular disease with susceptibility to stroke at a young age, renal dysfunction, corneal dystrophy, fever from anhidrosis due to sweat gland failure, cutaneous angiokeratomas, and pain in the extremities.[1,2] Gastrointestinal (GI) disturbance is one of the most common symptoms in these patients.[1] About 19% to 52% of patients report GI symptoms including nausea, vomiting, regurgitation, and abdominal pain. There is no known cure for this disease, and treatment is mainly directed toward management of symptoms such as pain in the extremities (acroparasthesias), hypertension, GI symptoms, hemodialysis (to remove and purify the blood), kidney transplantation for failed kidneys, and enzyme-replacement therapy. Patients without renal transplants often survive into adulthood, but are at increased risk of strokes, heart attack, and renal failure. Patients with renal transplants are reported to survive for more than six decades.[1–3]

Few articles have described the craniofacial manifestations of patients with this disorder.[2,4–6] Baccaglini et al[2] have provided the most comprehensive assessment from their review of 13 patients with Fabry's disease. They reported angiokeratomas on the palpebral and labial cutaneous tissues, intraoral and perioral angiokeratomas, telangiactasias of the labial mucosa and soft palate, cysts/pseudocysts of the maxillary sinus, diastemata in the anterior region, and bimaxillary prognathism. They also noted that xerostomia was present in almost half their patients.[2] The dental management of patients with Fabry's disease requires special considerations due to their susceptibility for renal disease, hypertension, and GI disturbances, xerostomia and the numerous medications often taken by these patients. Additional considerations for prosthodontic treatment include management of diastemata for esthetics and optimal occlusal scheme, management of bimaxillary prognathism and the accompanying "gummy smile." Presently, there are no reports in the literature describing the protocol for dental management of such patients.

Patients with generalized wear of dentition often present with multiple etiologies that are either mechanical, chemical, or a combination.[7–10] These etiologies indicate the patients'

previous habits, lifestyle, and any underlying medical condition. Several clinical reports have described fixed prosthodontic management of patients with generalized wear of dentition.[11–14] The patient's needs, finances, motivation, and time dictate prosthodontic treatment options for patients with generalized tooth wear. Close collaboration with other medical and dental specialists is often necessary.

The purpose of this clinical report is to describe the prosthodontic management of an American College of Prosthodontists Prosthodontic Diagnostic Index [15] (ACP PDI) class IV dentate patient with Fabry's disease. Unique features related to this patient's prosthodontic treatment include accommodation to complex medical problems, management of anterior diastemata, and choice of occlusal scheme.

CLINICAL REPORT

History

A 41-year-old Caucasian man presented to the prosthodontist requesting a comprehensive evaluation, in order to improve the esthetics and structure of teeth he recognized as being compromised (Fig 7.1). He was aware of his complex dental situation and desired a definitive solution. Evaluation of his medical history revealed he had been diagnosed with Fabry's disease during his childhood and presented with multiple conditions associated with his disorder. The patient's medical history included hypertension and bilateral renal failure followed by a renal transplant donated by his sibling. His medical condition resulted in a long history of GI disturbances including nausea, vomiting, and regurgitation. The patient's medications included immunosuppressants, antihypertensives, and drugs for enzyme replacement therapy. Of special consideration was Agalsidase Beta, an enzyme replacement drug administered to him intravenously once every 2 weeks. The patient's dental history revealed multiple teeth with large restorations in all four posterior quadrants. He stated that he had a history of excessive consumption of carbonated beverages many years ago, to stay hydrated during treatment for his renal condition. He also revealed that he was aware of his bruxism habits during the day and was unaware of any nocturnal habits. The patient led an active life and was not in any physical discomfort at the time of presentation.

Findings

Extraoral examination revealed multiple angiokeratomas in the perioral region including the lips (Fig 7.2). The intraoral soft tissues also showed angiokeratomas and telangiectasias in areas with nonkeratinized mucosa. The gingiva showed minimal inflammation, and the maximum probing depth was 3 mm. The patient did not had objective signs for xerostomia, but a predisposition was not ruled out due to his numerous medications and this characteristic being common in Fabry's

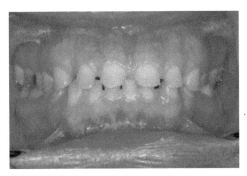

FIGURE 7.1 Pretreatment condition of the teeth in maximum intercuspation. Note the presence of diastemata only in the anterior region. Also note the angiokeratomas and telangiactasias of the alveolar and labial mucosa contributing to the reddish appearance.

disease patients.[2] The hard tissues revealed diastemata in the maxillary and mandibular anterior region only, a characteristic feature of patients with Fabry's disease.[2] Generalized severe attrition and erosion of the dentition was seen on the occlusal surfaces of all posterior teeth and lingual surfaces of maxillary anterior teeth (Fig 7.3). This was probably due to a combination of his GI condition and history of excessive consumption of carbonated beverages. The facial surfaces of mandibular premolars and lingual surfaces of maxillary premolars showed severe wear. The mandibular incisors showed minimal wear compared to the canines. Multiple amalgam restorations in the posterior region had loss of marginal integrity and were inadequate. All teeth responded positively to vitality testing of the pulp.

There was a 5-mm vertical overlap, with the mandibular incisors contacting the palatal tissues. Clinically, the crowns appeared short due to a combination of wear, altered passive eruption, and large jaw size. The patient presented with Angle's class I molar relationship; the malocclusion was primarily due to anterior spacing and generalized wear that had also resulted in a group function scheme of occlusion. The patient's maximum intercuspal position and centric occlusion were not coincident. Multiple laterotrusive and mediotrusive interferences were noted, which may have aggravated the patient's bruxism.[7] The patient's caries risk assessment revealed a high score due to the number of

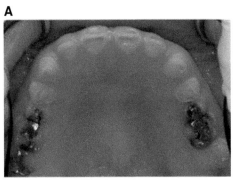

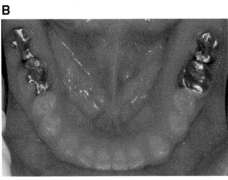

FIGURE 7.3 (A) Maxillary occlusal view showing generalized wear of teeth. Also note the large size of the maxilla, anterior diastemata, and multiple restored teeth. (B) Mandibular occlusal view showing generalized wear of teeth. Again, note the large size of the mandible, anterior diastemata, and multiple teeth with large restorations.

restored teeth and his predisposition to xerostomia related to his medical condition.[16,17] Based on clinical assessment, esthetics, and available freeway space, it was determined there was no loss in the patient's occlusal vertical dimension (OVD). Therefore, the patient met the criteria of category III described by Turner and Missirlian.[7] The patient also had excessive gingival display due to a combination of altered passive eruption, prognathic maxilla, and hypermobile maxillary lip. Radiographic examination showed acceptable crown-root ratios on all teeth and no bone loss (Fig 7.4).

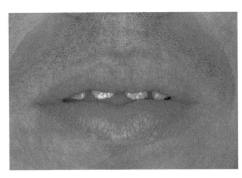

FIGURE 7.2 Angiokeratomas on the lips and perioral region.

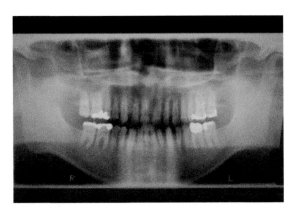

FIGURE 7.4 Pretreatment panoramic radiograph showing acceptable bone levels, crown-root ratios, and large restorations.

Diagnosis and Treatment Planning

The patient was under close medical supervision by his physician and nephrologist due to his disease and related symptoms. Based on his history and clinical, radiographic, and occlusal findings from mounted diagnostic casts, the patient was diagnosed as an ACP PDI class IV patient.[15] A multidisciplinary team of a prosthodontist, periodontist, orthodontist, and endodontist developed a treatment plan including complete crowns on all teeth except the mandibular incisors. Metal ceramic restorations (JP-1 Alloy; Jensen Dental, North Haven, CT) were planned on all teeth except the molars, which were to receive complete cast crowns made of high noble alloy (JC Alloy; Jensen Dental). Crown-lengthening procedures were planned for all teeth except the mandibular incisors to ameliorate clinical crown length and obtain better resistance form for the preparations. Elective endodontic treatment was planned for the maxillary right second premolar and mandibular left second molar, as the existing restorations were very close to the pulp. The patient refused to have his mandibular canines restored, as he deemed it to be too aggressive, and therefore the treatment plan was modified accordingly.

The treatment plan was presented for approval by the patient's nephrologist who recommended premedication with 2 gm of Amoxicillin, 1 hour prior to all procedures that would involve any bleeding, considering his renal transplant. Additional recommendations included avoidance of epinephrine-containing local anesthetics to prevent changes in hypertension and avoidance of all forms of nonsteroidal anti-inflammatory drugs, due to his renal condition. Therefore, acetaminophen was the recommended analgesic of choice. The patient was also prescribed 1.1% sodium fluoride topical dentifrice (Prevident 5000 Plus; Colgate-Palmolive, Morristown, NJ) for use twice daily. The patient was monitored by his nephrologist for systemic health, and his oral health and hygiene were closely monitored during the entire course of treatment.

Preprosthetic Treatment

The patient's maxillary incisal edge position was assessed by lip length, display of incisors with lips at repose, patient's age, esthetics, and phonetics.[18] The existing incisal edge positions were acceptable to the patient and clinician (Fig 7.2). A Lucia-type of acrylic resin jig[19] was fabricated over the mandibular incisors on the cast and was adjusted to correspond to a 2-mm increase in OVD at the incisors. Using this jig, a new centric relation record was obtained, and the casts were remounted on a semi-adjustable articulator (Hanau Wide Vue Arcon 183-2; Whip Mix Corp., Louisville, KY) at the planned OVD. Diagnostic waxing was then accomplished on the mounted casts. The patient requested that the diastemata in the maxillary anterior sextant be closed in

the final restorations, and the waxing was done accordingly. A partial group function occlusal scheme[21] was designed for the definitive restorations. After the patient approval of the diagnostic waxing, crown-lengthening procedures were accomplished by the periodontistin quadrants, over a series of four appointments. Scalloped vacuum-formed matrices prepared during the diagnostic waxing were used as guides for all crown-lengthening procedures. During the healing period, endodontic treatment on the two planned teeth was accomplished.

Prosthodontic Treatment

After 12 weeks of healing from crown lengthening, initial tooth preparations were accomplished, and interim prostheses were cemented. The interim prostheses were fabricated using the diagnostic waxing as a guide. The acrylic resin jig fabricated over the unprepared mandibular incisors acted as an aid to maintain the desired OVD increase of 2 mm. During subsequent periods of refinement of tooth preparations, a cast dowel and core was fabricated from high noble alloy and cemented on the maxillary right second premolar. The core of the mandibular left second molar was built using silver amalgam material, engaging undercuts in the pulp chamber and protruding 2 mm into the root canals.[20] For the remaining tooth preparations, all previous restorations were removed and not replaced. Presence of caries and demineralized dentin were checked with slow-speed round burs and a caries-detecting dye (Sable Seek; Ultradent Products, South Jordan, UT). Special attention was paid to ensure no undercuts existed in the tooth preparations. Grooves were incorporated to augment resistance form due to the short height of the prepared teeth. After refining final tooth preparations, the interim prostheses were relined and cemented accordingly (Fig 7.5). The interim prostheses had a partial group function occlusal scheme, where guidance was provided by the canines and both premolars in laterotrusive movements.[21]

The patient had the opportunity to experience the interim prostheses for 5 months. This allowed him to thoroughly evaluate his esthetics, function, and comfort and allowed the clinician a satisfactory assessment of the patient's tolerance

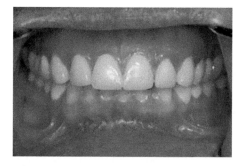

FIGURE 7.5 Teeth with interim prostheses, in centric occlusion. Note acceptable health of gingival tissues.

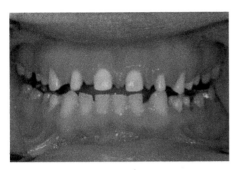

FIGURE 7.6 Finalized tooth preparations. Note "creation" of interdental papilla, once the diastemata were closed and contact was established between the incisors.

to the 2-mm OVD increase. Appropriate health of soft tissues was ensured prior to making final impressions (Fig 7.6). For the impression procedures, the patient was premedicated with 2 gm amoxicillin, and the gingiva was retracted using knitted cords (Ultrapak, Ultradent Products) of varying dimensions, soaked in 21.3% aluminum chloride (Hemodent; Premier Dental, Plymouth Meeting, PA). Thereafter, complete arch impressions of all tooth preparations were made using polyether impression material (Impregum Pentasoft, 3M ESPE, St. Paul, MN) in the maxillary and mandibular arches. The master cast and dies were prepared from these impressions to proceed with fabrication of the restorations (Fig 7.7). Thereafter, standard fixed prosthodontic principles[11–14] were followed, and the definitive restorations were fabricated. The prostheses were tried in the mouth, and minimal adjustments were made for esthetics and occlusion. The definitive restorations were then cemented with resin-modified glass ionomer cement (RelyX Luting Plus; 3M ESPE) (Fig 7.8). The partial group function occlusal scheme of the interim prostheses was emulated in the definitive restorations as well (Fig 7.9).

Posttreatment Therapy

After final cementation, new diagnostic impressions were made. An occlusal device was fabricated, and the patient was instructed to wear it at night. The patient was given detailed oral hygiene instructions and was advised to continue using the 1.1% sodium fluoride dentifrice for the rest of his life, due to his predisposition for xerostomia. He was also provided with a set of his new diagnostic casts to enable future monitoring of wear, especially on his unrestored mandibular incisors and canines. He was placed on 6-month recall for maintenance of oral health. At a 3.5-year recall, definitive restorations and health of the soft tissues remained stable. The patient remained satisfied with esthetics, function, and comfort of his prostheses (Fig 7.10). The patient's systemic health remained stable, and he continued his medical treatment with his nephrologist.

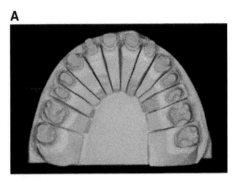

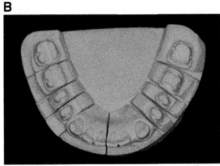

FIGURE 7.7 (A) Maxillary master cast with dies. Note that previous restorations in all posterior teeth were removed and incorporated as part of the tooth preparations. Grooves for resistance forms were placed wherever necessary. (B) Mandibular master cast with dies. Note that previous restorations in all posterior teeth were removed and incorporated as part of the tooth preparations. Grooves for resistance forms were placed wherever necessary.

DISCUSSION

From a prosthodontic treatment perspective, important factors in the management of this patient with Fabry's disease were: (1) complex medical history, (2) multiple medications taken by the patient, (3) limited choice of anesthetics and analgesics, (4) appointment durations and schedule, (5) management of anterior diastemata for esthetics, (6) partial group function occlusal scheme, and (7) patient's predisposition to xerostomia. It is unlikely that Fabry's disease had a direct bearing on the wear of this patient's dentition; however, it is important to note that he had a long history of GI disturbances including vomiting and regurgitation, history of excessive consumption of carbonated beverages to stay hydrated, and bruxism habits related to stress, all of which contributed to tooth wear. It is important that the prosthodontist ensure these patients have been thoroughly evaluated by a gastroenterologist torule out any premalignancy of the esophageal lining due to chronic vomiting and regurgitation.

The choice of restorative materials for this patient was based on a confluence of factors. Complete gold crowns cast in high noble alloy were used for all molar teeth, due to the patient's history of bruxism. Gold crowns are simple

A

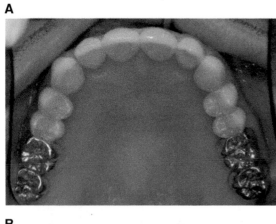

B

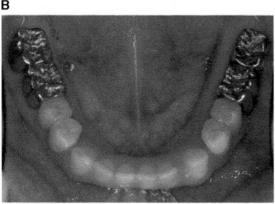

C

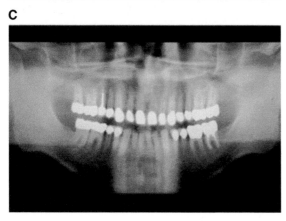

FIGURE 7.8   (A) Maxillary occlusal view showing the final metal ceramic and gold restorations. Note that diastemata have been closed only between central and lateral incisors; (B) mandibular occlusal view showing the final metal ceramic and gold restorations; (C) posttreatment panoramic radiograph showing acceptable bone levels, crown-root ratios, and definitive prostheses. Note that a cast dowel-core has been placed on tooth #4 and an amalgam coronal-radicular dowel and core on tooth #18.

monolithic restorations that require conservative tooth preparations and have proven longevity.[22,23] They have a lesser chance of fracture, making them an ideal choice of restoration for bruxism patients. The appearance of gold-colored teeth in the posterior region was not of an esthetic concern for

A

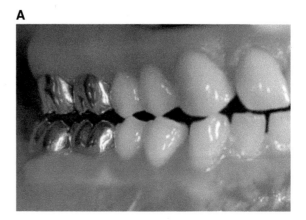

B

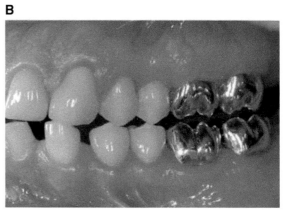

FIGURE 7.9   (A) Right laterotrusive image shows the developed partial group function scheme. The guidance was provided by the canines and premolars only. (B) Left laterotrusive image shows the developed partial group function scheme. The guidance was provided by the canines and premolars only.

this patient. Metal ceramic restorations were used in all the remaining teeth because of their long and successful clinical track record and their ability to appear esthetic with the help of skilled laboratory personnel.[24–27]

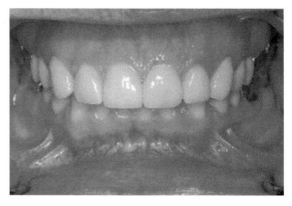

FIGURE 7.10   Frontal image taken at final follow-up, showing the posttreatment condition of the teeth in centric occlusion. The health of the gingival tissues is acceptable.

All-ceramic restorations were not considered in the anterior region because of patient's history of bruxism, need for additional tooth reduction, and difficulty of access for potential endodontic treatment in the future, which has been reported to be the primary complication of crowns in fixed prosthodontics.[28]

As the patient refused to have restorations on his partially worn mandibular canines, it was difficult to obtain a mutually protected articulation with canine guidance, given the positions of these teeth due to anterior diastemata. Addition of composite resin to the mandibular canines was not performed due to degradation of the dentin bond and potential fracture/accelerated wear from the opposing metal ceramic crowns. Group function is defined as "multiple contact relations between the maxillary and mandibular teeth in lateral movements on the working side whereby simultaneous contact of several teeth acts as a group to distribute occlusal forces."[29] In fixed prosthodontics, a complete group function with guidance provided by all posterior teeth may not be the preferred occlusal scheme; this is because forces are higher in the posterior region due to their proximity to the fulcrum of the mandible and hence, an anteriorly directed guidance is more favorable. Therefore, in this patient, a partial group function scheme was adopted, with guidance provided only by canines and both premolars in all laterotrusive movements.[21]

The mandibular incisors did not receive any prosthodontic treatment, as it was determined that the wear on these teeth was not significant enough to justify complete or partial coverage restorations. Furthermore, contact of the mandibular incisors with lingual surfaces of maxillary anterior crowns was successfully achieved in centric occlusion. The patient was cautioned that progressive wear of mandibular canines and incisors would warrant complete coverage restorations in the future.

Though it was clinically determined that the patient had no loss of OVD, a minimal increase of 2 mm at the incisors (about 1 mm in the molar region) was necessary to gain the needed space for restorations. This helped to achieve conservative tooth preparations in the molar regions for the planned gold restorations. Preprosthetic orthodontic treatment was offered as an option for the patient, but he refused it due to the duration of treatment. Therefore, the patient requested that the diastemata be closed through prosthodontic treatment only; however, the diastemata could be successfully closed only between the central and lateral incisors on each side. Closure of the diastema between the lateral incisors and canines could not be accomplished because of the increased space and to avoid violation of esthetic tooth proportions in the definitive restorations.

SUMMARY

This clinical report described the comprehensive fixed prosthodontic rehabilitation of a medically compromised ACP PDI class IV patient with a rare condition called Fabry's disease. Through an interdisciplinary team of dental specialists in close coordination with his nephrologist, a successful treatment protocol with special considerations was established and executed. Unique features related to this patient's prosthodontic treatment included management of anterior diastemata and use of a partial group function occlusal scheme. At a 3.5-year follow-up appointment, the patient's oral health and integrity of the restorations remained stable. Future prognosis will depend upon the patient's medical health, adherence to oral hygiene regimen, and motivation.

REFERENCES

1. Zarate YA, Hopkin RJ: Fabry's disease. *Lancet* 2008;372: 1427–1435.
2. Baccaglini L, Schiffmann R, Brennan MT, et al: Oral and craniofacial findings in Fabry's disease: a report of 13 patients. *Oral Surg Oral Med Oral Pathol Oral Radiol Endod* 2001;92:415–419.
3. National Institute of Neurological Disorders and Stroke. Fabry Disease Information Page. http://www.ninds.nih.gov/disorders/fabrys/fabrys.htm. Accessed on January 28, 2011.
4. Regattieri LR, Parker JL: Supernumerary teeth associated with Fabry-Anderson's syndrome. *Oral Surg Oral Med Oral Pathol* 1973;35:432–433.
5. Brindley HP, Archard HO, Alling CC, et al: Case 11, Part 2. Angiokeratoma corporis diffusum (Fabry's disease). *J Oral Surg* 1975;33:199–205.
6. Young WG, Pihlstrom BL, Sauk JJ Jr: Granulomatous gingivitis in Anderson-Fabry disease. *J Periodontol* 1980;51: 95–101.
7. Turner KA, Missirlian DM: Restoration of the extremely worn dentition. *J Prosthet Dent* 1984;52:467–474.
8. Verrett RG: Analyzing the etiology of an extremely worn dentition. *J Prosthodont* 2001;10:224–233.
9. Grippo JO, Simring M, Schreiner S: Attrition, abrasion, corrosion and abfraction revisited: a new perspective on tooth surface lesions. *J Am Dent Assoc* 2004;135:1109–1118.
10. Litonjua LA, Andreana S, Bush PJ, et al: Tooth wear: attrition, erosion, and abrasion. *Quint Int* 2003;34:435–446.
11. Stewart B: Restoration of the severely worn dentition using a systematized approach for a predictable prognosis. *Int J Periodontics Restorative Dent* 1998;18:46–57.
12. Potiket N: Fixed rehabilitation of an ACP PDI Class IV dentate patient. *J Prosthodont* 2006;15:367–373.
13. Michalakis KX: Fixed rehabilitation of an ACP PDI class III patient. *J Prosthodont* 2006;15:359–366.
14. Thongthammachat-Thavornthanasarn S: Treatment of a patient with severely worn dentition: a clinical report. *J Prosthodont* 2007;16:219–225.
15. McGarry TJ, Nimmo A, Skiba JF, et al: Classification system for the completely dentate patient. *J Prosthodont* 2004;13: 73–82.

16. Featherstone JD, Adair SM, Anderson MH, et al: Caries management by risk assessment: consensus statement, April 2002. *J Calif Dent Assoc* 2003;31:257–269.

17. Featherstone JD, Domejean-Orliaguet S, Jenson L, et al: Caries risk assessment in practice for age 6 through adult. *J Calif Dent Assoc* 2007;35:703–707, 710–713.

18. Spear FM, Kokich VG, Mathews DP: Interdisciplinary management of anterior dental esthetics. *J Am Dent Assoc* 2006;37:160–169.

19. Lucia VO: Centric relation. In Lucia VO (ed): Modern Gnathologic Concepts: Updated. Chicago, Quintessence, 1983, pp. 99–104.

20. Nayyar A, Walton RE, Leonard LA: An amalgam coronal-radicular dowel and core technique for endodontically treated posterior teeth. *J Prosthet Dent* 1980;43:511–515.

21. Fox CW Jr, Doukoudakis A, Fox SW, et al: A method for occlusal reshaping. *J Prosthodont* 1992;1:102–105.

22. Donovan TE, Simonsen RJ, Guertin G, et al: Retrospective clinical evaluation of 1,314 cast gold restorations in service from 1 to 52 years. *J Esthet Restor Dent* 2004;16:194–204.

23. Christensen GJ: The coming demise of the cast gold restoration? *J Am Dent Assoc* 1996;127:1233–1236.

24. Lindquist E, Karlsson S: Success rate and failures for fixed partial dentures after 20 years of service: part 1. *Int J Prosthodont* 1998;11:133–138.

25. Walton T: An up to 15-year longitudinal study of 515 metal-ceramic FDPs: part 1. Outcome. *Int J Prosthodont* 2002;15:439–445.

26. Holm C, Tidehag P, Tillberg A, et al: Longevity and quality of FPDs: a retrospective study of restorations 30, 20, and 10 years after insertion. *Int J Prosthodont* 2003;16:283–289.

27. De Backer H, Van Maele G, De Moor N, et al: An 18-year retrospective survival study of full crowns with or without posts. *Int J Prosthodont* 2006;19:136–142.

28. Goodacre CJ, Bernal G, Rungcharassaeng K, et al: Clinical complications in fixed prosthodontics. *J Prosthet Dent* 2003;90:31–41.

29. The glossary of prosthodontic terms. *J Prosthet Dent* 2005;94:10–92.

8

ANALYZING THE ETIOLOGY OF AN EXTREMELY WORN DENTITION

RONALD G. VERRETT, DDS, MS
Assistant Professor, Department of Prosthodontics, The University of Texas Health Science Center at San Antonio, San Antonio, TX

Keywords
Tooth wear; diagnosis; abrasion; attrition; erosion.

Correspondence
Dr. Ronald Verrett, Department of Prosthodontics-MSC 7912, The University of Texas Health Science Center, 7703 Floyd Curl Drive, San Antonio, TX 78229-3700. E-mail: Verrett@uthscsa.edu

Presented at the annual meeting of the American College of Prosthodontists, New York, NY, October 22, 1999, and at the annual meeting of the American Academy of Restorative Dentistry, Chicago, IL, February 25, 2001.

Accepted July 24, 2001

Published in *Journal of Prosthodontics* 2001; Vol. 10, Issue 4

doi:10.1053/jpro.2001. 28264

ABSTRACT

Patients requiring extensive restorative care frequently exhibit significant loss of tooth structure. Specific clinical findings in an extremely worn dentition may vary widely and are often confusing. Severe wear can result from a mechanical cause, a chemical cause, or a combination of causes. The location of the wear, the accompanying symptoms and signs, and information gained from the patient interview are essential components in determining the etiology. A diagnostic decision tree facilitates a systematic analysis and diagnosis of dental wear.

Patients seeking complex restorative care often exhibit clinical evidence of severe wear. This may be related to an aging patient population in which many individuals are retaining more teeth, but there is also compelling evidence to indicate that the incidence of wear is increasing in younger age groups.[1]

Tooth wear occurs as a physiologic process; normal ranges for specific populations have been reported.[2] Pathologic wear occurs when this normal rate is accelerated by unusual endogenous or exogenous factors. Severe tooth wear is frequently multifactorial and variable. To prevent further pathologic change, it is essential that the etiology of abnormal wear be determined, yet diagnosing the factors responsible for a severely worn dentition often presents a clinical conundrum. The purpose of this article is to review the clinical manifestations of tooth surface loss, to examine the predominant locations and clinical signs that accompany this pathology, and to describe an orderly approach to diagnosis.

INITIAL ASSESSMENT

The initial interview should include a thorough review of the patient's health history, an evaluation of the wear history, a discussion of the patient's dietary patterns, and an assessment of potential occupational factors and/or habits. The clinical examination should include an evaluation of the patient's dental status, observation of specific wear patterns, and, if possible, determination of the rate at which tooth structure has been lost. Serial bitewing or other radiographs, made in earlier years, may provide objective evidence of the rate of tooth surface loss. Casts made in earlier years may also prove useful in determining the progression of tooth wear.

Observing the patient's facial appearance provides information such as an apparent decrease in occlusal vertical dimension. With the teeth in occlusion, the patient may exhibit a diminished facial contour, thin lips with narrow vermilion borders, and drooping commissures (Fig 8.1).[3] Interocclusal space may appear excessive at the rest vertical dimension. Vertical dimension should be carefully evaluated using one of several techniques previously described.[4–9]

TERMINOLOGY

Four types of surface loss have been identified, distinguished by the differing causes of loss. *Attrition* describes mechanical wear resulting from mastication or parafunction, and is limited to the contacting surfaces of teeth.[10] *Abrasion* denotes the wearing away of structure through some unusual or abnormal mechanical process other than tooth-to-tooth contact.[10] *Erosion* indicates the progressive loss of tooth structure through chemical processes that do not involve bacterial action.[11] *Abfraction* connotes the pathologic loss of tooth structure attributed to mechanical loading and resulting in wedge-shaped defects in the cervical areas.[12,13]

Surface loss can be differentiated into three general causal categories: mechanical loss, which includes attrition and abrasion; chemical loss, which includes erosion; and finally, a proposed biomechanical category, described as abfraction by Grippo.[12] Abfraction lesions, in theory attributed to tooth flexure, remain controversial[12–14] and will not receive further attention in this article. Although categorization as mechanical or chemical constitutes a useful beginning toward understanding enamel wear, further exploration is necessary to determine specific etiologies.

DETERMINING ETIOLOGY

The diagnosis of severe wear is frequently clouded by the presence of multiple etiologic agents. The diagnostic challenge is to first correctly identify the signs of a severely worn dentition and then, using an orderly evaluation process, to arrive at an understanding of the etiology. It will be useful to begin the discussion of this process with a review of the general kinds of surface loss, including the developmental dysplasias that may contribute to the process.

First, it is important to distinguish between mechanical and chemical wear. Each has distinctive characteristics. Mechanical wear occurs between two or more moving surfaces. This type of surface loss occurs as teeth contact each other or are abraded by another source (Fig 8.2). With

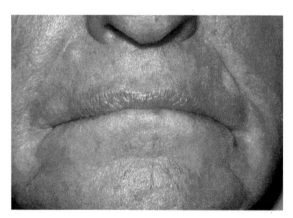

FIGURE 8.1   The appearance of the patient's face when the teeth are in maximum intercuspation may suggest a loss of vertical dimension. Diminished vermilion borders and drooping commissures are indications of a decreased occlusal vertical dimension.

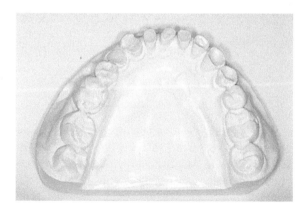

FIGURE 8.2   Mechanical wear has distinctive characteristics: wear facets with sharply defined line angles; restorations that wear at the same rate as adjacent enamel; asymptomatic teeth; and histories that include parafunctional habits.

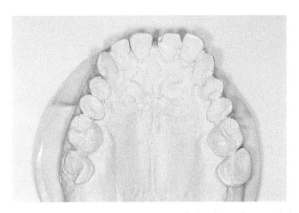

FIGURE 8.3 Chemical wear has distinctive characteristics: occlusal cupping and cratering with rounded margins; erosion lesions that do not articulate with opposing surfaces; elevated islands of restorative material, such as amalgam; and unstained but frequently hypersensitive teeth.

mechanical wear, restorations tend to wear at the same rate as adjacent tooth structure. Wear facets display sharply defined peripheries that can be matched on articulated diagnostic casts. Teeth with severe mechanical wear are frequently asymptomatic, and patients may report parafunctional habits.

Chemical erosion occurs when tooth surfaces experience prolonged exposure to acidic solutions (Fig 8.3), resulting in loss of structure and restorations that appear elevated, often termed "amalgam islands." Occlusal surfaces display cupping and cratering with rounded margins.[15] Such findings are pathognomonic for erosion. The teeth are frequently hypersensitive and, in most instances, are not stained. The cupping and cratering from erosion cannot be matched on opposing articulated diagnostic casts. The causative acid may come from within the body, from the diet, or from the environment, and a detailed history will often reveal the source.

Many reports have confirmed a multifactorial etiology associated with tooth surface loss. When considered as a single factor, location has not been shown to reliably indicate the cause of surface loss.[16] Limited population studies have attempted to identify factors associated with high-wear groups.[17–20] Johansson et al[21] examined 59 high-wear patients and found that men showed significantly more wear than women. Increased bite force was also positively correlated with increased wear. Analysis of saliva showed that a low buffering capacity and a diminished rate of secretion also were related to high wear rates.

An efficient diagnostic approach involves determining whether the cause of the surface loss is chemical or mechanical or a combination of both. The location of the loss and an interpretation of the accompanying signs and symptoms may then be used to guide the differential diagnostic process.

Finally, it must be noted that hereditary dysplasias, such as amelogenesis imperfecta and dentinogenesis imperfecta, compromise wear resistance and predispose teeth to accelerated surface loss from mechanical or chemical causes.[22]

Amelogenesis imperfecta, a local, systemic, or hereditary dysplasia affecting the quantity of enamel or the quality of calcification, results in enamel that is thinner and/or more friable, and thus more susceptible to chemical erosion and mechanical wear.

Dentinogenesis imperfecta, a hereditary dysplasia of the dentin affecting both primary and permanent dentitions,[22] results in teeth with a characteristic gray or brown opalescent appearance. A weak enamel-to-dentin bond results in the early loss of the enamel, rapid attrition, and increased susceptibility to caries.

DETERMINING THE CAUSE OF MECHANICAL WEAR

Once the mechanical nature of wear has been identified, the location or locations of surface loss should be analyzed. Several individual patterns of mechanical wear can be identified that tend to occur at predictable locations. In the first pattern, wear occurs primarily on the incisal surfaces of the anterior teeth. A second pattern displays occlusal wear throughout the arch, with progressively greater structural loss as one proceeds from the posterior teeth to the anterior teeth. A third wear pattern tends to occur on the facial surfaces of cuspids and premolars. Each of these patterns exhibits specific associated clinical signs and symptoms.

Pattern: Anterior Tooth Wear Greater Than Posterior Tooth Wear

Inadequate or unstable posterior support has been identified as a factor in severe anterior attrition and decreased occlusal vertical dimension.[23] The loss of posterior teeth has been reported as a major factor in the development of a traumatic anterior occlusion.[24] Posterior occlusal prematurities may also cause increased function on anterior teeth, resulting in increased wear (Fig 8.4).

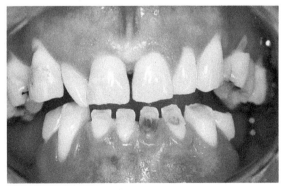

FIGURE 8.4 Mechanical wear affecting primarily the anterior teeth may result from posterior tooth loss, malposition, or interferences.

Pattern: Progressively Greater Wear on the Anterior Teeth

Mechanical wear resulting from bruxism often results in progressively greater wear toward the anterior teeth (Fig 8.5). An exception to this finding occurs in individuals with anterior open bite. Variations in mandibular movement may result in a wide variety of wear patterns in bruxing patients. As might be expected, bruxism produces surface loss, which is related to the duration and force of parafunction. A definitive diagnosis may be made by hand articulating diagnostic casts and matching wear facets. Additional intraoral findings may include grooving of the lateral borders of the tongue, evidence of cheek biting, and the presence of fractured porcelain restorations. Cupping or cratering of the occlusal surfaces can occur once the enamel has been perforated.

Pattern: Wear on Facial Surfaces of the Cuspids and Premolars

Excessive tooth brushing may produce noticeable wear on the facial surfaces of the cuspids and premolars, sometimes resulting in a "sandblasted" appearance with reduced anatomic detail (Fig 8.6).[25] Depending on the patient's oral hygiene habits, tooth brushing abrasion also may result in bizarre patterns of wear with notching or grooving of the teeth. The amount of surface loss will be affected by the individual's tooth brushing technique, the amount of time spent in brushing, the mechanical properties of the toothbrush, and the abrasiveness of the dentifrice.[26] A definitive diagnosis may be made by asking the patient to demonstrate his or her brushing technique. This may confirm that the location of the wear correlates with the source of the abrasion.

Pattern: Wear in Variable Locations, Primarily Occlusal and Incisal Surfaces

Variable wear on occlusal and incisal surfaces suggests some type of parafunctional habit as a causal factor. Such habits

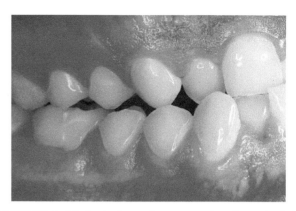

FIGURE 8.6 Mechanical wear that occurs primarily on the facial surfaces of cuspid and bicuspid teeth is often related to toothbrush/dentifrice misuse. Teeth may exhibit a loss of surface detail and a "sandblasted" appearance.

may be related to job requirements, habitual behaviors, or stress. Case reports document the destructive effects of foreign objects such as pipe stems, pins, needles, paper clips, sunflower seeds, and soft drink cans.[27] Wear is found primarily on the occlusal and incisal surfaces of the teeth (Fig 8.7).

Diagnostic Algorithm for Mechanical Wear

Mechanical wear can be unusual in appearance and difficult to diagnose. Using a three-tier decision tree can assist in categorizing the wear (Fig 8.8). First, identify the character of the pathologic wear, then the location, then evaluate the clinical signs and symptoms and discuss habit possibilities with the patient.

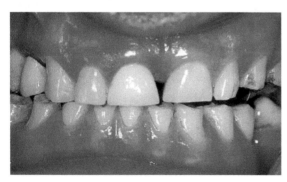

FIGURE 8.5 Mechanical wear that is progressively greater toward the anterior teeth and is characterized by extensive occlusal and incisal wear facets suggests chronic bruxism.

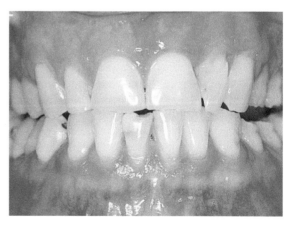

FIGURE 8.7 Mechanical wear can occur as a result of a variety of parafunctional habits, including biting on needles, pipe stems, hairpins, or paper clips, often resulting in notch-like defects at the occlusal or incisal surfaces.

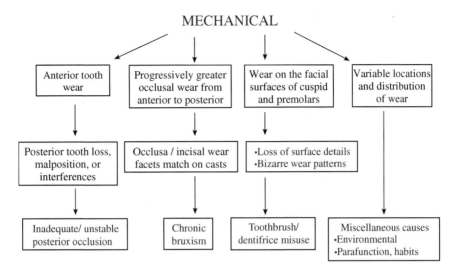

FIGURE 8.8   The etiology of pathologic wear resulting from mechanical causes can be determined by correlating the location of wear, other signs and symptoms, and information obtained during the patient interview.

DETERMINING THE CAUSE OF CHEMICAL EROSION

Pindborg[28] described "erosion" as loss of tooth structure resulting from a chemical process and not mediated by bacteria. Chemical erosion has been identified as a major cause of tooth surface loss. In a study of 100 patients referred for evaluation of tooth wear, 89% were determined to have erosion as a contributing cause.[29] Several population studies have shown an increasing prevalence of dental erosion in children. The largest of these studies, the United Kingdom Child Dental Health Survey of 1993, reported that 52% of the 5-year-olds surveyed showed evidence of significant erosion.[1] Awareness of the problem of erosion has increased in both the dental profession and in the general population for the past three decades.

The risk of dental erosion has been shown to increase with certain dietary habits, with gastric regurgitation or reflux, and in individuals with chronic self-induced vomiting.[12,30] Once the chemical cause of surface loss has been identified, the location should be assessed. Patterns of erosion with anterior tooth surface loss greater than posterior tooth surface loss or vs. can occur.

Pattern: Anterior Surface Loss Greater Than Posterior Surface Loss

Chemically mediated surface loss has been observed to occur in stages.[31] Lesions begin as smoothly glazed enamel and progress to concavities. As the erosion process continues, islands of restorative material become evident, and cupping of the enamel occurs. Chronic vomiting is the most common cause of severe erosion of the lingual surfaces of the

maxillary anterior teeth, although hiatal hernia and gastric reflux are also possible causes. Chemical erosion of the maxillary anterior teeth has been correlated with self-induced vomiting since 1937.[33] A diagnosis relating to chronic vomiting may be difficult to confirm because patients with eating disorders frequently deny such behavior.[32]

Chronic regurgitation can be recognized by the very specific pattern of surface loss (Fig 8.9).[33] As gastric contents, with a mean pH of 3.8,[34] rush past the teeth, the lingual surfaces of the maxillary anterior teeth are most severely affected. There is progressively greater erosive damage from posterior to anterior. Eroded palatal surfaces are very smooth, with the defects beginning at the gingival margins. The maxillary molars and premolars may have chamfer-like defects on the lingual surfaces. Mandibular teeth tend to

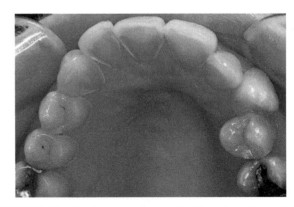

FIGURE 8.9   Erosion occurring on the lingual surfaces of the maxillary teeth is evidence of chronic regurgitation. The lingual surfaces of the maxillary premolars and molars may display chamfer margins.

be minimally affected because of the protection afforded by the tongue and the buccal mucosa.

Gastric reflux has also been shown to cause erosion on the lingual surfaces of the maxillary anterior teeth.[35–37] Erosion may occur as a localized phenomenon at other locations if the hydrochloric acid reflux solution is permitted to pool, as may happen, for example, when the patient is sleeping. Gastroesophageal reflux differs from vomiting both in the volume of acidic material to which the teeth are exposed, and in the lack of forceful expulsion, because muscular contraction of the diaphragm does not occur. Identification of gastroesophageal reflux disease, or GERD, is often suggested by the symptoms of belching, acidic tastes in the mouth, stomach aches on awakening, heartburn, and hyper-sensitivity of the affected teeth.[38] However, many patients with this disorder report no subjective symptoms, and ambulatory pH monitoring may be required to confirm this diagnosis.[38]

Alcoholism may lead to erosion resulting from chronic vomiting and regurgitation associated with gastritis. The lingual surfaces of the maxillary anterior teeth are primarily affected, with mandibular teeth minimally affected (Fig 8.10). Alcoholism is a relatively common condition in western countries, with an estimated incidence of as high as 10% in men.[39] Robb and Smith[40] found evidence of chemical erosion in 92% of a clinical sample of 37 inpatients admitted for the treatment of chronic alcoholism. They observed more severe wear in those who drank regularly as compared with binge drinkers (i.e., heavy alcohol consumption for up to 2 weeks with intervals of sobriety).

Citrus fruit sucking results in erosion on the facial surfaces of the maxillary anterior teeth (Fig 8.11). Severe erosion related to a prolonged history of eating or sucking lemons has been reported.[41] The location and severity of erosion is directly related to the manner in which the acidic food is consumed, the degree of its acidity, and the duration of exposure. In most instances, posterior teeth are spared the

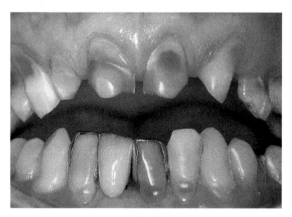

FIGURE 8.10   Chronic regurgitation related to alcoholism causes severe erosion of the maxillary teeth with minimal surface loss on the mandibular teeth.

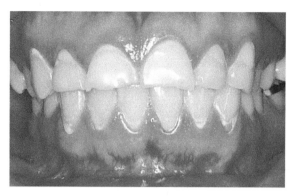

FIGURE 8.11   Citrus fruit sucking typically causes erosion on the facial surfaces of the maxillary anterior teeth, whereas the posterior teeth remain unaltered. The teeth contacted by the fruit and the manner of consumption determine the clinical presentation.

effects of the acid, and a marked transition from the eroded anterior teeth to the unaffected posterior teeth can be observed.

Pattern: Posterior Surface Loss Greater Than Anterior Surface Loss

The dietary causes of dental erosion have received widespread attention in case studies,[42–44] population surveys,[14,28,45,46] and in vitro testing.[47–50] As acidic food and drinks are consumed, the occlusal surfaces of the posterior teeth tend to display greater wear than the anterior teeth. Erosion resulting from extrinsic causes has been correlated with excessive consumption of low-pH carbonated beverages as well as fruits and juices with high citric acid contents. A study of 106 patients referred for evaluation of erosion, indicated a significant risk of surface loss occurred in patients who consumed citrus fruits more than twice a day or soft drinks at least once a day.[15]

Acidic beverages are widely consumed in our society. Larsen and Nyvad[51] studied the erosive potential of 18 acidic beverages and observed 3 distinct groupings: carbonated flavored soft drinks including colas; orange juices; and mineral water drinks. In general, enamel erosion was found to increase logarithmically as the pH decreased. Carbonated mineral waters were found to increase in pH by almost a half unit as they were poured, and the erosive effects on enamel were found to be minimal.

Chemical erosion in which posterior tooth surface loss is greatest at mandibular first molar and second premolar areas has been associated with holding carbonated soft drinks in the mouth and/or swishing (Fig 8.12). Erosion resulting from holding carbonated soft drinks in the mouth until the carbon dioxide bubbles have dissipated has been described.[52,53] Holding a low pH solution in the mandibular posterior area tends to produce a specific pattern of tooth surface loss. The buccal mucosa and the lateral borders of the tongue

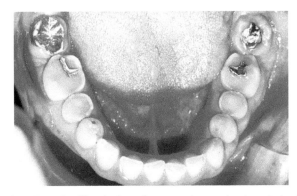

FIGURE 8.12 Chemical erosion occurring predominantly in the mandibular posterior region has been associated with holding and swishing soft drinks in the mouth. The low pH affects the occlusal surfaces of this area because of tongue position and gravity.

tend to limit the effects to the occlusal surfaces with the result that amalgam restorations on mandibular molars may appear as elevated islands. Cupping or cratering of the occlusal surface also may be present and may be severe. Maxillary teeth and mandibular anterior teeth are usually not affected.

Chemical erosion with surface loss evenly distributed on the occlusal surfaces of the maxillary and mandibular posterior teeth has been associated with chewing the pulp of citrus fruits (Fig 8.13). Eating citrus fruits more than twice a day has been observed to increase the risk of erosion 37-fold,[15] producing a specific pattern of wear similar to that resulting from habitually holding a carbonated soft drink in the mandibular posterior area. As the acidic citrus fruit pulp is mulled between the teeth, surface loss tends to occur on both maxillary and mandibular occlusal surfaces. Cupping and

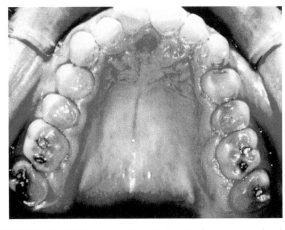

FIGURE 8.13 Uniform erosion of all posterior segments has been associated with the mulling of citrus fruits. The acidic fruit pulp contacts the opposing posterior occlusal surfaces and produces a wear pattern that may indicate a combination of mechanical and chemical wear.

cratering with smooth and rounded enamel edges is observed. This type of dental erosion has been associated with the increased intake of fruits in health-conscious individuals such as vegetarians.[43]

Pattern: Variable Locations, Miscellaneous Causes

Any medication that has an acidic pH and that is in frequent contact with tooth surfaces can cause erosion. Chewable vitamin C tablets,[54] chewable aspirin tablets,[55] and aspirin powders[56] have been associated with erosion on the occlusal surfaces of posterior teeth. Abuse of the illicit amphetamine drug, Ecstasy (3,4-methylene dioxymethamphetamine), has been associated with significant wear of the posterior occlusal surfaces when compared with age-matched, nondrug users.[57] In addition, the application of cocaine to the oral mucosa has been reported to produce cervical erosion on the facial surfaces of maxillary anterior and first premolar teeth.[58]

It should be noted that saliva plays an essential role in minimizing tooth surface loss from chemical erosion. Saliva dilutes, buffers, and neutralizes ingested acids and aids in remineralization by providing calcium and phosphate.[59] Therefore, xerostomia should be considered in evaluating the factors contributing to dental erosion.

Case reports and epidemiologic studies document erosion in factory workers related to occupational exposure to acidic fumes and aerosols.[60] Severe erosion affecting the facial surfaces of the anterior teeth has also been reported in professional wine tasters[61] and competitive swimmers.[62,63]

Because erosion lesions present a wide variety of appearances, a decision tree can be helpful in identifying chemically mediated surface loss patterns (Fig 8.14).

CONCLUSION

Organizing the evaluation of a severely worn dentition involves determining whether the character of the surface loss is chemical, mechanical, or both. In turn, identification of surface loss locations should be made and accompanying clinical signs and symptoms identified. These observations, along with information gained from the patient interview, can then be combined to guide the diagnostic process.

It is important to remember that surface loss may result from a combination of chemical and mechanical factors. Attrition from bruxism often can be identified in association with other causes. Patients may remain secretive about eating disorders and dietary habits. Establishing a diagnosis represents a challenge, but analysis and identification become more manageable if an orderly system of information gathering and analysis (Fig 8.15) is used to guide the process.

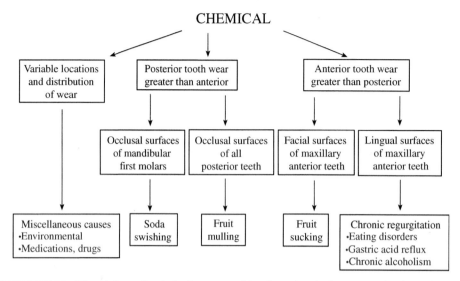

FIGURE 8.14   The etiology of pathologic wear resulting from chemical causes can be determined by correlating location of wear, the presenting signs and symptoms, and information obtained during the patient interview.

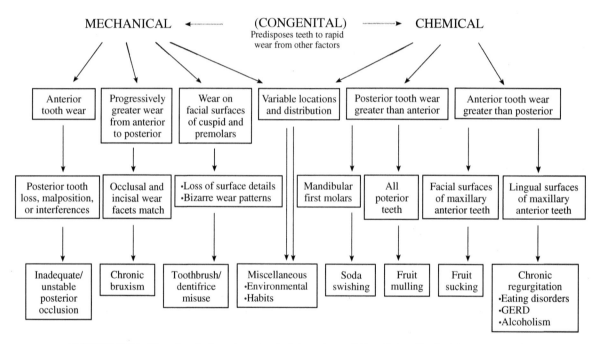

FIGURE 8.15   The chemical and mechanical branches of the diagnostic decision tree can be combined to provide a methodical framework for analyzing an extremely worn dentition.

ACKNOWLEDGMENTS

The author expresses gratitude to his mentor, Dr. Thomas C. Abrahamsen, who introduced the concepts and applied an orderly algorithm to understand the etiology of severe tooth wear. A special thanks is also extended to numerous prosthodontic colleagues who shared their clinical experiences and patient documentation resources.

REFERENCES

1. Shaw L, Smith AJ: Dental erosion—the problem and some practical solutions. *Br Dent J* 1998;186:115–118.
2. Lambrechts P, Braem M, Vuylsteke-Wauters M, et al: Quantitative in vivo wear of human enamel. *J Dent Res* 1989;68:1752–1754.
3. Rahn AO, Heartwell CM: *Textbook of Complete Dentures (ed 5)*. Media, PA, Lea and Febiger, 1993, p 253.

4. Boos RH: Intermaxillary relation established by biting power. *J Am Dent Assoc* 1940;27:1192–1199.

5. Silverman MM: Determination of vertical dimension by phonetics. *J Prosthet Dent* 1956;6:465–471.

6. Shanahan TES: Physiologic vertical dimension and centric relation. *J Prosthet Dent* 1956;6:741–747.

7. Thompson JR: The rest position of the mandible and its significance to dental science. *J Am Dent Assoc* 1946;33:151–180.

8. Wright WH: Use of intra-oral jaw relation wax records in complete dentures. *J Am Dent Assoc* 1939;26:542–557.

9. Pound E: Applying harmony in selecting and arranging teeth. *Dent Clin North Am* 1962;6:241–258.

10. Glossary of Prosthodontic Terms (ed 7). *J Prosthet Dent* 1999;81:48.

11. Glossary of Prosthodontic Terms. *J Prosthet Dent* 1999;81:70.

12. Grippo JO: Abfractions: a new classification of hard tissue lesions of teeth. *J Esthet Dent* 1991;3:14–19.

13. Lee WC, Eakle WS: Stress-induced cervical lesions: review of advances in past 10 years. *J Prosthet Dent* 1996;75:487–494.

14. Levitch LC, Bader JD, Shugars DA, et al: Non-carious cervical lesions. *J Dent* 1994;22:195–207.

15. Lussi A: Dental erosion. Clinical diagnosis and case history taking. *Eur J Oral Sci* 1996;104:191–198.

16. Jarvinen V, Rytömaa I, Meurman JH: Location of dental erosion in a referred population. *Caries Res* 1992;26:391–396.

17. Jarvinen VK, Rytomaa II, Heinonen OP: Risk factors in dental erosion. *J Dent Res* 1991;70:942–947.

18. Johansson A, Fareed K, Omar R: Analysis of possible factors influencing the occurrence of occlusal tooth wear in a young Saudi population. *Acta Odontol Scand* 1991;49:139–145.

19. Johansson AK, Johansson A, Birkhed D, et al: Dental erosion, soft-drink intake, and oral health in young Saudi men, and the development of a system for assessing erosive anterior tooth wear. *Acta Odontol Scand* 1996;54:369–378.

20. Milosevic A, Lennon MA, Fear SC: Risk factors associated with tooth wear in teenagers: A case control study. *Community Dent Health* 1997;14:143–147.

21. Johansson A, Kiliardis S, Haraldson T, et al: Covariation of some factors associated with occlusal tooth wear in a selected high-wear sample. *Scand J Dent Res* 1993;101:398–406.

22. Shafer WG, Hine MK, Levy BM, et al: *A Textbook of Oral Pathology (ed 4)*. Philadelphia, PA, Saunders, 1993, pp. 58–61.

23. Turner KA, Missirlian DM: Restoration of the extremely worn dentition. *J Prosthet Dent* 1984;52:467–474.

24. Akerly WB: Prosthodontic treatment of traumatic overlap of the anterior teeth. *J Prosthet Dent* 1977;38:26–34.

25. Milosevic A: Toothwear: Aetiology and presentation. *Dent Update* 1998;25:6–11.

26. Zero DT: Etiology of dental erosion—Extrinsic factors. *Eur J Oral Sci* 1996;104:162–177.

27. Ehrlich J, Hochman N, Yaffe A: Contribution of oral habits to dental disorders. *J Craniomandib Pract* 1992;10:144–147.

28. Pindborg JJ: *Pathology of the Hard Dental Tissues*. Philadelphia, PA, Saunders, 1970, pp. 294–311.

29. Smith BGN, Knight JK: A comparison of patterns of tooth wear with aetiological factors. *Br Dent J* 1984;157:16–19.

30. Scheutzel P: Etiology of dental erosion-intrinsic factors. *Eur J Oral Sci* 1996;104:178–190.

31. Eccles JD, Jenkins WG: Dental erosion and diet. *J Dent* 1974;2:153–159.

32. Kidd EA, Smith BG: Toothwear histories: A sensitive issue. *Dent Update* 1993;20:174–178.

33. Bargen JA, Austin LT: Decalcification of teeth as a result of obstipation with long continued vomiting. Report of a case. *J Am Dent Assoc* 1937;24:1271–1273.

34. Milosevic A, Brodie DA, Slade PD: Dental erosion, oral hygiene, and nutrition in eating disorders. *Int J Eat Disord* 1997;21:195–199.

35. Smith BGN, Robb ND: The prevalence of toothwear in 1007 dental patients. *J Oral Rehabil* 1996;23:232–239.

36. Bartlett DW, Evans DF, Anggiansan A, et al: A study of the association between gastro-oesophageal reflux and palatal dental erosion. *Br Dent J* 1996;181:125–131.

37. Gregory-Head BL, Curtis DA, Lawrence K, et al: Evaluation of dental erosion in patients with gastroesophageal reflux disease. *J Prosthet Dent* 2000;83:675–680.

38. Gregory-Head B, Curtis DA: Erosion caused by gastroesophageal reflux: Diagnostic considerations. *J Prosthodont* 1997;6:278–285.

39. Christen AG: Dentistry and the alcoholic patient. *Dent Clin North Am* 1983;27:341–361.

40. Robb ND, Smith BGN: Prevalence of pathological tooth wear in patients with chronic alcoholism. *Br Dent J* 1990;169:367–369.

41. Allan DN: Enamel erosion with lemon juice. *Br Dent J* 1967;122:300–302.

42. Asher C, Read MJF: Early enamel erosion in children associated with the excessive consumption of citric acid. *Br Dent J* 1987;162:384–387.

43. Linkosalo E, Markanen H: Dental erosions in relation to lactovegetarian diet. *Scand J Dent Res* 1985;93:436–441.

44. Gragg PP, Hudepohl NC, Baker BR, et al: Dental erosion associated with the use of imported, low-pH snacks. *Texas Dent J* 1998;115:7–13.

45. Johansson AK, Johansson A, Birkhed D, et al: Dental erosion, soft drink intake, and oral health in young Saudi men, and the development of a system for assessing erosive anterior tooth wear. *Acta Odontol Scand* 1996;54:369–378.

46. Al-Dlaigan YH, Shaw L, Smith A: Dental erosion in a group of British 14-year-old school children. Part II: Influence of dietary intake. *Br Dent J* 2001;190:258–261.

47. al-Hiyasat AS, Saunders WP, Sharkey SW, et al: The effect of a carbonated beverage on the wear of human enamel and dental ceramics. *J Prosthodont* 1998;7:2–12.

48. Maupome' G, Aguilar-Avila M, Medrano-Ugalde HA, et al: In vitro quantitative microhardness assessment of enamel with early salivary pellicles after exposure to an eroding cola drink. *Caries Res* 1999;33:140–147.

49. Meurman JH, Frank RM: Progression and surface ultra-structure of in vitro caused erosive lesions in human and bovine enamel. *Caries Res* 1991;25:81–87.

50. Dodds MW, Gragg PP, Rodriguez D: The effect of some Mexican citric acid snacks on in vitro tooth enamel erosion. *Am Acad Pediatr Dent* 1997;19:339–340.

51. Larsen MJ, Nyvad B: Enamel erosion by some soft drinks and orange juices relative to their pH, buffering effect and contents of calcium phosphate. *Caries Res* 1999;33:81–87.

52. High AS: An unusual pattern of dental erosion. A case report. *Br Dent J* 1977;143:403–404.

53. Harrison JL, Roeder LB: Dental erosion caused by cola beverages. *Gen Dent* 1991;39:23–24.

54. Giunta JL: Dental erosion resulting from chewable vitamin C tablets. *J Am Dent Assoc* 1983;107:253–256.

55. Sullivan RE, Kramer WS: Iatrogenic erosion of teeth. *J Dent Child* 1983;50:192–196.

56. McCracken M, O'Neal SJ: Dental erosion and aspirin headache powders: A clinical report. *J Prosthodont* 2000;9:95–98.

57. Redfearn PJ, Agrawal N, Mair LH: An association between the regular use of 3,4 methylenedioxy-methamphetamine (Ecstasy) and excessive wear of the teeth. *Addiction* 1998;93:745–748.

58. Kapila YL, Kashani H: Cocaine associated rapid gingival recession and dental erosion. A case report. *J Periodontol* 1997;68:485–488.

59. Moss SJ: Dental erosion. *Int Dent J* 1998;48:529–539.

60. Petersen PE, Gormsen C: Oral conditions among German battery factory workers *Community Dent Oral Epidemiol* 1991;19:104–106.

61. Wiktorsson A-M, Zimmerman M, Angmar-Månsson B: Erosive tooth wear: prevalence and severity in Swedish wine tasters. *Eur J Oral Sci* 1997;105:544–550.

62. Centerwall BS, Armstrong CW, Funkhouser LS, et al: Erosion of dental enamel among competitive swimmers at a gas chlorinated swimming pool. *Am J Epidemiol* 1986;123:641–647.

63. Filler SJ, Lazarchik DA: Tooth erosion: an unusual case. *Gen Dent* 1994;42:568–569.

9

FULL-MOUTH REHABILITATION OF A PATIENT WITH SEVERELY WORN DENTITION AND UNEVEN OCCLUSAL PLANE: A CLINICAL REPORT

ELNAZ MOSLEHIFARD, DDS, MSC,[1] SAKINEH NIKZAD, DDS, MSC,[2] FARIDEH GERAMINPANAH, DDS, MSC,[2] AND FARHANG MAHBOUB, DDS, MSC[1]

[1]Department of Prosthodontics, Faculty of Dentistry, Tabriz University of Medical Sciences, Tabriz, Iran
[2]Department of Prosthodontics, Faculty of Dentistry, Tehran University of Medical Sciences, Tehran, Iran

Keywords

Tooth wear; mini-implant; full-mouth rehabilitation; occlusal vertical dimension (OVD); occlusal plane.

Correspondence

Elnaz Moslehifard, Department of Prosthodontics, Faculty of Dentistry, Tabriz University of Medical Sciences, Golgasht Ave., Tabriz, Iran. E-mail: elnaz_moslehi@yahoo.com

Accepted January 24, 2011

Published in *Journal of Prosthodontics* January 2012; Vol. 21, Issue 1

doi: 10.1111/j.1532-849X.2011.00765.x

ABSTRACT

Severe tooth wear is frequently multifactorial and variable. Successful management is a subject of interest in dentistry. A critical aspect is to determine the occlusal vertical dimension (OVD) and a systematic approach that can lead to a predictable and favorable treatment prognosis. Management of patients with worn dentition is complex and difficult. Accurate clinical and radiographic examinations, a diagnostic wax-up, and determining OVD are crucial. Using mini-implants as orthodontic anchorage may facilitate orthodontic movement of teeth to improve their position, which is necessary for favorable prosthetic treatment. A 46-year-old man was referred for restoration of his worn and missing teeth. After diagnostic work-up, provisional removable prostheses were fabricated for both jaws, evaluated clinically, and adjusted according to esthetic, phonetic, and vertical dimension criteria. Clinical crown lengthening and free gingival graft procedures were performed in appropriate areas. Drifting of the left posterior mandibular teeth was corrected using mini-implants as orthodontic anchorage. Two conventional implants were inserted in the right mandibular edentulous area. After endodontic therapy of worn teeth, custom-cast gold dowels and cores were fabricated, and provisional removable prostheses were replaced with fixed provisional restorations. Metal ceramic restorations were fabricated, and a removable partial denture with attachments was fabricated for maxillary edentulous areas. An occlusal splint was used to protect the restorations. Full-mouth rehabilitation of the patient with severely worn dentition and an uneven occlusal plane was found to be successful after 3 years of follow-up. This result can encourage clinicians to seek accurate diagnosis and treatment planning to treat such patients.

Tooth wear is an increasingly important clinical problem in aging populations.[1,2] Many factors may combine to result in a worn dentition, and often the etiology of the wear remains unidentified. There is growing consensus that tooth wear observed in any individual may be the result of a combination of all the possible etiological factors over the lifetime of the dentition.[3] Tooth surface loss has been classified as erosion (dissolution of hard tissue by acidic substances), attrition (wear through tooth–tooth contact), abrasion (wear produced by interaction between teeth and other materials), and abfraction.[4–8] Abfraction has also been described as wedge-shaped defects,[9] noncarious cervical lesions,[10–13] and stress-induced cervical lesions.[14,15]

The management of tooth wear, especially attrition, is becoming a subject of increasing interest in the prosthodontic literature, from both a preventive and a restorative point of view.[16] Loss of occlusal vertical dimension (OVD) caused by physiologic tooth wear is usually compensated by continuous tooth eruption and alveolar growth.[17] In situations where tooth wear exceeds compensatory mechanisms, loss of OVD occurs; however, more commonly, the rate of tooth wear is slow, and compensatory eruption of the opposing teeth eliminates space for restoration.[18,19]

Management of patients with worn and missing teeth using fixed or removable prostheses is complex and difficult. Careful and comprehensive treatment planning is required for each individual case, and an assessment of the vertical dimension at rest and in occlusion is essential. Articulated study casts, together with a diagnostic wax-up, provide the necessary information required to evaluate the treatment options, and tolerance of changes to the OVD is usually confirmed with a diagnostic splint or prosthesis.[20,21]

The inclusion of implants as anchor units dramatically alters the balance between anchorage and active segments and can be managed in ways that offer significant advantages to the practitioner. Implants have proven to be reliable and effective sources of orthodontic anchorage, so much so that a new category of anchorage has arisen.[22] One treatment option that employs implants in anchorage is defined as "indirect anchorage," the enhanced anchorage using an implant to stabilize dental units, which in turn serve as the anchor units. This employs an implant in a location other than a dental one, such as the retromolar region or mid-palatal area joined to a tooth or teeth by virtue of a rigid connector. This article presents an approach to rehabilitating a worn dentition with metal ceramic restorations (MCR), a removable partial denture (RPD), and use of implants for anchorage and regaining the space for dental implants in addition to the restoration.

CLINICAL REPORT

A 46-year-old man was referred to the Department of Prosthodontics, Faculty of Dentistry, Tehran University of Medical Sciences, Tehran, Iran, for prosthetic restoration of his worn anterior teeth, as well as replacement of missing teeth. The patient was in good general health, and the medical and dental history indicated no contraindications for dental treatment. Clinical and radiographic examinations revealed severe tooth surface loss on the maxillary anterior teeth and to some degree on the mandibular anterior teeth. Other teeth had drifted into edentulous areas. Inappropriate spacing between the teeth, a remaining root of maxillary right first premolar, and an uneven occlusal plane were observed (Figs 9.1–9.6). No signs and symptoms were found in the temporomandibular joints, and the patient reported no parafunctional habits. A periodontal examination revealed that the attached gingiva around the mandibular left second molar was inadequate, no mobility was noted, and the furcation was involved in the right maxillary first molar (Fig 9.7).

DIAGNOSTIC PROCEDURES

The differential diagnosis included mechanical attrition of anterior teeth, possibly resulting from inadequate posterior occlusion. The patient had acceptable oral hygiene. The vertical dimension was assessed clinically. Physiologic

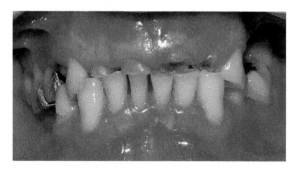

FIGURE 9.1   Frontal view of the dentition before treatment.

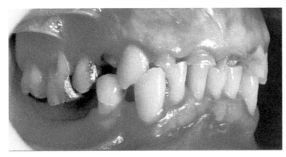

FIGURE 9.2   Right lateral view of the dentition before treatment.

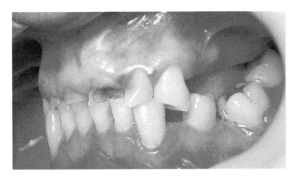

FIGURE 9.3   Left lateral view of the dentition before treatment.

rest position was determined by facial measurements and confirmed by phonetics.[23,24] The interocclusal distance was judged to be approximately 4 mm, and the OVD could be restored by increasing it approximately 1 mm. In addition, the wear resulted in protrusive deviation of the mandible. By guiding the mandible into centric relation, there was some space in the anterior region for rehabilitation.[25] Prior to definitive treatment, diagnostic casts (Moldano, Bayer, Leverkusen, Germany) were obtained from primary impressions (Alginate, Tropicalgin, Zhermack, Rovigo, Italy).

The bite registration procedure was accomplished using an acrylic anterior programming device (Duralay, Reliance Dental Mfg Co., Worth, IL) in the anterior region and baseplate wax (Cavex Setup Regular Modelling Wax, Cavex Holland BV, Haarlem, The Netherlands) supported by the acrylic baseplate (Acropars 200, Marlic, Tehran, Iran) in the posterior region when the mandible was guided into centric relation (CR) by bimanual manipulation technique. To confirm the record, a small amount of zinc oxide–eugenol paste (Luralite, Kerr Corp., Orange, CA) was placed on the wax over each indented area, and the mandible was held in CR until the paste set. Using this record and an arbitrary facebow (Dentatus Facebow; Dentatus AB, Stockholm, Sweden), the casts were mounted on a semiadjustable articulator (Dentatus ARH-Type; Dentatus AB). The incisal pin was adjusted for a

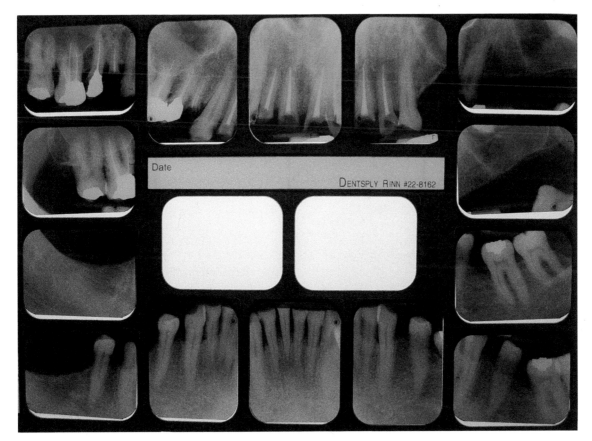

FIGURE 9.4   Periapical radiographs before treatment.

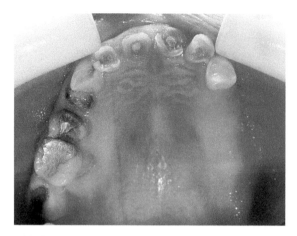

FIGURE 9.5   Maxillary occlusal view before treatment.

1 mm opening. After a primary wax-up, the interim prostheses were fabricated at this new OVD. The patient used these prostheses for 3 months to check the proposed vertical dimension. After 3 months the patient was satisfied with this new OVD without any signs and/or symptoms.

The hinge axis was determined using a pantograph (Denar, Denar Corp., Anaheim, CA), and a second series of diagnostic casts obtained from impressions (Alginate, Tropicalgin) was mounted on a fully adjustable articulator (Denar D5A Series; Waterpik Technologies, Ft. Collins, CO) using an interocclusal registration in CR when the mandible was guided into CR using the bimanual manipulation technique as mentioned before.

The condylar guidance of the articulator was set using the tracing. The curves of Spee and Wilson as well as the orientation of the occlusal plane were determined using a Broadrick occlusal plane analyzer. A diagnostic waxing of this plane revealed that the left mandibular third molar was above the ideal plane, and the spaces for replacement of the left first molar and the right first premolar in the mandible were insufficient. In addition, the width-to-length ratio in the maxillary incisors was 3:2 instead of the ideal 4:5. It was determined that this ratio was inappropriate esthetically.[26]

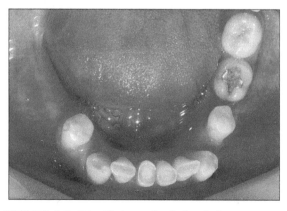

FIGURE 9.6   Mandibular occlusal view before treatment.

The patient was categorized as class IV according to the classification system for partial edentulism developed by the American College of Prosthodontists.[27] Therefore, a treatment plan was developed with the aim of improving occlusion, restoring masticatory function, and improving the patient's appearance. During the following visit, treatment options were discussed with the patient, including root canal therapy (RCT) of the right maxillary second premolar and the right first molar, extraction of the right maxillary first premolar, periodontal therapy (including treating the furcation involvement of the first maxillary molar and performing a free gingival graft in the left mandibular second molar), crown lengthening of maxillary incisors for better esthetic results, orthodontic therapy to regain space, implant placement in suitable areas, and prosthetic treatment (MCR and RPD). Because of pneumatization of the left maxillary sinus, sinus lifting surgery was needed in this area for fixed prosthetic rehabilitation, but the patient did not accept this surgery, and construction of an RPD was planned. The patient accepted the treatment plan.

PREPROSTHETIC PROCEDURES

After RCT and periodontal therapy, the orthodontic treatment plan was scheduled. The space analysis for the right mandibular first premolar and the left mandibular first molar was completed; 5 and 4 mm were required in the right and left, respectively. Three 12 mm long and 2 mm wide mini-implants (Jelenko Co., Armonk, NY) were placed between the right mandibular canine and second premolar, distal to the left mandibular second premolar and distobuccal to the left mandibular second molar simultaneous with third molar extraction. During surgery, a 0.009 ligature wire was extended out of the retromolar area for force application. After 2 weeks, loads were applied by coil spring and then an elastic chain on the second molar and a customized wire on the second mandibular right premolar (Figs 9.8 and 9.9).

DENTAL IMPLANT PLACEMENT

Using the panoramic film and by considering the amount of distal bodily movement of the second mandibular right premolar, the position of the right mandibular implants was estimated, and a radiographic stent was fabricated with drill holes coated with barium sulfate (Barium Sulfate, Daroupakhsh Co., Tehran, Iran); cone-beam CT scan (Picasso Trio, E-WOO Technology, Gyeonggi-Do, South Korea) was used for meticulous evaluation of dental implant position to restore the right mandibular molars. After determining that no correction was needed, implant placement surgery was scheduled. This stent was used during implant surgery, and two implants were placed in the right

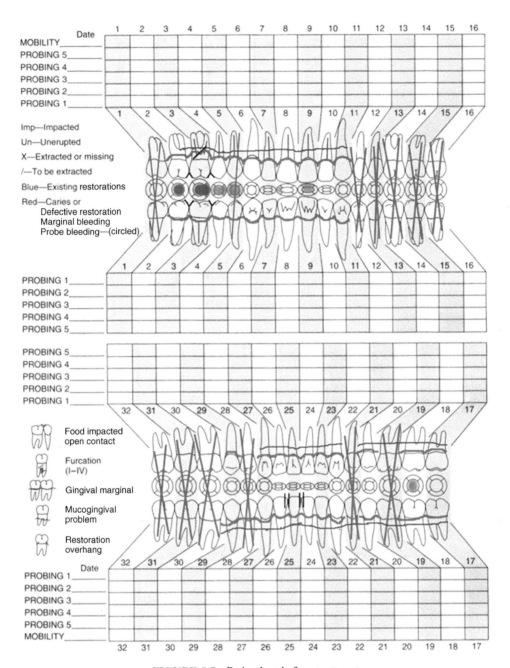

FIGURE 9.7   Perio chart before treatment.

mandibular segment to replace the mandibular right first and second molars (ITI Implants, 4.1 mm diameter, 10 mm long, Straumann AG, Waldenburg, Switzerland).

ENDODONTIC AND PERIODONTAL PROCEDURES AND RESTORATION OF TEETH

During the healing phase after implant placement, mandibular incisors were prepared using the diagnostic wax-up index, and it was determined that the right and left mandibular central incisors and the left lateral incisor required endodontic therapy because of pulp exposure during tooth preparation according to the putty index obtained from the wax-up. After completion of RCT, custom-cast gold dowels and cores (Degubond 4; DeguDent, Hanau, Germany) were fabricated for the right and left mandibular central incisors and the left lateral incisor. Tooth preparation with a circumferential shoulder-bevel margin configuration was performed on the mandibular anterior teeth. Interim prostheses were fabricated and cemented with noneugenol zinc oxide cement (Temp-Bond NE; Kerr Corp.). Next, maxillary anterior custom-cast

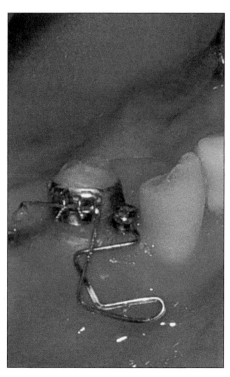

FIGURE 9.8   Mini-implants used as orthodontic anchorage; the load was applied on the second mandibular premolar using a customized wire.

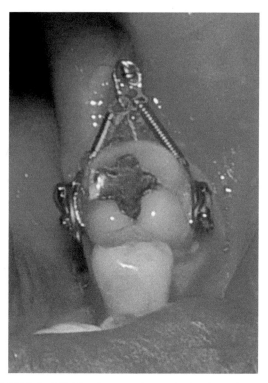

FIGURE 9.9   Mini-implants used as orthodontic anchorage; the load was applied on the second mandibular left molar using a coil spring.

gold dowels and cores were fabricated, and tooth preparation was performed.

In this stage, esthetic crown lengthening of the maxillary anterior segment was performed using a vacuum shell guide according to the diagnostic wax-up. After 1 week, the interim prostheses were adjusted according to the new margin. During 2 months of gingival healing, the already delivered interim removable prosthesis was relined with resilient lining material (Soft Liner, Kerr Dental, Romulus, MI) to fulfill the functional needs of the patient. The preparation of mandibular posterior teeth with a chamfer margin configuration was then performed.

A period of healing is necessary before applying load to conventional dental implants. This period varies from 4 to 6 months in humans. After 4 months, the dental implants were ready for loading. According to the wax-up index and ideal occlusal plane, the implant abutment heights were determined (two solid abutments, 7 mm height, Straumann AG). The abutments were tightened with a torque wrench to 35 N cm, and interim prostheses were cemented with temporary cement (TempBond NE).

Custom-cast gold dowels and cores were fabricated for the right maxillary posterior teeth, and the preparation was performed with shoulder-bevel margins in the buccal and chamfer margin in the palatal aspects. For the occlusal plane correction, the maxillary second molar was prepared for an

onlay restoration, and interim prostheses were cemented (TempBond NE). After completion of the preparations, irreversible hydrocolloid impressions (Alginate, Tropicalgin) for interim prostheses were made and mounted on the articulator with the facebow record index and interocclusal registration. The wax-up for interim prostheses was performed.

New laboratory-processed interim prostheses (Tempron, GC Corp., Tokyo, Japan) and interim removable prostheses were fabricated by the laboratory and delivered. The canine-protected articulation was established bilaterally (Figs 9.10 and 9.11). After adjusting and cementing these interim prostheses, hydrocolloid impressions of the restorations were made, the stone casts were mounted on the articulator, and the anterior guide table was customized (Duralay) (Fig 9.12).

FINAL REPLACEMENT OF MISSING TEETH

The orthodontic treatment took 2 months to complete. The retention period for orthodontic therapy was completed in 3 months. Then, preparation of the teeth was completed. The mini-implants were removed simply by unscrewing in the opposite direction. The final impressions were made with light body silicone impression material (Speedex, Coltene

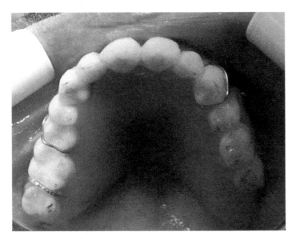

FIGURE 9.10   Occlusal view of maxillary interim prostheses.

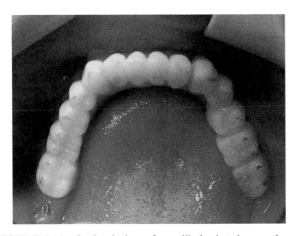

FIGURE 9.11   Occlusal view of mandibular interim prostheses.

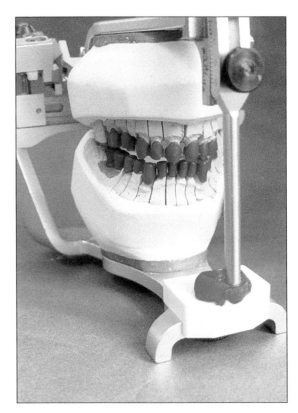

FIGURE 9.12   Working casts on the articulator.

AG, Altstatten, Switzerland) in a custom acrylic tray (Acropars 200), and the casts were mounted on the articulator using interocclusal registrations, which recorded CR by guiding the mandible using bimanual manipulation using an anterior programming device and record bases with wax occlusion rims in the posterior.

A full contour wax-up was accomplished for the MCRs. A nonrigid connector (Interlock type cylindrical, Bredent, Seden, Witzighausen, Germany) was inserted in the distal of the pier abutment (the left mandibular second premolar). The rest seats were carved on the cingulums of both canines, the mesial occlusal of the maxillary premolar, and the distal occlusal of the right maxillary molar; in addition, guide planes were created using a surveyor. For esthetic reasons, two extracoronal castable attachments (Rhein 83, Bologna, Italy) were placed on the distal side of both maxillary canines using a surveyor to eliminate the need for clasp arms in the labial aspect. Then cut-back was performed according to the index, and the precious metal frameworks (Degudent U, Degudent GmbH) were fabricated.

The frameworks were evaluated radiographically and intraorally for fit, occlusion, retention, and stability (Fig 9.13). Porcelain (Ceramco, Dentsply Ceramco, Burlington, NJ) was applied to complete the crowns. The lingual contours of the maxillary incisors were adjusted according to the anterior guide table. The MCRS were provisionally cemented using temporary cement, and the onlay was bonded using an adhesive luting agent (Panavia F 2.0, Kurary, Osaka, Japan) (Fig 9.14).

To begin the RPD phase of treatment, an impression of the maxilla (Wash, Speedex) was made in a custom acrylic tray (Acropars 200) after border molding (Impression Compound, Richter & Hoffmann, Harvard Dental Gmbh, Berlin, Germany). The framework was cast from Ni–Cr material (Verabond II, Aalba Dent, Cordelia, CA), and the fit was checked intraorally. The keyways of the attachments (pink cap, soft retention) were placed in the RPD framework. Then the acrylic heat-processed teeth (SR Orthosit PE, Ivoclar Vivadent, Amherst, NY) were arranged in occlusion, and canine-protected articulation was adjusted. The RPD was completed; occlusal contacts were adjusted, and the RPD delivered to the patient (Figs 9.15 and 9.16).

A hard acrylic resin occlusal splint (Acropars) was fabricated for night use to prevent parafunctional occlusal wear. Minor adjustments were required at four postinsertion visits. After 2 months, the temporary cement was changed with poly-carboxylate cement (Hoffmann's, Berlin, Germany),

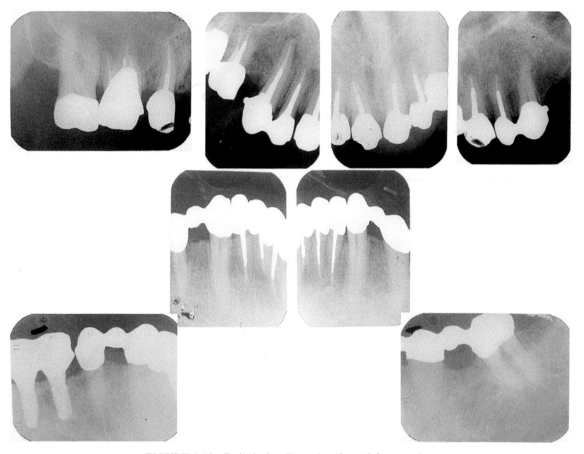

FIGURE 9.13 Periapical radiographs of metal frameworks.

and the patient was placed on a 6-month recall. The 3-year evaluation of the esthetics and function of the restorations showed no evidence of temporomandibular joint problems, fractures in the teeth, or MCRs.

DISCUSSION

Tooth surface loss has been classified[28] into erosion, attrition, abrasion, and abfraction. Tooth wear has a multifactorial

cause[29] and may be generalized throughout the dentition, but is often localized to incisors and canines. Niswonger, cited by Tallgren,[30] found that 80% of severe tooth wear patients have a normal interocclusal rest space. The distribution of wear in the dentition is not even, as is evidenced by the difference between the anterior and posterior teeth. Inadequate or unstable posterior support has been identified as a factor

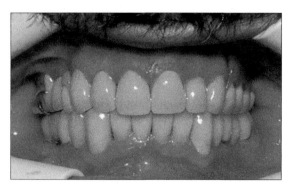

FIGURE 9.14 Frontal view of the completed treatment with MCRs and RPD.

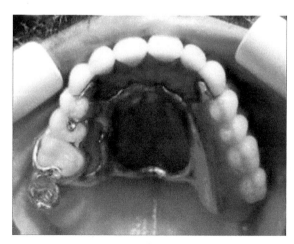

FIGURE 9.15 Occlusal view of the maxillary arch after treatment.

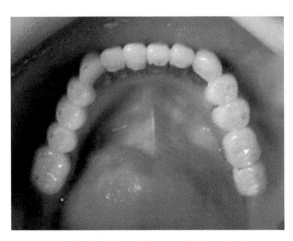

FIGURE 9.16   Occlusal view of the mandibular arch after treatment.

in severe anterior attrition and decreased OVD.[31] Posterior occlusal prematurities, too, may cause increased function on anterior teeth, resulting in increased wear.

Clinical judgment plays a major role in the assessment of this important component in rehabilitation. A variety of techniques, such as phonetics, interocclusal distance, swallowing, and patient preferences, have been proposed to determine measurements for the correct OVD.[32-34]

Interocclusal rest space can be generated by the following methods:

1. Occlusal adjustment if necessary.
2. Reduction of the opposing teeth. Periodontal crown lengthening surgery can increase the clinical crown height, thereby allowing further tooth reduction.
3. Increasing the OVD by restoring the posterior teeth in one or both jaws.
4. Elective endodontic treatment, followed by dowel-retained restorations.
5. Orthodontic movement of teeth to create interocclusal space.[35]

It is important to establish the cause of wear before intervention to help improve the effectiveness of any preventive and restorative care.[29] Standard dental implants as the anchorage for orthodontic treatment have drawbacks such as the difficulty of selecting proper implant sites in most patients, the need to wait for osseointegration before force loading, the invasiveness of the surgical procedure, difficulty of maintaining oral hygiene, and high cost.[36] Also these implants can only be placed in limited sites, such as the retromolar and edentulous areas. Removable osseointegrated titanium mini-implants have been successfully used as anchorage. The Ti–6Al–4V alloy was used instead of commercially pure Ti due to its superior strength.[37] In this case mini-implants were used for anchorage. The mini-implants generally do not move during treatment. At the end of

orthodontic treatment, or when the anchorage is no longer needed, the screw is simply removed under local anesthesia, using a screwdriver. The oral mucosa around the surgical site will usually recover within 10 to 14 days.[38] Contrary to other methods, in this method the tooth moves bodily, and it is not necessary to apply interarch stabilization to minimize side effects. Simultaneous molar intrusion can be performed, eliminating the need for occlusal reduction.[39]

In this case the cone-beam CT was used to evaluate the meticulous placement of the implants because of low dose radiation during CT scan; however, CT examinations are expensive and deliver a relatively high radiation dose to the patient. The most recently introduced imaging modality is cone beam volumetric tomography (CBVT), which seems very promising with regard to preimplant imaging. CBVT generally delivers a lower radiation dose to the patient compared to CT and provides reasonably sharp images with 3D information. Recent studies indicate that CBVT images have sufficient accuracy to be used for preimplant assessments.[40,41] It has been demonstrated that the error in measurements obtained from CBVT scans is less than 0.5 mm.[42] The low exposure parameters of CBVT result in poor soft-tissue contrast compared with CT.[43,44] Reports indicate that low-dose CT protocols result in significantly less exposure than previously thought, without compromising image quality significantly.[45]

CONCLUSION

Management of patients with a worn dentition is complex and difficult. Accurate clinical and radiographic examinations, a diagnostic wax-up, and determining OVD are crucial. Using mini-implants as orthodontic anchorage may facilitate orthodontic movement of teeth to improve their position, which is necessary for favorable prosthetic treatment. Full-mouth rehabilitation of the patient with severely worn dentition and an uneven occlusal plane was found to be successful after 3 years of follow-up. This result can encourage clinicians to seek accurate diagnosis and treatment planning to treat such patients.

REFERENCES

1. Smith BG, Knight JK: An index for measuring the wear of teeth. *Br Dent J* 1984;156:435–438.
2. Bartlett D, Phillips K, Smith B: A difference in perspective—the North American and European interpretations of tooth wear. *Int J Prosthodont* 1999;12:401–408.
3. Crothers AJR: Tooth wear and facial morphology. *J Dent* 1992;20:333–341.
4. Glossary of prosthodontic terms. *J Prosthet Dent* 1999;81: 39–110.

5. Barbour ME, Rees GD: The role of erosion, abrasion and attrition in tooth wear. *J Clin Dent* 2006;17:88–93.

6. Bardsley PF: The evolution of tooth wear indices. *Clin Oral Investig* 2008;12:15–19.

7. Mwangi CW, Richmond S, Hunter ML: Relationship between malocclusion, orthodontic treatment, and tooth wear. *Am J Orthod Dentofacial Orthop* 2009;136:529–535.

8. Spear F: A patient with severe wear on the anterior teeth and minimal wear on the posterior teeth. *J Am Dent Assoc* 2008;139:1399–1403.

9. Litonjua LA, Bush PJ, Andreana S, et al: Effects of occlusal load on cervical lesions. *J Oral Rehabil* 2004;31:225–232.

10. Gallien GS, Kaplan I, Owens BM: A review of noncarious cervical ental lesions. *Compendium* 1994;11:1366–1372.

11. Levitch LC, Bader JD, Shugars DA, et al: Non-carious cervical lesions. *J Dent* 1994;22:195–207.

12. Grippo JO: Noncarious cervical lesions: the decision to ignore or restore. *J Esthet Dent* 1992;4:55–64.

13. Lambert RL, Lindenmuth JS: Abfraction—a new name for an old entity. *J Colo Dent Assoc* 1994;72:31–33.

14. Lee WC, Eakle WS: Possible role of tensile stress in the etiology of cervical erosive lesions of teeth. *J Prosthet Dent* 1984;52:374–380.

15. Braem M, Lambrechts P, Vanherle G: Stress-induced cervical lesions. *J Prosthet Dent* 1992;67:718–722.

16. Spijker AV, Kreulen CM, Creugers NHJ: Attrition, occlusion, (dys)function, intervention: a systematic review. *Clin Oral Impl Res* 2007;18:117–126.

17. Murphy T: Compensatory mechanisms in facial height adjustment to functional tooth attrition. *Aust Dent J* 1959;4:312–323.

18. Berry DC, Poole DF: Attrition: possible mechanisms of compensation. *J Oral Rehabil* 1976;3:201–206.

19. Faigenblum M: Removable prostheses. *Br Dent J* 1999;186: 273–276.

20. Hemmings KW, Howlett JA, Woodley NJ, et al: Partial dentures for patients with advanced tooth wear. *Dent Update* 1995;2:52–59.

21. Ibbetson RJ, Setchell DJ: Treatment of the worn dentition: 2. *Dent Update* 1989;16:305–307.

22. Celenza F: Implant-enhanced tooth movement: indirect absolute anchorage. *Int J Periodontics Restorative Dent* 2003;23:533–541.

23. Zarb GA, Bolender CL, Carlsson GE: *Boucher's Prosthodontic Treatment for Edentulous Patients* (ed 11). St. Louis, Mosby, 1997, p. 210.

24. Rivera-Morales WC, Mohl ND: Restoration of the dimension of occlusion in the severely worn dentition. *Dent Clin North Am* 1992;36:651–664.

25. Milosevic A: Toothwear: management. *Dent Update* 1998;25: 50–55.

26. Blitz N: Anterior crowns in re-establishing vertical dimension of occlusion: overcoming fear of heights. *Oral Health* 1997;87: 23–24.

27. McGarry TJ, Nimmo A, Skiba JF, et al: Classification system for partial edentulism. *J Prosthodont* 2002;11:181–193.

28. Addy M, Shellis RP: Interaction between attrition, abrasion and erosion in tooth wear. *Monogr Oral Sci* 2006;20:17–31.

29. Bartlett DW, Shah P: A critical review of non-carious cervical (wear) lesions and the role of abfraction, erosion and abrasion. *J Dent Res* 2006;85:306–312.

30. Tallgren A: Changes in adult face height due to aging, wear and loss of teeth and prosthetic treatment. *Acta Odontol Scand* 1957;15 (suppl): 1–112.

31. Turner KA, Missirlian DM: Restoration of the extremely worn dentition. *J Prosthet Dent* 1984;52:467–474.

32. Tjan AHL, Miller GD, The JG: Some esthetic factors in a smile. *J Prosthet Dent* 1984;51:24–28.

33. Halperin AR, Graser GN, Rogoff GS, et al: *Mastering the Art of Complete Dentures* (ed 1). Chicago, Quintessence, 1988, pp. 94–97.

34. Lundquist DO, Luther WW: Occlusal plane determination. *J Prosthet Dent* 1970;23:489–498.

35. Hemmings KW, Darbar UR, Vaughan S: Tooth wear treated with direct composite restorations at an increased vertical dimension: results at 30 months. *J Prosthet Dent* 2000;83:287–293.

36. Bae SM, Park HS, Kyung HM, et al: Clinical application of micro-implant anchorage. *J Clin Orthod* 2002;36:298–301.

37. Morais LS, Serra GG, Muller CA, et al: Titanium alloy mini-implants for orthodontic anchorage: immediate loading and metal ion release. *Acta Biomaterialia* 2007;3:331–339.

38. Gianocotti A, Muzzi F, Santini F, et al: Miniscrew treatment of ectopic mandibular molars. *J Clin Orthod* 2003;37:380–383.

39. Park HS, Kyung HM, Sung JH: A simple method of molar uprighting with micro-implant anchorage. *J Clin Orthod* 2002;36:592–596.

40. Pinsky HM, Dyda S, Pinsky RW, et al: Accuracy of three-dimensional measurements using cone-beam CT. *Dentomaxillofac Radiol* 2006;35:410–416.

41. Ludlow JB, Laster WS, See M, et al: Accuracy of measurements of mandibular anatomy in cone beam computed tomography images. *Oral Surg Oral Med Oral Pathol Oral Radiol Endod* 2007;103:534–542.

42. Marmulla R, Wortche R, Muhling J, et al: Geometric accuracy of the NewTom 9000 cone beam CT. *Dentomaxillofac Radiol* 2005;34:28–31.

43. Scarfe WC, Farman AG, Sukovic P: Clinical applications of conebeam computed tomography in dental practice. *J Can Dent Assoc* 2006;72:75–80.

44. Katsumata A, Hirukawa A, Noujeim M, et al: Image artefact in dental cone-beam CT. *Oral Surg Oral Med Oral Pathol Oral Radiol Endod* 2006;101:652–657.

45. Ekestubbe A: Conventional spiral and low-dose computed mandibular tomography for dental implant planning. *Swed Dent J Suppl* 1999;138:1–82.

10

IMPLANT-SUPPORTED PROSTHETIC REHABILITATION OF A PATIENT WITH LOCALIZED SEVERE ATTRITION: A CLINICAL REPORT

ISIL CEKIC-NAGAS, DDS, PHD AND GULFEM ERGUN, DDS, PHD

Department of Prosthodontics, Faculty of Dentistry, Gazi University, Ankara, Turkey

Keywords

Full-mouth rehabilitation; dental implant; vertical dimension; attrition.

Correspondence

Dr. Isil Cekic-Nagas, Servi Sokak 6A/7, Kolej, Ankara, Turkey. E-mail: isilcekic@gazi.edu.tr, isilcekic@gmail.com

This study was presented at the 37 Annual Congress of the EPA and 41ˢᵗ Annual Meeting of the SSPD in Turku, Finland, on August 21–24, 2013.

The authors deny any conflicts of interest.

Accepted March 23, 2014

Published in *Journal of Prosthodontics* June 2015; Vol. 24, Issue 4

doi: 10.1111/jopr.12211

ABSTRACT

Patients usually adapt to their existing occlusal vertical dimension (OVD). It is essential to resolve each of the problems associated with decreased vertical dimension as a result of attrition. This report describes the multidisciplinary dental treatment of a 40-year-old male patient who had severe tooth wear, resulting in reduced vertical dimension. After clinical evaluations, extraoral examination showed a reduction of the lower facial height, drooping, and overclosed commissures. Ten dental implants were placed into the maxillary and mandibular alveolar processes. During the osseointegration period, an interim removable partial denture was made at increased OVD to use in the first stage of rehabilitation. It was used for 3 months as a guide for preparing the definitive restorations. The patient's adaptation to the increased OVD was evaluated. During this period, he was asymptomatic. Following the evaluation period, the provisional fixed restoration was used for 3 months. Then, full-mouth definitive prostheses supported by a combination of implants and teeth were fabricated to upper and lower jaws. Osseointegration of the implants, peri-implant mucosa health, prosthesis function, and esthetics were assessed after 1 week and 1, 3, and 6 months. After 3 years of follow-up, no functional or esthetic difficulties with the implants and restorations were noted.

Dental wear could be a potential chronic problem for dentition, since it is multifactorial and is generally a combination of abrasion, attrition, and erosion.[1–3] Although several factors affect the type and rate of wear, attrition could be a physiologic process that occurs by the loss of tooth tissue due to friction between opposing teeth.[3,4] In addition, pathologic wear occurs when the normal rate of physiologic process is accelerated by endogenous or exogenous factors. The etiology of wear should be diagnosed properly to prevent these pathological changes.[5] The tooth wear process might lead to destruction of the stomatognathic system with severe tooth surface loss and is associated with decreased occlusal vertical dimension (OVD).[6–8] Since alterations in OVD could cause adaptable reactions in the temporomandibular joint (TMJ), periodontium, and tooth surfaces, some patients do not always need their stomatognathic system with decreased vertical dimension to be restored.[9] However, in some severe cases, decreased vertical dimension with worn teeth could result in an unesthetic appearance, decreased masticatory efficiency, loss of muscle tone, dentin hypersensitivity, and pulpitis.[10,11] Therefore, for managing a complete oral rehabilitation, a systematic approach should be followed by increasing the vertical dimension progressively. Thus, occlusal splints or fixed or removable partial dentures (RPDs) might be the treatment options for situations where loss of OVD has occurred.[12–15]

The use of dental implants integrated into the living tissues of the jaws to replace a single tooth or multiple adjacent missing teeth is a predictable procedure in consideration of optimal esthetic characteristics and long-lasting stability.[11,16] Furthermore, the size of the edentulous space between existing teeth might be critical for the subsequent implant placement.[17,18] To improve treatment success, a multidisciplinary approach with collaboration between the maxillofacial surgeon and prosthodontist for implant planning and placement should be considered.[19]

The aim of this clinical report is to illustrate the restorative treatment of a patient with worn anterior dentition by a sequence of treatment, including surgical and prosthetic multidisciplinary approaches.

CLINICAL REPORT

A 40-year-old man was referred to Gazi University, Department of Prosthodontics with a chief complaint concerning inability to chew and unpleasant esthetics, because of his worn anterior teeth and loss of posterior teeth. He reported that he had lost his posterior teeth 3 years ago because of periodontal disease. The patient's general medical history was not significant, and he had no temporomandibular disorder or pain in the mastication muscles. Extraoral examination showed a reduction of the lower facial height, protuberant lips, wrinkles, drooping and overclosed commissures,

and an unpleasant smile caused by collapsed OVD. The general standard of oral hygiene and gingival situation were not satisfactory. In addition, periodontal condition and soft-tissue examination showed no pocket depth over 2 mm or mobility of any remaining teeth; however, there was loss of gingival papillae between the maxillary right and left central teeth (#11 and #21), possibly due to maxillary and mandibular incisor contact resulting in loss or cratering of the interdental alveolar crest. Radiographic evaluation demonstrated adequate bone support for the remaining teeth. Clinically, the patient demonstrated partial edentulism, and localized severe attrition was seen, especially in the right anterior teeth (Fig 10.1). In addition, the intraoral and radiographic examination verified that maxillary left and right first premolars, second premolars, first molar, maxillary left second molar, mandibular right and left first premolars, second premolar, and first and second molars were lost (#14–16, #24–27, #34–37, and #44–47; Fig 10.1). A treatment plan was formulated that required communication between the surgeon and the prosthodontist. To assist the interdisciplinary consultation process, a diagnostic setup was prepared by the prosthodontist. The patient's casts were mounted on a semiadjustable articulator (Stratos 200; Ivoclar Vivadent, Schaan, Liechtenstein) using a facebow record and an interocclusal record made with the aid of a Lucia jig and poly(vinyl siloxane) occlusal registration material (Exabite II; GC Corp., Tokyo, Japan). After careful assessment, it was determined that a 6 mm loss of OVD had occurred. To restore the lost OVD, the occlusion, function, and esthetics of the patient, increasing the OVD by interim removable partial prosthesis, interim fixed prosthesis, and full-mouth rehabilitation with implant-teeth-supported metal ceramic restorations were planned. Informed consent was obtained from the patient before beginning the treatment.

Surgical Procedure

Decisions regarding implant length and width were based on an examination of periapical and panoramic radiographs of the maxillary and mandibular bone. In total, ten implants (five in the maxilla, five in mandible) were planned by the prosthodontist. Mounted diagnostic casts were used to fabricate a guide for implant placement by the surgeon. The implant surgery was undertaken under local anesthesia and following the guidelines determined by the manufacturer. The surgical procedure started with an intraoral crestal incision followed by subperiosteal dissection of the mucoperiosteum. Flattening of the alveolar crest was performed with a bur and under copious sterile saline irrigation. At the insertion stage, the implants were placed at a depth according to the guidelines given by the manufacturer (Standard Plus Implants; Straumann AG, Basel, Switzerland). Five implants were placed in both the maxilla and mandible (Table 10.1).

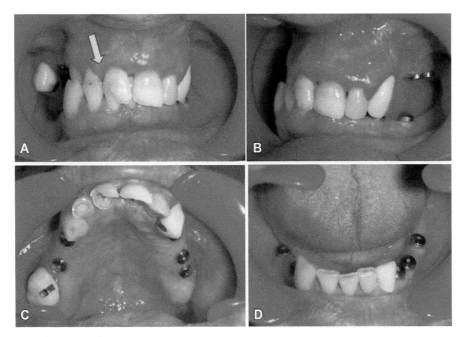

FIGURE 10.1   Intraoral view of the patient before treatment. (A) Facial aspect. (B) From left side. (C) View of maxilla. (D) View of mandible. Arrow indicating the main attrition (#11, #12, #21).

TABLE 10.1   Region and Type of Implants

Region	#14, #24, #35, #26	#16, #27, #34, #44	#37, #46
Type	4.1 mm in diameter, 12 mm total length	4.1 mm in diameter, 10 mm total length	4.1 mm in diameter, 8 mm total length

Postoperative treatment consisted of standard analgesics, chlorhexidine 0.2% mouthrinses, antibiotics, and non-steroidal analgesics for three consecutive days. Sutures were removed 1 week after surgery. After a bone-healing period of 6 months, a second-stage surgery was undertaken; the healing abutments were connected and left in place for 3 weeks for peri-implant soft-tissue healing. Standard oral hygiene instructions, including brushing of the healing abutments, were given to the patient.

Prosthetic Stage

The new OVD was set to increase by approximately 6 mm in the incisal guidance pin of the articulator. Then, the maxillary right and left central incisor and right lateral incisor and canine (#11, #12, #13, #21) had root canal therapy and postcore restorations. An RPD was made at the increased OVD to use at the first stage of the rehabilitation (Fig 10.2). This interim removable denture was used for 3 months as a guide for the definitive oral rehabilitation. The patient's adaptation to the increased OVD was evaluated. During this period, the patient's functions, muscle sensitivity, mastication, TMJ discomfort, swallowing, speech, and anterior and posterior speaking space were assessed. No muscle tenderness or temporomandibular discomfort was found, and the patient was asymptomatic. Development in facial esthetics, speech, and mastication showed the patient's tolerance capacity.

The proper OVD was determined using the physiologic rest position of the mandible as a guide and noting the existing interocclusal distance. It was decided that all of the teeth should be restored with full-mouth rehabilitation to restore lost vertical dimension. After preparation of the remaining teeth (Fig 10.3), the provisional crowns were fabricated (autopolymerizing acrylic resin, ALIKETM; GC America, Alsip, IL) using a vacuum-formed matrix (Drufolen H; Dreve Dentamid GmbH, Unna, Germany). The interim fixed restoration was cemented with temporary cement (Temp Bond NETM; Kerr, Salerno, Italy).

The previous interim removable denture made at increased OVD was adapted to the interim fixed prostheses. These interim prostheses were used for 3 months as a guide for the definitive oral rehabilitation. In addition, protrusive contact, canine guidance, esthetics, and phonetics of the interim prosthesis were assessed, and 1-, 2-, and 3-month check-ups were performed.

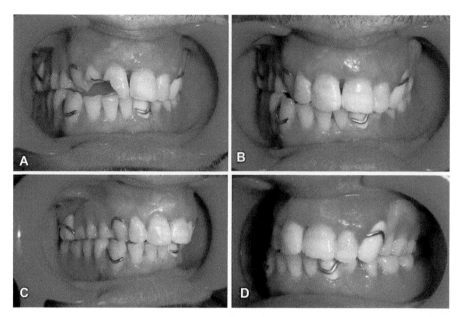

FIGURE 10.2 (A) The increased vertical dimension by RPD. (B) Intraoral view of the patient at increased vertical dimension after postcore restorations of right central and lateral teeth. (C) View from right side. (D) View from left side.

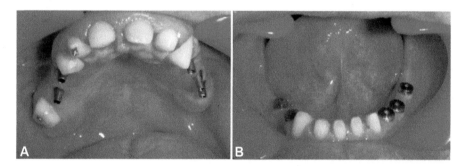

FIGURE 10.3 Intraoral view after preparation of the teeth (A) maxilla (B) mandible.

After 3 months, the impression copings were placed. Definitive impressions of the maxillary and mandibular teeth and abutments were made with a polyether impression material (Impregum; 3M ESPE, Seefeld, Germany). The impression copings were fixed onto the abutment analog. Then, cement-retained prostheses were completed on abutment level models from a base metal alloy (Master-Tec; Ivoclar Vivadent AG, Schaan, Liechtenstein) and porcelain (VITA VM 13, VITA Zahnfabrik, Bad Sackingen, Germany; Fig 10.4).

Centric occlusion, protrusive contacts, and canine guidance were assessed in the definitive anterior restoration. The scheme of occlusion was mutually protected articulation. The right lateral tooth (#12), which was below the plane of occlusion, created a reverse occlusal plane. To offset this reverse occlusal curve, the incisal guidance was increased. As a result, a flat mandibular plane of occlusion was established (Fig 10.4). The occlusal plane and esthetics were used as a guide to establish anterior guidance.

Phonetics was assessed using the closest speaking space technique. The technique, suggested by Silverman, was reported to give constant and reproducible results. The closest speaking space was considered to be between the lower centric occlusion line and the upper closest speaking line.[20] Finally, the definitive restoration was cemented with temporary cement (Temp Bond NETM). Oral hygiene and regular check-up were emphasized. Following evaluation of the patient after 24 hours, 48 hours, and 1 week, occlusal corrections were made. Once the occlusal adjustments, speech, and esthetics seemed satisfactory, all restorations were cemented definitely with zinc polycarboxy-late cement (Adhesor® Carbofine, Kerr, Salerno, Italy; Fig 10.4). Compared with the pretreatment profile (Fig 10.5A), the post-treatment profile photographs (Fig 10.5B) showed a marked improvement in the facial profile (Fig 10.6). Following the definitive cementation of all restorations, a protective occlusal splint was manufactured to protect the restorations. Routine radiographs consisted of panoramic radiographs

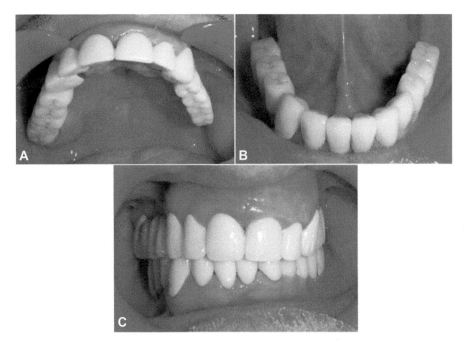

FIGURE 10.4   Posttreatment intraoral views showing restored teeth (A) maxilla, (B) mandible, (C) maxilla and mandible from facial aspect.

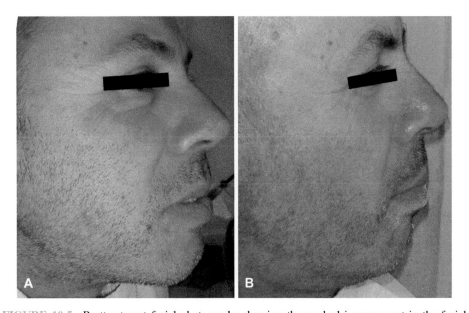

FIGURE 10.5   Posttreatment facial photographs showing the marked improvement in the facial profile (A) before treatment (B) after treatment.

taken preoperatively, after placement of implants, at the time of prosthetic loading, and annually thereafter until the end of follow-up (Fig 10.7).

Follow-Up Period

Routine clinical assessments were made after 1 and 4 weeks, 3 and 6 months, and 1, 2, and 3 years with visual and radiographic examinations. Criteria for success included functional harmony, absence of pain, no tension or tiredness in facial and masticatory muscles, and phonetic and esthetic satisfaction. The patient acknowledged having improved function and esthetics and was pleased with the results.

DISCUSSION

Loss of tooth substance or even severe tooth wear might be a contributing factor to dental occlusion problems.[14] Patients with these problems often seek treatment because of an

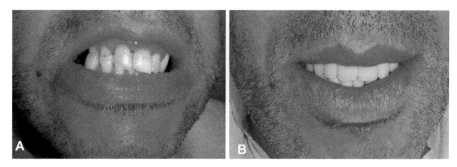

FIGURE 10.6   (A) Pretreatment smile of the patient, (B) posttreatment smile of the patient.

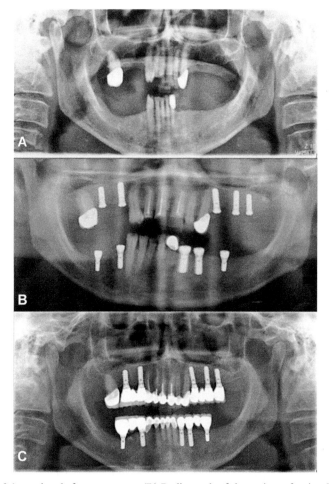

FIGURE 10.7   (A) Radiograph of the patient before treatment. (B) Radiograph of the patient after implant surgery. (C) Radiograph of the patient after treatment.

unpleasant appearance, impaired mastication, and speech difficulties. In addition, the lack of uniformity of the occlusal plane, supereruption, loss of vertical dimension, and bone morphology in edentulous areas may cause prosthodontic challenges.[11] When there is tooth loss, to maintain the oral functions properly, the oral system should be reestablished.[21] In this case, severe dental wear was seen in the right anterior maxilla. This could be related to the malocclusion problems associated with the loss of posterior teeth. Once the anterior

teeth attrited, the anterior guidance was lost. Furthermore, the position of the remaining teeth in the dental arch was altered, as well as in relation to the antagonist teeth.

Tooth surface loss associated with decreased OVD could be recovered by continuous tooth eruption and alveolar bone growth in some cases. Moreover, the treatment might include surgical crown lengthening or orthodontic movements.[8] If tooth wear could not be compensated by dentoalveolar growth, and the loss of OVD is severe or associated with short worn teeth, then progressive increase in OVD with interim prostheses for 2 to 6 months could be used as an appropriate approach.[8,12] Previous studies recommended the use of RPDs as interim prostheses for patients with attrition of anterior teeth and multiple missing anterior teeth.[13,14,22,23]

In this case, the attrition was severe in the right anterior region, and the patient had a concave profile (Figs 10.1 and 10.5A). Following the determination of 6 mm loss of OVD, the interim RPD was made to be used for about 3 months for restoring the lost OVD. Since provisional crowns had been prepared from autopolymerizing acrylic resin, they might demonstrate dimensional degeneration and marginal accuracy problems in long-term use.[24] In addition, use of a fixed interim prosthesis on prepared teeth might cause pulpitis or periodontal problems in the long term. Therefore, initially an RPD was chosen to restore loss of OVD.[25] Then, a fixed interim prosthesis was used for 3 months. During the 3-month period, to evaluate temporomandibular discomfort, wear, and muscle fatigue, the restorations were cemented temporarily, and no complication occurred.

To restore lost OVD, the multidisciplinary team should be in close collaboration in terms of planning the immediate, transitory, and long-term phases of treatment.[16,26] To rehabilitate these patients with esthetics and for functional success, prosthetic, orthodontic, and surgical collaboration might be required. The use of dental implants in supporting fixed prosthetic rehabilitations can provide high success when certain conditions are met during the manufacture of the implant, in its placement, in its eventual functional loading, and in its maintenance.[15,17] In this report, because of the long treatment period and the difficulty of the treatment procedure, surgical/orthodontic/prosthodontic treatment was not preferred by the patient. Therefore, to restore the missing teeth, surgical/prosthodontic multidisciplinary rehabilitation was planned, and a total of ten implants were placed in the maxilla and mandible.

Mutually protected articulation is described as an occlusal scheme in which the posterior teeth prevent excessive contact of the anterior teeth in maximum intercuspation, and the anterior teeth disengage the posterior teeth in all mandibular excursive movements.[27] In this report, a mutually protected occlusal scheme was used to prevent the destruction of the provisional and definitive restorations. Furthermore, the patient had an end-to-end incisor relationship in right anterior maxilla and concave facial profile at the beginning of the treatment (Figs 10.5A and 10.6A). At the end of the prosthetic rehabilitation, both the facial appearance and the occlusion were improved (Figs 10.5B and 10.6B).

CONCLUSION

Restoring lost OVD by RPD and full-mouth rehabilitation should be done progressively and carefully for maintaining the health and structure of the masticatory system in the patient who has severely worn teeth. In addition, these prosthetic rehabilitations play a major role in the patient's physical attractiveness and social confidence.

ACKNOWLEDGMENT

The authors wish to thank Asst. Prof. Suleyman Bozkaya for his great effort and expert in surgical part of this case report.

REFERENCES

1. Sierpinska T, Konstantynowicz J, Orywal K, et al: Copper deficit as a potential pathogenic factor of reduced bone mineral density and severe tooth wear. *Osteoporos Int* 2014;25:447–454.
2. Abrahamsen TC: The worn dentition-pathognomonic patterns of abrasion and erosion. *Int Dent J* 2005;55(4 Suppl 1):268–276.
3. Carlsson GE, Johansson A, Lundqvist S: Occlusal wear. A follow-up study of 18 subjects with extensively worn dentitions. *Acta Odontol Scand* 1985;43:83–90.
4. Malkoc MA, Sevimay M, Yaprak E: The use of zirconium and feldspathic porcelain in the management of the severely worn dentition: a case report. *Eur J Dent* 2009;3:75–80.
5. Verrett RG: Analyzing the etiology of an extremely worn dentition. *J Prosthodont* 2001;10:224–233.
6. Dawson PE: *Evaluation, Diagnosis and Treatment of Occlusal Problems* (ed 2) St. Louis, Mosby, 1989.
7. Turner KA, Missirlian DM: Restoration of the extremely worn dentition. *J Prosthet Dent* 1984;52:467–474.
8. Chu FC, Siu AS, Newsome PR, et al: Restorative management of the worn dentition: 4. Generalized toothwear. *Dent Update* 2002;29:318–324.
9. Cura C, Saraçoğlu A, Oztürk B: Prosthetic rehabilitation of extremely worn dentitions: case reports. *Quintessence Int* 2002;33:225–230.
10. Guttal S, Patil NP: Cast titanium overlay denture for a geriatric patient with a reduced vertical dimension. *Gerodontology* 2005;22:242–245.
11. Ergun G, Cekic-Nagas I: Implant-prosthetic rehabilitation of a patient with nonsyndromic oligodontia: a clinical report. *J Oral Implantol* 2012;38:497–503.
12. Song MY, Park JM, Park EJ: Full mouth rehabilitation of the patient with severely worn dentition: a case report. *J Adv Prosthodont* 2010;2:106–110.
13. Sato S, Hotta TH, Pedrazzi V: Removable occlusal overlay splint in the management of tooth wear: a clinical report. *J Prosthet Dent* 2000;83:392–395.
14. Windchy AM, Morris JC: An alternative treatment with the overlay removable partial denture: a clinical report. *J Prosthet Dent* 1998;79:249–253.

15. Listgarten MA, Lang NP, Schroeder HE, et al: Periodontal tissues and their counterparts around endosseous implants. *Clin Oral Implants Res* 1991;2:1–19.

16. Lee RL, Gregory GG: Gaining vertical dimension for the deep bite restorative patient. *Dent Clin North Am* 1971;15: 743–763.

17. Worsaae N, Jensen BN, Holm B, et al: Treatment of severe hypodontia-oligodontia–an interdisciplinary concept. *Int J Oral Maxillofac Surg* 2007;36:473–480.

18. Ergun G, Egilmez F, Cekic-Nagas I, et al: Effect of platelet-rich plasma on the outcome of early loaded dental implants: a three year follow-up study. *J Oral Imp* 2013;39:256–263.

19. Ng DY, Wong AY, Liston PN: Multidisciplinary approach to implants: a review. *N Z Dent J* 2012;108:123–128.

20. Silverman MM: The comparative accuracy of the closet-speaking-space and the freeway space in measuring vertical dimension. *J Acad Gen Dent* 1974;22:34–36.

21. Okeson JP: Occlusion and functional disorders of the masticatory system. *Dent Clin North Am* 1995;39:285–300.

22. Chu FC, Yip HK, Newsome PR, et al: Restorative management of the worn dentition: I. Aetiology and diagnosis. *Dent Update* 2002;29:162–168.

23. Ganddini MR, Al-Mardini M, Graser GN, et al: Maxillary and mandibular overlay removable partial dentures for the restoration of worn teeth. *J Prosthet Dent* 2004;91:210–214.

24. Burns DR, Beck DA, Nelson SK: A review of selected dental literature on contemporary provisional fixed prosthodontic treatment: report of the Committee on Research in Fixed Prosthodontics of the Academy of Fixed Prosthodontics. *J Prosthet Dent* 2003;90:474–497.

25. Brännström M: Reducing the risk of sensitivity and pulpal complications after the placement of crowns and fixed partial dentures. *Quintessence Int* 1996;27:673–678.

26. Ergun G, Kaya BM, Egilmez F, et al: Functional and esthetic rehabilitation of a patient with amelogenesis imperfecta. *J Can Dent Assoc* 2013;79:157–162.

27. The glossary of prosthodontic terms. *J Prosthet Dent* 2005;94: 10–92.

11

RESTORATION OF THE OCCLUSAL VERTICAL DIMENSION WITH AN OVERLAY REMOVABLE PARTIAL DENTURE: A CLINICAL REPORT

PIERO ROCHA ZANARDI, MD, MAYARA SILVA SANTOS, ROBERTO CHAIB STEGUN, MD, PHD, NEWTON SESMA, MD, PHD, BRUNO COSTA, MD, PHD, AND DALVA CRUZ LAGANÁ, MD, PHD
Department of Prosthodontics, School of Dentistry, University of São Paulo, São Paulo, Brazil

Keywords
Dental occlusion; occlusal vertical dimension; removable partial denture.

Correspondence
Piero Rocha Zanardi, Department of Prosthodontics, School of Dentistry, University of São Paulo, Av. Prof. Lineu Prestes 2227, Zip Code 05508-000 Cidade Universitária – São Paulo – SP, Brazil. E-mail: pierozndl@gmail.com.br

Zanardi Piero Rocha ORCID ID http://orcid.org/0000-0003-4690-0074.

The authors deny any conflict of interest.

Accepted March 15, 2015

Published in *Journal of Prosthodontics* September 2015

doi: 10.1111/jopr.12351

ABSTRACT

The process of tooth loss throughout life, associated with severe occlusal wear, may pose a challenge in the rehabilitation of partially edentulous arches. In these cases, many therapeutic procedures are necessary because each tooth must be restored to obtain the correct anatomical contour and recover the occlusal vertical dimension (OVD). A removable partial denture (RPD) with occlusal/incisal coverage, also known as an overlay RPD, is an alternative treatment option with fewer interventions, and, consequently, lower cost. This clinical report reviews the principles involved in the clinical indication for an overlay RPD, as well as the necessary planning and execution, to discuss the feasibility and clinical effectiveness of this treatment, identifying the indications, advantages, and disadvantages of this procedure through the presentation of a clinical case. The overlay RPD can be an alternative treatment for special situations involving partially edentulous arches in patients who need reestablishment of the OVD and/or realignment of the occlusal plane, and it can be used as a temporary or definitive treatment. The main advantages of this type of treatment are its simplicity, reversibility, and relatively low cost; however, further studies are needed to ensure the efficacy of this treatment option.

Occlusal dental wear is a physiological process that can be aggravated by pathological conditions such as bruxism. The type of food ingested can also have an effect, as harder, more acidic foods can accelerate tooth wear.[1] However, in terms of the physiological question, the amount of tooth wear can be used to estimate age with a high level of accuracy.[1,2] With respect to the area that suffers the largest amount of loss, anterior tooth wear is greater than that in the posterior region, involving not only physiologic, but also esthetic alterations.[3] The body response to tooth wear seems to have two paths according to the alterations in the occlusal vertical dimension (OVD). The former supports the notion of bone compensation, especially in the lower jaw. In this way, occlusal bone remodeling and growth would promote passive tooth eruption while there is wear.[4] The latter indicates that the bone would not be remodeled,[5] leading to a loss in the OVD and facial alterations. With these two situations in mind, the first step in oral rehabilitation involving severe tooth wear is to determine whether the OVD is appropriate. The initial diagnosis of any type of alteration is fundamentally important to the choice of treatment, because the clinical procedures may vary. If the OVD concept is correct, rehabilitation planning should consider periodontal surgical corrections associated with restorative treatment[6] to restore the correct contour and crown length in the gingival way, assuming that the occlusal limit is correct; however, if there is OVD loss, the periodontal surgical procedures may not be necessary, because restorative treatment resolves the clinical symptoms (Fig 11.1).

Regardless of the need for periodontal surgical procedures, worn teeth need to undergo a restorative procedure. The most important issue is correct diagnosis. Thus, the OVD reestablishment procedures involve very similar steps that may be repeated for different patients such as the wax-up and provisional stages. There seems to be no consensus regarding the best choice of long-term treatment, which can range from direct composite resin restoration or laminated veneers to

metal ceramic crowns.[7] Unfortunately, these treatment options still pose a financial challenge for the patient once many dental elements are involved. Some alternative must be considered to correctly plan the treatments. The overlay removable partial denture seems to be cost-effective.[8]

CLINICAL REPORT

A 62-year-old white man with good general health was referred to the Removable Partial Denture Clinic at the School of Dentistry, University of São Paulo, São Paulo, Brazil, for treatment. His chief complaint was to replace some lost teeth in the posterior inferior region and restore the anterior worn teeth. During the clinical exam, no pain was reported during muscle and joint palpation. The patient reported that his wife hears some "strange noise as if something was scraping" during the night. The intraoral exam revealed moderate wear in the inferior arch with good and healthy periodontal insertion and a complete denture in the maxilla (Fig 11.2). The OVD reduction could be seen because of the thin aspect of the lower lip. The tooth wear reduced the clinical crown to half its size, resulting in dentin exposure on the cervical region. The first and second molars were absent on both sides. The left second premolar migrated to a distal position, creating a space for a hypothetical "third" premolar.

Because of the number of support teeth present in the mandible and the necessity for reestablishing OVD to treat the moderate dental wear, we suggested dental implants for the missing tooth, laminated veneers for the anterior teeth and a porcelain overlay for the posterior region. Due to the high cost of the treatment, the patient requested an alternative option; as a result, an overlay removable partial denture (ORPD) was indicated. Once the patient agreed on the cost, the treatment began.

The first step was to create impressions of the maxillary and mandibular arches using irreversible hydrocolloid; then,

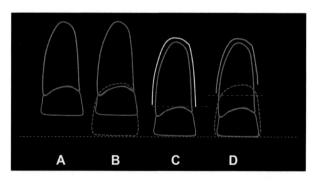

FIGURE 11.1 Classical situations involving tooth wear: (A) initial conditions of tooth wear and OVD loss; (B) restorative solution for case A; (C) initial condition of tooth wear without OVD loss; and (D) periodontal surgical procedures and restorative treatment for correction.

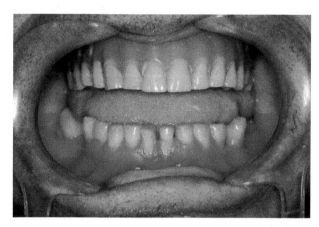

FIGURE 11.2 Intraoral view of the patient's initial condition.

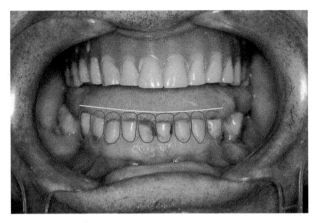

FIGURE 11.3   Virtual planning performed to assist in the predictability of the restorative procedure.

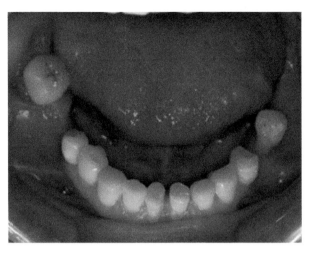

FIGURE 11.4   Incisal restoration of the anterior teeth and the occlusal rest seat.

the casts were assembled in a semi-adjustable articulator for initial evaluation. The Willis gauge was used to obtain the correct OVD. The apparatus was positioned at the pupil and in the junction of the lips. From the initial measurement, 3 mm was reduced, respecting the interocclusal space posteriorly, as verified by the Silverman phonetic test. The final measurement was transposed to the subnasion to the gnathion in the correct OVD, which in turn was 2 mm higher than that presented by the patient's occlusion. The second step was to acquire intraoral photographs to apply the digital smile design concept[9] as an auxiliary diagnosis method to facilitate the diagnosis and communication with the laboratory (Fig 11.3).

Basic periodontal procedures were used at the start of the clinical treatment. The incisal surfaces were restored with composite resin, providing the anterior teeth with a regular surface. A modified back-action circumferential clasp was used on #35 and the circumferential clasp on #34, #45, and #47. After tripoding the casts, the survey line was drawn, and a critical analysis of the components was selected according to the need for axial recontouring. A resin guide, made on the cast by milling a resin block adapted over the dental crown of the supports, inscribed the path of insertion when reduced to the gypsum surface, outlined those areas where a reduction was necessary, and indicated the extent and location on the tooth; however, the measured undercut was obtained on the buccal surface of the abutments (#34, #35, #45, and #47), where the retentive potential was less than 0.25 mm (Fig 11.4).

After mouth preparation, a working cast was obtained with an alginate impression on which the framework was directly outlined. The cast Co–Cr clasp assembly was fit onto the patient, and minor discrepancies were removed with a round bur (Fig 11.5).

After the appropriate framework seating was achieved, the acrylic resin teeth were assembled. Each tooth was worn out

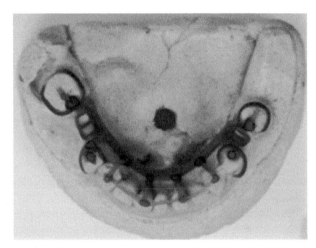

FIGURE 11.5   Framework wax-up with a simple occlusal retention for the acrylic resin.

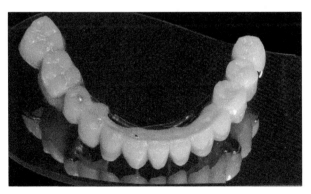

FIGURE 11.6   ORPD final aspect.

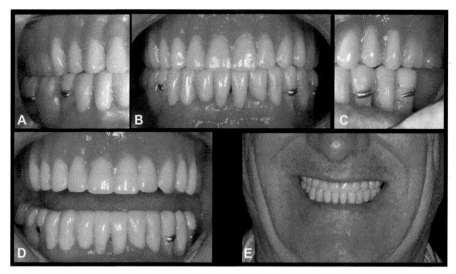

FIGURE 11.7   (A) Right lateral view. (B) Frontal view. (C) Left lateral view. (D) Occlusal plane view. (E) Final esthetic result.

until it became like a veneer for the anterior teeth and could act as an overlay for the posterior teeth. The goal in this case was to recover the incisal loss and cover the buccal area, allowing for tooth uniformity to promote a better esthetic result. The mandibular tooth mounting followed an ideal Curve of Spee. Once this contour was corrected, the new complete denture was constructed on the maxilla. After the initial analysis and with the patient's agreement, the piece was polymerized with two colors: the overlay area was polymerized with heat-polymerizing acrylic resin in the same color as the teeth, and the other areas were subjected to the regular procedures (Fig 11.6).

During the installation of the prosthesis, the patient was informed about correct hygienic procedures, as this type of prosthesis may accumulate more detritus because of its large contact area with the teeth. Since the Curve of Spee was respected, it was possible to have an appropriate occlusion with the new complete denture (Figs 11.7A–11.7D). Patient satisfaction was immediate regarding the final esthetic result (Fig 11.7E). The patient did not report any pain or discomfort during the weekly follow-up.

DISCUSSION

Clinicians can use a variety of tools to assist with the start point determination[9] and make the treatment more predictable. Oral rehabilitation must follow some specific steps that are very similar, regardless of the type of the definitive prosthesis. The best restorative treatment option for the patient with tooth wear is not clear, and the ORPD is not mentioned as a definitive treatment.[7] Because of its low cost, this type of treatment can be indicated for solving several tooth situations that require only one prosthesis.[8]

The following are three ways to perform an ORPD: (I) with occlusal metallic covering and complete resin or ceramic veneer;[8,10,11] (II) with an occlusal resin covering and partial resin veneer;[12] and (III) with an occlusal resin covering and a complete buccal veneer, as described in this article. Types I and III are very similar with respect to the final esthetics once there is a color and contour pattern: they lack a visible line between the worn tooth and the prosthetic tooth. However, this type of buccal covering may not be acceptable in all patients due to the level of tooth wear and the possibility of an increase in the buccal volume. Treatment workflow was favored by the maxilla. All these alterations were made easier because once the mandible was corrected it was only necessary to fabricate a new complete denture on the maxilla.

CONCLUSION

The overlay RPD treatment seems to be satisfactory, restoring the OVD and esthetics and providing greater muscle comfort for the patient with low cost and shorter working time. Further randomized clinical trials are suggested to compare the long-term effectiveness of different treatment options for the worn teeth associated with OVD loss.

REFERENCES

1. Liu B, Zhang M, Chen Y, et al: Tooth wear in aging people: an investigation of the prevalence and the influential factors of incisal/occlusal tooth wear in northwest China. *BMC Oral Health* 2014;14:65.

2. Telang LA, Patil K, Mahima VG: Age estimation of an Indian population by using the Kim's scoring system of occlusal tooth wear. *J Forensic Dent Sci* 2014;6:16–24.

3. Pigno MA, Hatch JP, Rodrigues-Garcia RC, C et al: Severity, distribution, and correlates of occlusal tooth wear in a sample of Mexican-American and European-American adults. *Int J Prosthodont* 2001;14:65–70.

4. Levartovsky S, Matalon S, Sarig R, C et al: The association between dental wear and reduced vertical dimension of the face: a morphologic study on human skulls. *Arch Oral Biol* 2015;60:174–180.

5. Varrela J, Varrela TM: Dental studies of a Finnish skeletal material: a paleopathologic approach. *Tandlaegebladet* 1991;96:283–290.

6. Davarpanah M, Jansen CE, Vidjak FM, C et al: Restorative and periodontal considerations of short clinical crowns. *Int J Periodontics Restorative Dent* 1998;18:424–433.

7. Muts EJ, vanPelt H, Edelhoff D, C et al: Tooth wear: a systematic review of treatment options. *J Prosthet Dent* 2014;112:752–759.

8. Ganddini MR, Al-Mardini M, Graser GN, C et al: Maxillary and mandibular overlay removable partial dentures for the restoration of worn teeth. *J Prosthet Dent* 2004;91:210–214.

9. Coachman C, Calamita M: Digital smile design: a tool for treatment planning and communication in esthetic dentistry. *Quintessence Dent Technol* 2012:103–112.

10. Alfadda SA: A conservative and reversible approach for restoring worn teeth: a clinical report. *J Prosthet Dent* 2014;112: 18–21.

11. Fonseca J, Nicolau P, Daher T: Maxillary overlay removable partial dentures for the restoration of worn teeth. *Compend Contin Educ Dent* 2011;32: I 12, 14–20 (quiz 21, 32).

12. Bataglion C, Hotta TH, Matsumoto W, et al: Reestablishment of occlusion through overlay removable partial dentures: a case report. *Braz Dent J* 2012;23:172–174.

PART III

MANAGEMENT OF CONGENITAL DISORDERS

12

FULL-MOUTH REHABILITATION OF A HYPOHIDROTIC ECTODERMAL DYSPLASIA PATIENT WITH DENTAL IMPLANTS: A CLINICAL REPORT

AFSANEH SHAHROKHI RAD, DMD, MSC,[1] HAKIMEH SIADAT, DDS, MSC,[2] ABBAS MONZAVI, DDS, MSC,[2] AND AMIR-ALI MANGOLI[3]

[1]Dental Research Center, Tehran University of Medical Sciences, Tehran, Iran; Prosthodontics Department, School of Dentistry, Qazvin University of Medical Sciences, Qazvin, Iran
[2]Department of Prosthodontics and Dental Implants, School of Dentistry and Dental Research Center, Tehran University of Medical Sciences, Tehran, Iran
[3]Dental Technician, Tehran, Iran

Keywords
Implant; osseointegration; overdenture; reconstruction; hypohidrotic ectodermal dysplasia.

Correspondence
Afsaneh Shahrokhi Rad, DMD, MSc, Dental Research Center, School of Dentistry Building, Tehran University of Medical Sciences, Ghods Street, Keshavarz Boulevard, Tehran, Iran 141555583. E-mail: ashahrokhi@tums.ac.ir

Accepted November 22, 2005

Published in *Journal of Prosthodontics* May-June 2007; Vol. 16, Issue 3

doi: 10.1111/j.1532-849X.2006.00173.x

ABSRACT

Prosthodontic treatment in patients with ectodermal dysplasia (ED) is difficult to manage because of the oral deficiencies typical in this disorder and because afflicted individuals are quite young when they are evaluated for treatment. This clinical report describes an 18-year-old patient with hypohidrotic ED treated with dental implants. Treatment included a maxillary implant overdenture and a mandibular hybrid prosthesis supported by osseointegrated implants. At the 1-year follow-up, the patient presented significant improvements in oral function and psychosocial activities.

The ectodermal dysplasias (EDs) are a group of genetic disorders involving congenital defects of two or more ectodermal structures; that is, the skin, hair, nails, nerve cells, sweat glands, and parts of the eye and ear.[1,2] Oral findings often are significant and can include multiple abnormalities of the dentition (such as anodontia, hypodontia, or malformed and widely spaced peglike teeth), loss of occlusal vertical dimension, protuberant lips, and lack of normal alveolar ridge development.[3,4] With little or no dental support, a hypoplastic maxilla and mandible result in bite collapse and narrowing of the alveolar ridges.

ED is inherited as an X-linked recessive trait, and has two major types: (1) hypohidrotic or anhidrotic (decreased number or total absence of sweat glands or their abnormal function resulting in a reduced level or lack of perspiration) and (2) hidrotic EDs. The most common condition among the EDs is hypohidrotic ectodermal dysplasia (HED).[5,6] HED is the more severe form and is associated with hypodontia or anodontia, hypotrichosis (fine, sparse blond hair, including a decreased density in both eyebrows and eyelashes), and hypohidrosis or anhidrosis.[7,8]

Conventional prosthodontic treatment for an ED patient has consisted of various combinations of overdentures, complete or partial removable prostheses, or fixed prostheses.[9,10] In recent years, endosseous dental implants have been recognized as an important alternative for ED patients to support, stabilize, and retain the prosthesis.[11–13]

The placement of endosseous dental implants in locations favorable for supporting subsequent restorations may be difficult, however, and may require bone grafting.[11,14]

The present article describes the using of osseointegrated dental implants to rehabilitate an HED patient with cleft palate who presented with maxillary oligodontia, mandibular anodontia, and severe atrophy of the residual alveolar crest.

CLINICAL REPORT

An 18-year-old male patient with HED was referred for dental treatment. The chief complaint was the unaesthetic appearance and lack of function of his dentition.

The patient was under medical care for severe dry eye (xerosis), hearing loss, respiratory problems, and abnormal skin. There were no other medical complications for this patient.

Extraoral examination revealed generalized trichodysplasia (fine sparse hair, scant eyelashes and eyebrows), onchodysplasia (abnormal nails), frontal bossing, a depressed nasal bridge, lip thickening, decreased lower facial height, a prominent chin, and a resultant concave facial profile. The intraoral examination in turn showed partial maxillary (Fig 12.1) and total mandibular edentulism (Fig 12.2), unilateral open cleft palate, and severe maxillary and mandibular atrophy with a small, thin underdeveloped alveolar ridge. Carious lesions, dental plaque, and calculus deposits were observed on the existing maxillary teeth.

Closure of the congenital complete unilateral cleft lip had been performed at 6 months of age and closure of the complete unilateral cleft palate at the age of 6 years. The surgery was unsuccessful and, as a result, secondary repair surgery and a bone graft using free iliac crest was performed at the age of 17 years. Mandibular and maxillary osteoplasty was performed at the same time to correct prognathic

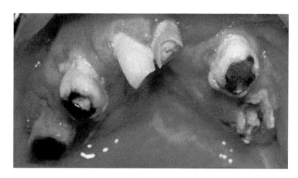

FIGURE 12.1   Intraoral view of maxillary remaining dentition.

appearance. Again, the surgical procedure for the closure of the palatal cleft was considered unsuccessful.

Orthopantomography (Fig 12.3) and computed spiral tomography revealed extreme maxillary atrophy with little remnant bone. The permanent central incisors and the first and second molars were judged to have a poor prognosis due to severe alveolar bone loss.

The remaining maxillary teeth were considered for extraction because of their poor prognosis and advanced periodontal disease. Complete dentures were fabricated as a provisional restoration.

The definitive treatment plan included fabrication of a maxillary implant-supported overdenture (RP-4 according to Misch) and a mandibular implant-supported fixed prosthesis (FP-3 according to Misch).[15]

Preliminary impressions were made using irreversible hydrocolloid impression material (Alginoplast, Heraeus Kulzer, South Bend, IN), and final impressions were made with vinyl polysiloxane impression material (Affinis, Coltene AG, Feldwiesenstrasse Altstatten, Switzerland). Casts were mounted using an arbitrary facebow (Dentatus, Dentatus USA Ltd., New York, NY), and a centric relation record obtained with polyether bite registration material (Ramitec, 3MESPE, St. Paul, MN) on a semiadjustable articulator (Dentatus ARH, Dentatus USA Ltd.). Tooth setup was accomplished on the mounted casts from which a

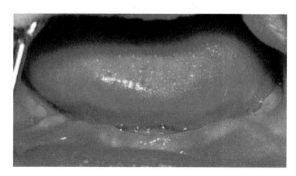

FIGURE 12.2   Intraoral view of mandibular residual ridge.

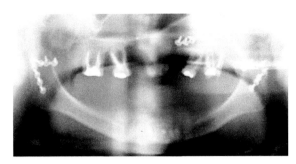

FIGURE 12.3   Preoperative panoramic radiograph.

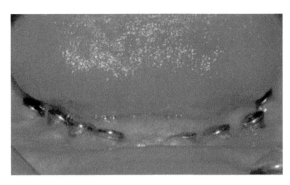

FIGURE 12.5   Intraoral view of implants in the mandibular arch.

radiographic template with metallic balls and a surgical template were fabricated.

Orthopantomography with these radiographic templates was performed to determine proper implant locations. No metallic balls were considered for the alveolar cleft region.

At the appointment for delivery of the complete dentures, the patient was instructed to wear the prosthesis during healing, following extraction of the teeth.

The surgical procedure was performed under general anesthesia. Eight ITI SLA implants (Institute Straumann AG, Waldenburg, Switzerland) with regular platforms were placed in the maxilla, and the same number were placed in the mandibular arch according to the locations of the metallic balls on the radiographic template and the positions of sleeves in the surgical template. Ten days following the surgical procedure, sutures were removed, and the interim complete dentures relined with soft liner (UFI Gel P, Voco, Cuxhaven, Germany).

Six months after the procedure, clinical and radiographic examinations confirmed the osseointegration of all 16 implants (Figs 12.4–12.6). This observation has been made in other reports of patients with ED who received edentulous implants.[8,11,12]

Preliminary impressions for implant-supported restorations were made with silicone impression material (Speedex, Coltène AG), and new diagnostic casts were obtained.

Custom trays for making final impressions were fabricated on these casts. Screw-retained impression copings (Institute Straumann AG) were placed into the implant bodies, and final impressions were made with polyether (Impregum F, 3M ESPE) using an open tray technique.[16]

To obtain accurate centric relation records, screw-retained record bases were fabricated on the master casts.[16] Casts were mounted on a semiadjustable articulator (Denar Mark II, Teledyne Water Pik, Fort Collins, CO) using centric relation and an arbitrary facebow record (Denar Slidematic, Teledyne Water Pik).

The existence of an open cleft palate and oral hygiene maintenance problems, as well as speech and esthetic difficulties, contraindicated fixed prosthesis treatment planning. As a result, an implant-supported overdenture was selected as the optimal treatment option for the maxillary arch. A hybrid prosthesis was the treatment of choice for the mandibular arch.

Abutment selection was performed on the master cast, and superstructures were fabricated according to the diagnostic setup. Eight ball attachments (Rhein 83, Bologna, Italy) were placed on the maxillary superstructure to retain the overdenture. Superstructures were tried-in to ensure passive fitness (Figs 12.7 and 12.8). Periapical radiographs confirmed complete adaptation of the superstructures over the implant abutments.

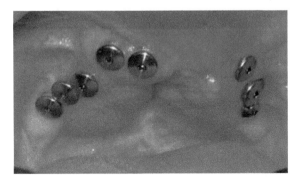

FIGURE 12.4   Intraoral view of maxillary implants with cover screws in place.

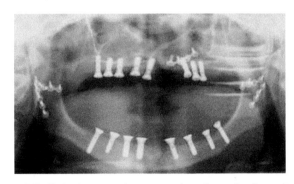

FIGURE 12.6   Postoperative panoramic radiograph of osseointegrated implants.

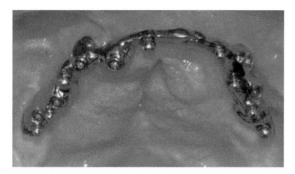

FIGURE 12.7 Maxillary overdenture superstructure with ball attachments for overdenture retention.

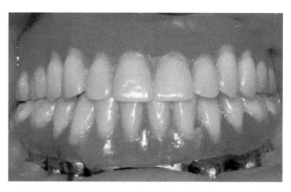

FIGURE 12.9 Clinical view of maxillary implant-supported overdenture and mandibular fixed prosthesis.

Tooth setup was completed with the superstructures in place. After esthetic try-in, confirmation of centric relation and making protrusive and lateral check bite records, the implant fixed prosthodontic occlusion concept (i.e., mutually protected occlusion) was applied.[17] At delivery, abutment screws and superstructure screws were tightened with controlled torque (35 and 15 N/cm^2, respectively), and a clinical remount was performed to refine the occlusion (Fig 12.9). The access holes were filled with a light-cured composite resin (Tetric Ceram, Ivoclar Vivadent AG, Schaan, Leichtenstein). Oral hygiene instructions were provided to the patient.

Follow-ups were performed after the first week, first month, sixth month, and first year, following prostheses insertion. No complications such as speech impairment, esthetic problems, screw loosening and/or fracture, or implant mobility were detected. The patient reported improvements in oral function and self-confidence.

DISCUSSION

ED presents a group of patients with severe congenital and developmental anomalies. Hypodontia and anodontia are the most common oral characteristics of ED. These anomalies affect esthetic and functional activities, which in turn can bring about psychosocial problems for the patient.

The dentist may be the first person to identify ED in young patients. Rapid growth in early life dictates the use of removable partial or complete dentures for these patients. When full growth is reached, treatment planning may include dental implants to retain, support, and stabilize prostheses.[6,11,13,18] Osseointegrated implants offer an alternative that will provide major improvement in the long-term prognosis for oral rehabilitation.

In treatment planning for implant dentistry in these patients, extra care must be taken to determine whether adequate bone level to receive the implants is present and whether there is adequate vertical dimension of bone to support the implants. Diminished bone volume may limit the success of implants, especially in the maxilla.[11]

This article describes full-mouth rehabilitation of an ED patient using osseointegrated dental implants. A maximum of eight osseointegrated implants were used for each arch to compensate for diminished alveolar ridge height, and the resultant reduced length of implant bodies. This would be especially advisable because some of the implants may fail over time. Further, because of the necessity of using general anesthesia and the fact that such surgeries would be very difficult to be carried out in future, an increased number of osseointegrated implants (eight) were used. A maxillary overdenture was fabricated to facilitate the hygiene maintenance of the open cleft palate region. Prosthodontic treatment improved the patient's esthetic and functional condition and increased his psychosocial confidence and activities.

CONCLUSION

To conclude, this case suggests that the use of dental implants in the rehabilitation of ED patients can provide excellent support for dental rehabilitation, both functionally and esthetically.

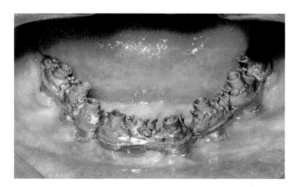

FIGURE 12.8 Mandibular superstructure for FP-3 prosthesis tried-in the mouth.

ACKNOWLEDGMENTS

We thank Dr. Hamid Mahmoudhashemi for his surgical expertise and Dr. Zahra Tahouri for her great help.

REFERENCES

1. Hickey A, Vergo JR TJ: Prosthetic treatments for patients with ectodermal dysplasia. *J Prosthet Dent* 2001;86: 364–368.
2. National Foundation for Ectodermal dysplasia. http://www.nfed.org/.
3. Guckes AD, Scurria MS, King TS, et al: Prospective clinical trial of dental implants in persons with ectodermal dysplasia. *J Prosthet Dent* 2002;88:21–25.
4. Dhanrajani PJ, Jiffry AO: Management of ectodermal dysplasia: a literature review. *Dent Update* 1998;25:73–75.
5. NaBadalung DP: Prosthodontic rehabilitation of an anhidrotic ectodermal dysplasia patient: a clinical report. *J Prosthet Dent* 1999;81:499–502.
6. Pigno MA, Blackman RB, Cronin RJ, et al: Prosthodontic management of ectodermal dysplasia: a review of the literature. *J Prosthet Dent* 1996;76:541–545.
7. Blattner RJ: Hereditary ectodermal dysplasia. *J Pediatr* 1968;73:444–447.
8. Davarpanah M, Moon JW, Yang LR, et al: Dental implants in the oral rehabilitation of a teenager with hypohidrotic ectodermal dysplasia: report of a case. *Int J Oral Maxillofac Implants* 1997;12:252–258.
9. Bolender CL, Law DB, Austin LB: Prosthodontic treatment of ectodermal dysplasia. A case report. *J Prosthet Dent* 1964;14:317–325.
10. Snawder KD: Considerations in dental treatment of children with ectodermal dysplasia. *J Am Dent Assoc* 1976;93:1177–1179.
11. Guckes AD, Brahim JS, McCarthy GR, et al: Using endosseous implants for patients with ectodermal dysplasia. *J Am Dent Assoc* 1991;122:59–62.
12. Smith R, Vargervik K, Kearns G, et al: Placement of an endosseous implant in a growing child with ectodermal dysplasia. *Oral Surg Oral Med Oral Pathol* 1993;75:669–673.
13. Rashedi B: Prosthodontic Treatment with implant fixed prosthesis for a patient with ectodermal dysplasia: a clinical report. *J Prosthodont* 2003;12:198–201.
14. Graber LW: Congenital absence of teeth: a review with emphasis on inheritance pattern. *J Am Dent Assoc* 1978;96:266–275.
15. Misch CE: Prosthetic option in implant dentistry. In Misch CE (ed): *Dental Implant Prosthetics*. St. Louis, MO, Mosby, 2005, pp 43–52.
16. Hobo S, Ichida E, Garcia LT: *Osseointegration and Occlusal Rehabilitation*. Chicago, Quintessence, 1989, pp. 153–55.
17. Misch CE: Maxillary denture opposing an implant prosthesis: hydroxyapatite augmentation and modified occlusal concepts. in Misch CE (ed): *Contemporary Implant Dentistry* (ed 2) St. Louis, MO, Mosby, 1999, pp 629–645.
18. Penarrocha-Diago M, Uribe-Origone R, Rambla-Ferrer J, et al: Fixed rehabilitation of a patient with hypohidrotic ectodermal dysplasia using zygomatic implant. *Oral Surg Oral Med Oral Pathol* 2004;98:161–165.

13

PROSTHETIC REHABILITATION WITH COLLAPSIBLE HYBRID ACRYLIC RESIN AND PERMANENT SILICONE SOFT LINER COMPLETE DENTURE OF A PATIENT WITH SCLERODERMA-INDUCED MICROSTOMIA

KUNWARJEET SINGH, BDS, MDS,[1] NIDHI GUPTA, BDS, MDS,[2] RIDHIMAA GUPTA, BDS, MDS,[1] AND DEX ABRAHM[3]

[1]Department of Prosthodontics, Dental Materials and Implantology, Institute of Dental Studies and Technologies, Modinagar, Ghaziabad, India
[2]Department of Pedodontics and Preventive Dentistry, Institute of Dental Studies and Technologies, Modinagar, Ghaziabad, India
[3]Department of Conservative Dentistry, Institute of Dental Studies and Technologies, Modinagar, Ghaziabad, India

Keywords
Collapsible complete denture; scleroderma; microstomia; permanent silicone soft liner; Molloplast B.

Correspondence
Kunwarjeet Singh, Institute of Dental Studies and Technologies—Prosthodontics, Dental Materials and Implantology, NH-58, Delhi-Meerut Road, Modinagar, Ghaziabad, Uttar Pradesh 201010, India. E-mail: drkunwar@gmail.com

The authors deny any conflict of interest.

Accepted July 31, 2013

Published in *Journal of Prosthodontics* July 2014; Vol. 23, Issue 5

doi: 10.1111/jopr.12127

ABSTRACT

Scleroderma is an autoimmune multisystem rheumatic condition characterized by fibrosis of connective tissues of the body, resulting in hardening and impairment of the function of different organs. Deposition of collagen fibers in peri-oral tissues causes loss of elasticity and increased tissue stiffness, resulting in restricted mouth opening. A maximal oral opening smaller than the size of a complete denture can make prosthetic treatment challenging. Patients with microstomia who must wear removable dental prostheses (RDPs) often face the difficulty of being unable to insert or remove a conventional RDP. A sectional-collapsible denture is indicated for the prosthetic management of these patients, but reduced manual dexterity often makes intraoral manipulation of the prosthesis difficult. A single collapsible complete denture is a better choice for functional rehabilitation of these patients. This clinical report describes in detail the prosthodontic management of a maxillary edentulous patient with restricted mouth opening induced by scleroderma with a single collapsible removable complete denture fabricated with heat-polymerized silicone soft liner and heat-cured acrylic resin. The preliminary and secondary impressions were made with moldable aluminum trays by using putty and light-body poly(vinyl siloxane) elastomeric impression material. The collapsed denture can be easily inserted and

removed by the patient and also provides adequate function in the mouth.

Scleroderma, also known as systemic sclerosis, dermatosclerosis, or hidebound disease, is an autoimmune disorder of unknown etiology characterized by vasomotor disturbance, fibro-sis of connective tissue, overproduction of normal collagen fibers,[1] subsequent atrophy of the skin, subcutaneous tissues, muscles, and internal organs (kidney, lungs, heart, alimentary tract, etc.) with associated immunologic disturbances. Increased deposition of collagen fibers in tissues is a characteristic feature of scleroderma. It may begin in children or young adults, although the greatest incidence is between 30 and 50 years of age, females being affected more often than males (3–6:1). It is a chronic, debilitating, connective-tissue disease resulting in the hardening and tightening of the skin and mucosa.[1,2]

Scleroderma can have a significant adverse effect upon the health of the mouth. A wide variety of different problems can arise that may result in increased susceptibility to dental decay, gingivitis, and difficulty with dentures. These oral problems, in particular xerostomia (mouth dryness), microstomia (limited mouth opening), and decreased mucosal resiliency, can reduce the quality of life of affected individuals.

Microstomia (small oral orifice) is observed in 70% to 80% of patients with systemic scleroderma.[3] It is probably the most significant oral consequence of scleroderma, giving rise to limited mouth opening and, as a result, difficulty with eating and sometimes speech. The limited mouth opening also makes it difficult for affected individuals to insert and remove the prosthesis.

Deposition of collagen fibers in peri-oral tissues results in loss of elasticity and hardening of the skin, resulting in a decreased oral opening. The lips become thin and rigid, and skin folds are lost around the mouth, giving a mask-like appearance and lack of expression. Due to the sclerotic changes, the tongue may become hard and board-like, making speaking and swallowing difficult.[4] The involvement of the temporomandibular joint further increases the narrowing of the oral opening. Due to a restricted mouth opening, these patients are unable to wear a conventional removable prosthesis, as they often face difficulty in inserting and removing the prosthesis.[5]

Sectional,[6,7] collapsible,[8,9] or sectional–collapsible[10,11] are types of prostheses proposed for prosthodontic management of patients with limited intraoral access. The two segments of sectional dentures can be fixed using various systems such as clasp retainers, stud attachments, a telescope system, magnetic attachments, swing-lock attachments, or

pins. Various techniques recommended for making preliminary impressions for patients with microstomia have included the stock impression trays of each half of the mouth for sectional impressions with heavy- and light-body silicone impression materials and flexible impression trays made with silicone putty. The sectional custom trays can be connected with hinges, plastic building screws, orthodontic expansion screws, or locking levers.[5]

Scleroderma patients suffer dry mouth (xerostomia) due to fibrosis of salivary gland ducts and a decrease in resiliency of oral mucosa due to deposition of collagen fibers. Both conditions make the oral mucosa vulnerable to trauma from the denture. These patients often suffer from denture-induced mucosa soreness. The viscoelastic and elastic properties of the permanent silicone soft liner permits wide and even distribution of forces. Its cushioning effect helps in absorption of impact forces involved in functional and parafunctional movements, thereby minimizing the trauma of underlying supporting tissues.

Microstomia presents some difficulties in prosthetic rehabilitation of these patients by conventional approaches. Denture fabrication by traditional techniques is complicated by a limited oral opening, which must be modified. Due to reduced manual dexterity and reduced mouth opening, these patients have problems with insertion and removal of the prosthesis. Hence, there is a necessity for fabricating complete dentures that are different from conventional ones.

This article describes an alternative innovative technique for the fabrication of a collapsible maxillary complete denture with a heat-cured permanent silicone soft liner and heat-cured acrylic resin to treat a patient with scleroderma-induced microstomia.

CLINICAL REPORT

A 55-year-old female patient with restricted mouth opening was referred to our dental center for prosthetic rehabilitation. She had a limited mouth opening with a diameter around 23 mm (Fig 13.1) caused by scleroderma. The patient had the symptoms of scleroderma in her hands and face (Fig 13.2) characterized by finger deformities, restricted hand movement, stretched facial skin, and an expressionless face. She was not able to move her left hand.

The intraoral examination revealed a partially edentulous maxilla and mandible with few remaining teeth (#6, #7, and #15) in the maxillary arch, and all mandibular teeth were

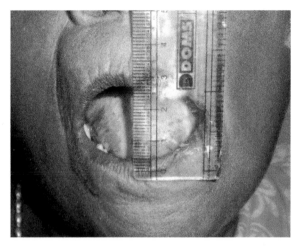

FIGURE 13.1   Patient with restricted mouth opening (23 mm).

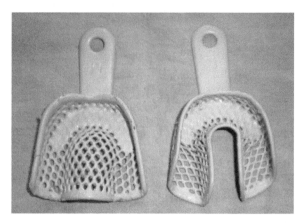

FIGURE 13.3   Stock trays showing change in dimensions.

present except #24, #25, #26, and #27. She also suffered dry mouth, potentially due to fibrosis of the salivary glands. The patient wore an ill-fitting maxillary denture and a mandibular removable partial denture with shortened flanges. The patient had concerns about sectional collapsible dentures, which are most often recommended for prosthetic rehabilitation of patients with microstomia. Therefore, a hybrid collapsible maxillary denture with heat-cured acrylic resin and permanent silicone soft liner and a cast partial removable dental prosthesis with short extension up to the first premolar to replace the missing mandibular incisor were fabricated.

Fabrication Technique

Preliminary impressions were made with moldable aluminum stock trays (Fig 13.3) with poly(vinyl siloxane) (PVS) elastomer of putty consistency (Aquasil soft putty/regular set; Dentsply DeTrey, Konstanz, Germany). After the over-extended maxillary impression was trimmed, the secondary impression was made with light-body PVS impression material (Aquasil LV; Dentsply DeTrey) over the primary impression. Before the impressions were made, the single visit intentional root canal treatment of the remaining three

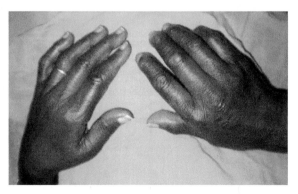

FIGURE 13.2   Hand and finger deformities.

maxillary teeth was completed and prepared as overdenture abutments, except #27, which was circumferentially covered by soft liner of the prosthesis to improve the retention.

The impressions were then poured with dental stone (Kalstone; Kalabhai Karson Pvt. Ltd., Mumbai, India) to obtain the master cast. To establish occlusal vertical dimension (OVD) and to record the centric relation, the temporary record denture base was made of thermoplastic sheets (Star™ Soft Eva Sheets; Andent Pvt. Ltd., Delhi, India), 1.5-mm thick. Jaw relation records were obtained with the use of occlusion rims oriented to the established OVD, the anatomic occlusal plane, and the patient's centric relation. The wax rim was sectioned in the canine–premolar region for easy insertion into the patient's mouth. Then, the master casts were mounted on a semiadjustable articulator (Hanau™ Wide-Vue Arcon Articulator; Whip Mix Corp., Louisville, KY), and artificial teeth (Cosmo HXL, Dentsply DeTrey) were arranged.

After try-in, the flasking and dewaxing was completed. The thermoplastic resin record base (Star™ Soft Eva Sheets) was cleaned and again readapted on the master cast to create space for a permanent soft liner. The thickness of spacer should be 1 to 2 mm, and it can be fabricated from a thermoplastic resin sheet or acrylic resin trimmed to the required thickness. The separating medium was then applied on the mold, except the teeth, and on the master cast.

The heat-cured acrylic resin (Lucitone 199 Denture Base Material; Dentsply DeTrey) was mixed according to manufacturer's instruction and packed in dough stage into a lukewarm flask. Prior to pressing, a polyethylene (PE) foil was placed between the acrylic and spacer for easy separation of flask parts at trial closure. The flask was pressed for 10 to 15 minutes at 100 kp under hydraulic press. The flask was opened, and PE foil and excess acrylic were removed. Also, acrylic was cut from half of the palatal surface (Fig 13.4) to create space for the soft liner. A thin cut (slit) was made with a surgical scalpel in the canine–premolar region of the acrylic

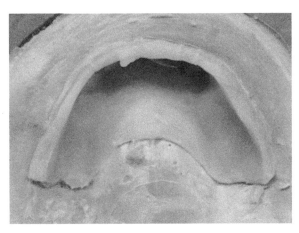

FIGURE 13.4 Excess as well as half the acrylic resin from the palatal surface was cut off.

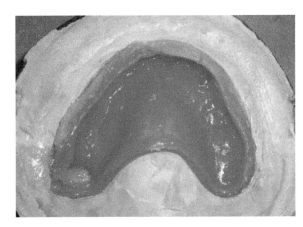

FIGURE 13.6 Permanent soft liner denture base after trial closure.

resin before it attained sufficient stiffness to prevent any deformation during packing of soft liner over it. This cut, along with soft liner, allows flexion of the prosthesis for easy insertion into the mouth.

Again, the flask was closed with spacer and PE foil and put into a clamp. The clamp was tightened, placed in cold water, and brought to boil for approximately 30 minutes. Then, the flask was cooled. This prepolymerization prevents possible reaction of the soft liner with the acrylic monomer and also allows acrylic resin to gain adequate stiffness to avoid deformation by the permanent soft liner (Molloplast B; Detax GmbH and Co, Ettlingen, Germany) material during pressing. The flask was then removed from the clamp and opened carefully. The PE foil and spacer were removed.

Molloplast B needs no mixing. It is available in a dough-like consistency in a jar. The required amount of material was dispensed with a clean spatula from the jar and packed onto the prepressed acrylic in the flask (Fig 13.5). A new PE foil was

placed between the permanent soft liner and counter of the flask. The flask was closed and prepressed in intervals at 100 kp. The flask was opened, and PE foil and excess soft liner were removed (Fig 13.6). The flask was again closed and pressed for approximately 10 to 15 minutes at 100 kp. The flask was then placed in the clamp, and the whole assembly was placed in cold water and heated slowly to 100 °C. The polymerization was done in boiling water at 100 °C for approximately 2 hours. The flask was cooled slowly. After the flask was opened, the prosthesis was retrieved, finished, and polished. The acrylic was polished normally. The excess soft liner was cut with scissors, and polishing was done over rough areas with a polishing disc. The definitive hybrid prosthesis fabricated from acrylic resin and soft liner is quite collapsible (Fig 13.7). A conventional noncollapsible prosthesis is difficult to insert into the oral cavity of a microstomia patient (Fig 13.8). This collapsible hybrid prosthesis can be easily inserted and removed from the oral cavity even by a patient with limited manual dexterity (Fig 13.9). After occlusal adjustments, the prosthesis was delivered to the patient.

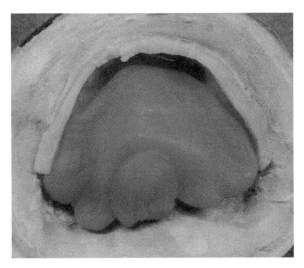

FIGURE 13.5 Permanent soft liner packed onto the partially prepolymerized acrylic resin.

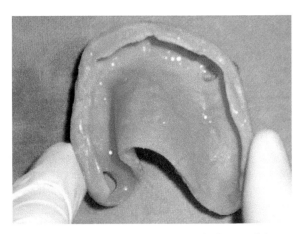

FIGURE 13.7 Collapsible permanent soft liner and heat-cure acrylic resin denture.

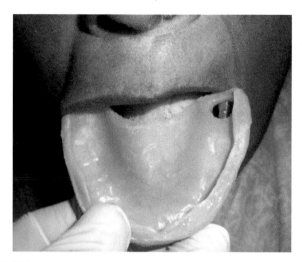

FIGURE 13.8   Normal size of prosthesis greater than maximum oral opening.

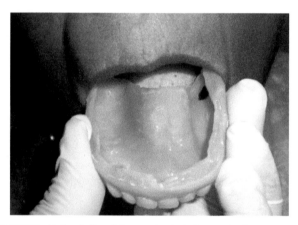

FIGURE 13.9   Collapsible prosthesis being easily inserted into the oral cavity.

During the first 2 years follow-up, the patient was quite satisfied with the prosthesis.

DISCUSSION

Fabrication of a single hybrid collapsible denture with acrylic resin and permanent silicone soft liner for a patient with microstomia and limited manual dexterity is a better choice, because it can be easily inserted and removed by the patient and also minimizes the trauma of underlying supporting tissues. It also maintains intimate contact with tissues and increases prosthesis retention.

An implant-supported prosthesis can also be considered as a viable treatment option, but chronic use of corticosteroids, which are often used for treatment of scleroderma, has been cited as an absolute contraindication or relative contraindication for the placement of dental implants.[12,13] Several reports showed loss of osseointegration in patients with chronic use of corticosteroids.[14,15]

Saving a few remaining teeth to be used as overdenture abutments has a great advantage for the scleroderma patient, as this seems to help compensate for the patient's decreased manual dexterity by keeping flanges short with improved retention. The first difficulty in prosthetic rehabilitation starts with impression making. For this purpose, flexible and sectional stock trays[16,17] have been proposed. In this report, flexible moldable aluminum trays were used for making preliminary impressions with putty-consistency PVS elastomeric impression material. After trimming the excess, the same impression was used for making a secondary impression with light-body PVS.

When the oral opening is limited, joining the segments of a sectional denture intraorally may be difficult for these patients. Keeping in mind the patient's concerns, we fabricated the collapsible hybrid maxillary denture with a combination of silicone soft liner and heat-cured acrylic resin. The silicone soft liner (Molloplast B) is a heat-activated silicone supplied in dough consistency. The use of soft liner has been advocated in the literature for the management of edentulous patients who suffer from chronic pain, soreness, or discomfort due to prolonged contact between the rigid denture base and underlying tissues. Heat-activated permanent silicone soft liners have high resilience and prolonged elasticity, which enables them to maintain their cushioning effect for a longer period of time. Scleroderma patients suffer from xerostomia and decreased mucosal resiliency, making them prone to trauma from the dentures. The cushioning effect of the soft liner minimizes the trauma of underlying supporting structures.

The most challenging aspect in the use of the soft liner is its tendency to support microorganism growth. The maintenance of good oral and denture hygiene can effectively minimize the microbial/fungal colonization of liners and prolong their life. Molloplast B has an antiplaque effect (according to manufacturer), which minimizes plaque deposition. Even so, the patient must be instructed about proper oral and denture hygiene. The soft liner should be cleaned with a soft brush in conjunction with a very mild detergent or wiped with cotton under cold water.

The hybrid acrylic resin and permanent silicone soft liner collapsible denture is an innovative prosthesis, which can be successfully used for functional rehabilitation of scleroderma-induced microstomia, oral submucuos fibrosis, cleft lip, burns, maxillofacial trauma, surgical treatment of orofacial neoplasm, and radiotherapy. The patient was able to insert and remove the prosthesis easily because of its collapsible posterior section of soft liner and a slit created in the acrylic denture base in the canine–premolar region. The esthetic aspect was not good because of perioral tissue rigidity and fullness created by the denture flange, but retention and stability of the prosthesis was good. During the initial phase of denture insertion, the patient complained about difficulty in speaking and chewing but within 6 to 8 weeks, she was satisfied with these aspects, as found on the follow-up visits.

CONCLUSION

This clinical report suggests that hybrid collapsible acrylic resin and permanent silicone soft liner denture is an innovative treatment modality for functional prosthetic rehabilitation of a scleroderma patient with limited mouth opening and manual dexterity to insert and remove the prosthesis. The patient was satisfied and adapted to the prosthesis well.

REFERENCES

1. Suzuki Y, Abe M, Hosoi T, et al: Sectional collapsed denture for a partially edentulous patient with microstomia: a clinical report. *J Prosthet Dent* 2000;84:256–259.

2. Cura C, Cotert HS: User A: fabrication of a sectional impression tray and sectional complete denture for a patient with microstomia and trismus: a clinical report. *J Prosthet Dent* 2003;89:540–543.

3. Marmary Y, Glaiss R, Pisanty J: Scleroderma: oral manifestations. *Oral Surg Oral Med Oral Pathol* 1981;52:32–37.

4. Dhanasomboon S, Kiatsiriroj K: Impression procedure for a progressive sclerosis patient: a clinical report. *J Prosthet Dent* 2000;83:279–282.

5. Prithiviraj DR, Ramaswamy S, Ramesh S: Prosthetic rehabilitation of patients with microstomia. *Indian J Dent Res* 2009;20:483–486.

6. Al-Hadi LA: A simplified technique for prosthetic treatment of microstomia in a patient with scleroderma: a case report. *Quintessence Int* 1994;25:531–533.

7. McCord JF, Tyson KW, Blair IS: A sectional complete denture for a patient with microstomia. *J Prosthet Dent* 1989;61:645–647.

8. Benetti R, Zupi A, Toffain A: Prosthetic rehabilitation for a patient with microstomia: a clinical report. *J Prosthet Dent* 2004;92:322–327.

9. Yenisey M, Külünk T, Kurt S, et al: A Prosthodontic management alternative for scleroderma patients. *J Oral Rehabil* 2005;32:696–700.

10. Moghadam BK: Preliminary impression in patients with microstomia. *J Prosthet Dent* 1992;67:23–25.

11. Watanabe I, Tanaka Y, Ohkubo F C et al: Application cast magnetic attachments to sectional complete dentures for a patient with microstomia: a clinical report. *J Prosthet Dent* 2002;88:573–577.

12. Fonseca RJ, Davis WH: *Reconstructive Preprosthetic Oral and Maxillofacial Surgery*. Philadelphia, Saunders, 1986.

13. Smiler DG. Implants: evaluation and treatment planning. *CDA J* 1987;15:35–41.

14. Cranin AN: Endosteal implants in a patient with corticosteroid dependence. *J Oral Implantol* 1991;17:414–417.

15. Smith RA, Berger R, Dodson TB: Risk factors associated with dental implants in healthy and medically compromised patients. *Int J Oral Maxillofac Implants* 1992;7:367–372.

16. Naylor WP, Manor RC: Fabrication of a flexible prosthesis for the edentulous scleroderma patient with microstomia. *J Prosthet Dent* 1983;50:536–538.

17. Luebke RJ: Sectional impression tray for patients with constricted oral opening. *J Prosthet Dent* 1984;52:135–137.

14

NASOALVEOLAR MOLDING AND LONG-TERM POSTSURGICAL ESTHETICS FOR UNILATERAL CLEFT LIP/PALATE: 5-YEAR FOLLOW-UP

PRAVINKUMAR G. PATIL, MDS,[1] SMITA P. PATIL, MDS,[2] AND SOUMIL SARIN, MDS[3]

[1]Department of Prosthodontics, Government Dental College and Hospital, Nagpur, India
[2]Department of Orthodontics and Dentofacial Orthopedics, Swargiya Dadasaheb Kalmegh Smruti Dental College and Hospital, Nagpur, India
[3]Department of Prosthodontics, Postgraduate Institute, Chandigarh, India

Keywords
Cleft lip and palate; nasoalveolar molding; presurgical orthopedics.

Correspondence
Pravinkumar G. Patil, Room No. 121, Department of Prosthodontics, Government Dental College and Hospital, GMC Campus, Nagpur, Maharashtra, 440003, India. E-mail: pravinandsmita@yahoo.co.in.

Accepted August 3, 2011

Published in *Journal of Prosthodontics* October 2011; Vol. 20, Issue 7

doi: 10.1111/j.1532-849X.2011.00782.x

ABSTRACT

The nasoalveolar molding (NAM) technique has been shown to significantly improve the surgical outcome of the primary repair in cleft lip and palate patients. A 6-day-old female infant was managed with the presurgical NAM technique. Periodic adjustments of the appliance were continued every week to mold the nasoalveolar complex into the desired shape for the next 5 months. The 13 mm of alveolar cleft width was reduced to 1.5 mm. The depressed nostril on the cleft side was molded into the normal anatomy. The nose and upper lip were surgically repaired at the age of 5 months. The second stage surgery of palatal closure was performed at the age of 18 months. The patient was followed up regularly at 6-month intervals for the next 5 years.

The basic goal of any approach to cleft lip, alveolus, and palate repair, whether for the unilateral or bilateral anomaly, is to restore normal anatomy. Ideally, deficient tissues should be expanded, and malpositioned structures repositioned prior to the surgical correction. This provides a foundation for a less-invasive surgical repair. An approach of presurgical nasoalveolar molding (NAM) therapy includes not only reduction of the size of the intraoral alveolar cleft through the molding of the bony segments, but also the active molding and positioning of the surrounding soft tissues affected by the cleft, including the deformed soft tissue and cartilage in the cleft nose. NAM was developed at the

Institute of Reconstructive Plastic Surgery at New York University Medical Center.[1] However, the pioneering research on neonatal molding of the nasal cartilage was performed by Matsuo et al.[2–4] The objective of NAM is to reduce the size of the intraoral cleft and to actively mold and position the surrounding tissues affected by the cleft before surgical intervention.[5–7] The resultant tissue positioning by NAM improves postsurgical esthetics better than previously described presurgical orthopedic techniques in the cleft lip/palate do.[5] The purpose of this article is to describe a long-term (5-year) developmental and esthetic soft- and hard-tissue response after NAM and surgical repair of the unilateral cleft lip/palate.

CLINICAL REPORT

A 6-day-old female infant was referred to the Department of Prosthodontics for presurgical NAM. A general physical check-up was done under the supervision of the physician, and consent was obtained to start the active molding therapy within the first week of birth. Initial examination revealed unilateral cleft lip and cleft palate on the right side (Fig 14.1). The distance between the two alveolar segments was 13 mm. The medical and family history of the parents was non-contributory. The complete procedure of NAM, along with the recall appointment schedule was described to the parents. The tentative timetable of the subsequent surgical appointments was also described.

The initial intraoral impression was obtained with a heavy-bodied polyvinylsiloxane impression material (Reprosil; Dentsply, York, PA) as described by Brecht et al.[6] For fast setting of the impression material, two parts of base material can be mixed with one part of the catalyst with clinically acceptable properties.[6] The infant was held in an inverted position during impression making to prevent the tongue from falling back and to allow fluids to drain out of the oral cavity. The impression was made in the hospital setting with facilities to manage an airway emergency and with a surgeon present as part of the impression team.[6,8] High-volume evacuation was also ready at all times in the case of regurgitation of the stomach contents. Once the impression material was set, the tray was removed, and the oral cavity was examined for residual impression material. The impression was then poured with dental stone (Kalstone; Kalabhai Karson, Mumbai, India) to obtain an accurate cast (definitive cast). One more cast was obtained from the same impression and preserved as a permanent patient record. All the undercuts and the cleft space were blocked on the definitive cast with the baseplate wax (Modeling wax; Deepti Dental Products, Ratnagiri, India). The molding prosthesis (2–3 mm thick) was fabricated using heat-polymerizing clear acrylic resin (DPI heat cure-clear; Dental Products of India, Mumbai, India). A retention button was fabricated and positioned anteriorly at an angle of 40° to the palate. The appliance was then secured extraorally to the cheeks and bilaterally by surgical tapes with orthodontic elastic bands (Fig 14.2). The use of skin barrier dressing-tapes (Tegaderm; 3M ESPE, St. Paul, MN) was advocated to

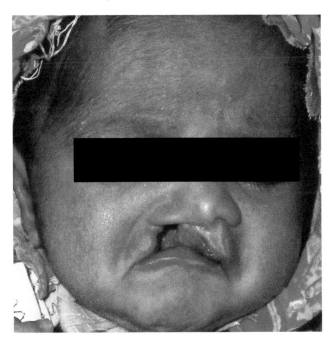

FIGURE 14.1   Pretreatment view of the infant with cleft lip and palate at the age of 6 days.

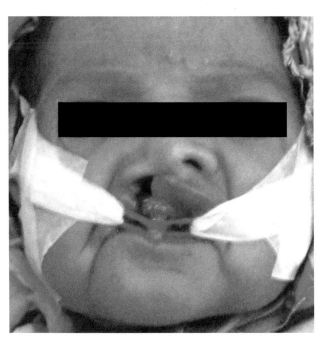

FIGURE 14.2   NAM appliance without nasal stent in position.

reduce irritation on the cheeks. The surgical tape elastic was looped on the retention arm of the molding prosthesis, and the tape was secured to the cheeks. The elastics (inner diameter 0.25 inch, wall thickness heavy) were stretched to approximately two times their resting diameter, for a proper activation force of approximately 100 g. The patient's parents were instructed to keep the plate in the mouth at all times, except removing once daily for cleaning. The periodic recall appointments were scheduled at 1-week intervals. During each appointment, the intraoral examination was carefully carried out to check for ulcerations, inflammation, or swelling due to the active molding forces by the appliance. Sequential selective addition of 1 mm of the soft resilient liner material (Permasoft; Dentsply) on the palatal aspect of the lesser segment and buccal aspect of the greater segment and trimming on the palatal aspect of the greater segment and buccal aspect of the lesser segment was carried out during recall appointments at 2- to 3-week intervals.[6] Periodic measurement of the interalveolar distance was made either directly in the mouth or on the casts prepared at the 1-month recall appointment.

Once the width of the alveolar gap was reduced to about 5 mm, the NAM appliance nasal stent component was incorporated (Fig 14.3).[6] This addition was delayed because with the reduced alveolar gap, the base of the nose and the lip segment alignment was improved. The stent, made of 0.36 inch, round stainless steel wire, takes the shape of a "swan neck" (Fig 14.4).[6-8] The swan-neck shape provides access to tape the lip across the cleft.[6-8] The stent was attached to the labial flange of the molding prosthesis, near the base of the retention arm. A small loop was created to retain the intranasal hard acrylic component of the nasal stent. The hard acrylic component was shaped into a kidney-shaped bi-lobed form. A layer of soft denture liner was added to the hard acrylic for patient comfort. The upper lobe was inserted inside the nose and gently lifted forward of the dome until a moderate amount of tissue blanching was evident

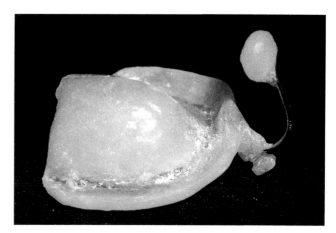

FIGURE 14.4 Complete NAM appliance with swan-neck-shaped nasal stent.

(Fig 14.5). The lower lobe of the stent lifted the nostril apex and defined the top of the columella. Periodic examination of the tissues and adjustment of the appliance was continued every week to mold the nasoalveolar complex into the desired shape. After 5 months, the width of the cleft between two alveolar segments at the crestal level was approximately 1.5 mm (Figs 14.6 and 14.7). A 1.5 cm intercrestal distance ensures a clinically desirable approximation of the base of the alveoli of the opposing segments. Thus, the NAM procedure was completed, and the patient was referred to the plastic surgeon for the surgical repair.

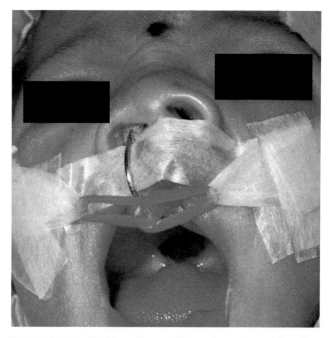

FIGURE 14.5 NAM appliance with nasal stent in position. Note the position of intranasal position of the nasal stent and horizontal lip banding.

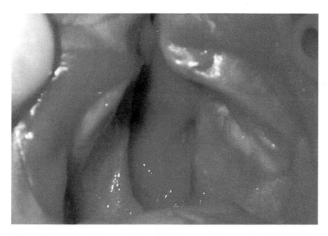

FIGURE 14.3 Two months of active molding reduced the intersegmental width from 13 to 5 mm.

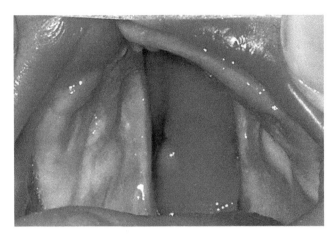

FIGURE 14.6 Four months of active NAM reduced the intersegmental width to 1.5 mm.

General physical examination was carried out again, and the patient was found to be healthy for the surgery. Surgical closure of the lip and nose was performed at 5 months of age (Fig 14.8). The surgical technique was modified to take advantage of the NAM preparation. The approximation of the alveolar segments permits the surgeon to easily perform palatal and alveolar closure. At 18 months of age, a second surgery of palatal closure was performed in which both palatal and alveolar segments were closed (Fig 14.9). The patient was then followed regularly at 6-month intervals for the next 5 years. Soft- and hard-tissue examination was carried out during each appointment. The palate was closed completely with the second surgery, and no palatal perforation was observed as the patient grew. The lip and nose repair scars were minimal and less identifiable, giving the patient a normal facial esthetic appearance.

The last recall visit of the patient was at the age of 5 years. A complete set of primary teeth were erupted, except the right lateral incisor (in the cleft region) (Fig 14.10). Radiographic examination revealed that the right lateral incisor was congenitally missing. Mild lingual inclination of all erupted primary teeth on the right side (smaller segment side) was observed. The palate was well healed with normal anatomical

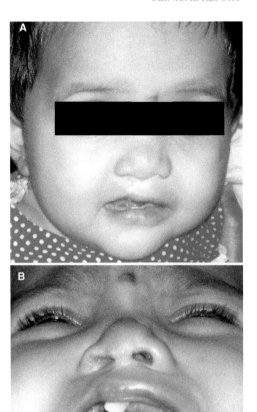

FIGURE 14.8 (A) Postsurgical esthetic outcome after first-stage surgery of lip and nose repair at the age of 12 months. (B) Inferior view of the face showing the repaired nose and lip.

contour (Fig 14.10). The cleft defect was found to have increased at the alveolar crestal region, without oronasal fistula formation (Fig 14.11). The alveolar defect was planned to be reconstructed with another surgical intervention to prevent the further increase in defect size and restore

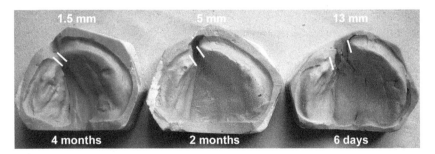

FIGURE 14.7 Casts prepared at the age of 6 days, 2 months, and 4 months as the patient's intersegmental distance reduced from 13 to 5 to 1.5 mm, respectively. Note the two parallel white lines on each cast indicating the intersegmental distance.

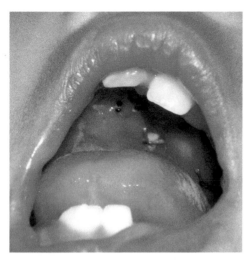

FIGURE 14.9 Second-stage surgery of palatal closure at the age of 18 months.

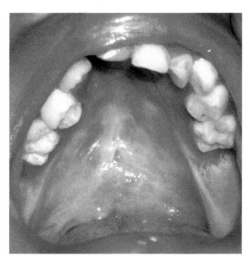

FIGURE 14.10 Intraoral view of the patient at the age of 5 years, showing completely repaired cleft palate with desired anatomical form.

normal anatomical contour of the entire maxillary arch. An interdisciplinary treatment approach regarding the palatal expansion and correction of the lingual tilting of the teeth on smaller segment will be considered with the orthodontist. Improved esthetic appearance of the patient in the nostril region and upper lip was observed, and thus overall facial appearance was well appreciated (Figs 14.11 and 14.12). The parents were pleased with the overall esthetic outcome.

DISCUSSION

The goal of NAM in the orofacial orthopedic treatment of unilateral lip and palate clefts is to align and approximate the maxillary hemialveolar segments while simultaneously supporting and molding the deformed nasal cartilages, correcting

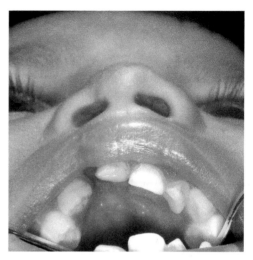

FIGURE 14.11 Inferior view of the patient's face showing completely repaired cleft lip/palate along with normal nasal form. Note a small defect in the alveolar segment that can be repaired by another surgical intervention.

and centering the nasal tip projection, and lengthening the deficient cleft-side columella in early infancy, before primary reparative lip surgery.[6–8] As in the case of neonatal auricular cartilage, active molding and repositioning of the nasal cartilages take advantage of the plasticity of cartilage in the newborn infant.[5,9] The temporary plasticity of nasal cartilage in the neonatal period is believed to be caused by high levels of hyaluronic acid, a component of the proteoglycan intercellular matrix, found circulating in the infant for several weeks after birth.[5,9] The NAM technique in the treatment of cleft lip and palate deformity presents several

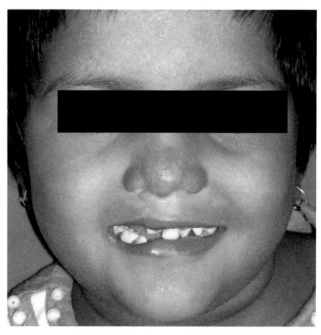

FIGURE 14.12 Posttreatment esthetic outcome at the age of 5 years.

benefits. The reduction in the size of the cleft gap facilitates the repair of the entire lip–nose–alveolus complex in one surgical procedure. Long-term studies of NAM therapy indicate that the change in nasal shape is stable with less scar tissue and better lip and nasal form.[10] In the presented case, the shape of the repaired nostril was identical to that of the opposite-side normal nostril, giving a symmetrical facial appearance when examined at the age of 5 years, indicating a stable nasal shape. Also, the scars on the upper lip were almost nonidentifiable. Future surgical interventions to correct the deformities to achieve soft-tissue esthetics can be minimized due to such improvement. Permanent teeth also can be expected to erupt in normal position.[7] In this clinical report, a well-aligned full complement of deciduous dentition was completely erupted (except the right lateral incisor, which was congenitally missing) at the age of 5 years with slight palatal inclinations of the teeth on the smaller segment of the alveolus. This will facilitate the alignment of the permanent dentition in a desirable position. Reduced need for alveolar bone grafting by NAM has been suggested by some authors.[11,12] In a bilateral cleft patient, NAM, along with columellar elongation, eliminates the need for columellar lengthening surgery.[13] Thus, NAM frequently simplifies surgeons' reconstruction in cleft lip and palate. Modified surgical techniques like gingivoperiosteoplasty followed by NAM ensures long-term postsurgical esthetics.[6,14] Lee et al[14] studied the long-term effect of NAM followed by gingivoperiosteoplasty on mid-face growth at prepuberty and concluded that the growth was not affected by NAM. Pai et al[15] assessed nostril symmetry and alveolar cleft width in infants with unilateral cleft lip and palate following NAM and found that NAM improved symmetry of the nose in width, height, and columella angle, compared to their presurgical status with some relapse of nostril shape in width (10%), height (20%), and angle of columella (4.7%) at 1 year of age. Nasal conformers were recommended by Liou et al[16] and can be placed for 4 to 6 months to compensate for relapse and the differential growth. A nasal stent plays an important role in such reshaping of the alar cartilage. The swan-neck shape of the stent provides the access to tape the lip across the cleft and allows controlled activation of the nasal stent to apply a gentle forward and upward molding vector to the dome of the lower lateral alar cartilage and a reciprocal alveolar molding vector on the medial hemialveolar segment.[6–8]

Prahl et al[17] studied the effect of infant orthopedics on maxillary arch form and position of the alveolar segments and concluded that infant orthopedics does not prevent collapse and can be abandoned as a tool to improve maxillary arch form. Prahl et al[18] similarly conducted a randomized clinical trial on the effect of infant orthopedics on facial appearance. They concluded that infant orthopedics have no effect on facial appearance; however, in both studies the effect of passive maxillary plates, instead of active tissue molding like NAM, were evaluated. Bongaarts et al[19]

evaluated the effect of infant orthopedics on maxillary arch dimensions in the deciduous dentition in patients with unilateral cleft lip and palate and concluded that infant orthopedics had no observable effect on maxillary arch dimensions or on the contact and collapse scores in the deciduous dentition at the ages of 4 and 6 years. In the presented case, lingual tilting of the deciduous teeth on the right side segment could not be prevented. Speech intelligibility is one of the important criteria to evaluate the early functional outcomes in cleft lip and palate patients. Van Lierde et al[20] determined the intelligibility (words, sentences, storytelling), as judged by their parents, of 43 children (mean age 4.9 years) with unilateral cleft lip and palate who received a Wardill–Kilner palatoplasty, and concluded there was no significant difference in intelligibility for storytelling between children with cleft palate and the normative data. The locked segment, nostril expansion, tissue ulceration, failure to retain the appliance, failure to tape the lip segment, and exposure of primary teeth are common complications that can be encountered throughout the molding procedure.[6] Parent cooperation is critical to success of the NAM procedure.

Though presurgical infant orthopedic devices remain controversial, numerous studies have shown that NAM provides safe, effective, and long-lasting improvements to the esthetics of the nasolabial complex in infants with cleft deformities.[10,13,14,21,22] Deng et al[23] performed NAM in 38 infants with cleft lip and palate and concluded that the NAM procedure can improve nasal profile and decrease the width of alveolar cleft. Similar results have been achieved in our case. Nakamura et al[24] evaluated the short-term postoperative nasal forms after NAM followed by primary lip repair for children with complete unilateral cleft lip and palate and concluded that following NAM the lip closure procedure provide good nasal forms; however, long-term follow-up will be necessary to clarify effects on the growth of nasal tissues reconstructed in infancy. This clinical report illustrated the long-term (over 5 years) follow-up to indicate the effects of growth on the reconstructed cleft lip and palate and found the therapy to be effective in maintaining the stability of the growing nasoalveolar complex. According to Aminpour and Tollefson[25], maxillary appliances have been used for 50 years; however, nasal molding is a relatively recent development that has shown progress but not without stalwart criticism. Hence, more specific and longitudinal research is still needed to end the controversy about NAM and its clinical efficacy.

CONCLUSION

Long-term postsurgical esthetic results can be achieved in cleft lip/palate patients following the NAM procedure. Frequent surgical intervention to achieve the desired esthetic results can be avoided by presurgical NAM.

REFERENCES

1. Grayson BH, Cutting C, Wood R: Preoperative columella lengthening in bilateral cleft-lip and palate. *Plast Reconstr Surg* 1993;92:1422–1423.

2. Matsuo K, Hirose T: Nonsurgical correction of cleft lip nasal deformity in the early neonate. *Ann Acad Med Singapore* 1988;17:358–365.

3. Matsuo K, Hirose T, Otagiri T, et al: Repair of cleft lip with nonsurgical correction of nasal deformity in the early neonatal period. *Plast Reconstr Surg* 1989;83:25–31.

4. Matsuo K, Hirose T: Preoperative non-surgical over-correction of cleft lip nasal deformity. *Br J Plast Surg* 1991;44:5–11.

5. Grayson BH, Cutting CB: Presurgical nasoalveolar orthopedic molding in primary correction of the nose, lip and alveolus of infants born with unilateral and bilateral clefts. *Cleft Palate Craniofac J* 2001;38:193–198.

6. Brecht LE, Grayson BH, Cutting CB: Nasoalveolar molding in early management of cleft lip and palate. In: Taylor TD (ed): *Clinical Maxillofacial Prosthetics*. Chicago, Quintessence, 2000, pp. 63–84.

7. Grayson BH, Shetye PR: Presurgical nasoalveolar moulding treatment in cleft lip and palate patients. *Indian J Plast Surg* 2009;42:S56–S61.

8. Suri S: Design features and simple methods of incorporating nasal stents in presurgical nasoalveolar molding appliances. *J Craniofac Surg* 2009;20:1889–1894.

9. Matsuo K, Hirose T, Tonomo T: Nonsurgical correction of congenital auricular deformities in the early neonate: a preliminary report. *Plast Reconstr Surg* 1984;73:38–50.

10. Maull DJ, Grayson BH, Cutting CB, et al: Long-term effects of nasoalveolar molding on three-dimensional nasal shape in unilateral clefts. *Cleft Palate Craniofac J* 1999;36:391–397.

11. Santiago PE, Grayson BH, Cutting CB, et al: Reduced need for alveolar bone grafting by presurgical orthopedics and primary gingivoperiosteoplasty. *Cleft Palate Craniofac J* 1998;35:77–80.

12. Pfeifer TM, Grayson BH, Cutting CB: Nasoalveolar molding and gingivoperiosteoplasty versus alveolar bone graft: an outcome analysis of costs in the treatment of unilateral cleft alveolus. *Cleft Palate Craniofac J* 2002;39:26–29.

13. Grayson BH, Santiago PE, Brecht LE, et al: Presurgical nasoalveolar molding in infants with cleft lip and palate. *Cleft Palate Craniofac J* 1999;36:486–498.

14. Lee CT, Grayson BH, Cutting CB, et al: Prepubertal midface growth in unilateral cleft lip and palate following alveolar molding and gingivoperiosteoplasty. *Cleft Palate Craniofac J* 2004;41:375–380.

15. Pai BC, Ko EW, Huang CS, et al: Symmetry of the nose after presurgical nasoalveolar molding in infants with unilateral cleft lip and palate: a preliminary study. *Cleft Palate Craniofac J* 2005;42:658–663.

16. Liou EJ, Subramanian M, Chen PK, et al: The progressive changes of nasal symmetry and growth after nasoalveolar molding: a three-year follow-up study. *Plast Reconstr Surg* 2004;114:858–864.

17. Prahl C, Kuijpers-Jagtman AM Van't Hof MA, et al: A randomized prospective clinical trial of the effect of infant orthopedics in unilateral cleft lip and palate: prevention of collapse of the alveolar segments (Dutchcleft). *Cleft Palate Craniofac J* 2003;40:337–342.

18. Prahl C, Prahl-Andersen B, van't Hof MA, et al: Infant orthopedics and facial appearance: a randomized clinical trial (Dutchcleft). *Cleft Palate Craniofac J* 2006;43:659–664.

19. Bongaarts C, van't Hof M A, Prahl-Andersen B, et al: Infant orthopedics has no effect on maxillary arch dimensions in the deciduous dentition of children with complete unilateral cleft lip and palate (Dutchcleft). *Cleft Palate Craniofac J* 2006;43:665–672.

20. Van Lierde KM, Luyten A, Van Borsel J, et al: Speech intelligibility of children with unilateral cleft lip and palate (Dutch cleft) following a one-stage Wardill-Kilner palatoplasty, as judged by their parents. *Int J Oral Maxillofac Surg* 2010;39:641–646.

21. Yang S, Stelnicki EJ, Lee MN: Use of nasoalveolar molding appliance to direct growth in newborn patient with complete unilateral cleft lip and palate. *Pediatr Dent* 2003;25:253–256.

22. Kirbschus A, Gesch D, Heinrich A, et al: Presurgical nasoalveolar molding in patients with unilateral clefts of lip, alveolus and palate. Case study and review of the literature. *J Cranio-maxillofac Surg* 2006;34 (Suppl): 45–48.

23. Deng XH, Zhai JY, Jiang J, et al: A clinical study of presurgical nasoalveolar molding in infants with complete cleft lip and palate. *Zhonghua Kou Qiang Yi Xue Za Zhi* 2005;40:144–146.

24. Nakamura N, Sasaguri M, Nozoe E, et al: Postoperative nasal forms after presurgical nasoalveolar molding followed by medial-upward advancement of nasolabial components with vestibular expansion for children with unilateral complete cleft lip and palate. *J Oral Maxillofac Surg* 2009;67:2222–2231.

25. Aminpour S, Tollefson TT: Recent advances in presurgical molding in cleft lip and palate. *Curr Opin Otolaryngol Head Neck Surg* 2008;16:339–346.

15

INTERDISCIPLINARY CARE FOR A PATIENT WITH AMELOGENESIS IMPERFECTA: A CLINICAL REPORT

CATHERINE MILLET, DDS, PHD,[1,2] JEAN-PIERRE DUPREZ, DDS, PHD,[2,3] CHRISTINE KHOURY, DDS,[3] LAURENT MORGON, DDS, PHD,[4] AND BÉATRICE RICHARD, DDS, PHD[3,5]

[1]Department of Prosthodontics, Faculty of Dentistry, Université Lyon 1, Lyon, France
[2]Oral Manifestations of Rare Diseases Center, Hospices Civils de Lyon, F-69365, Lyon, France
[3]Department of Pediatric Dentistry, Faculty of Dentistry, Université Lyon 1, Lyon, France
[4]Department of Orthodontics, Faculty of Dentistry, Université Lyon 1, Lyon, France
[5]Department of Biological Sciences, Faculty of Dentistry, Université Lyon 1, Lyon, France

Keywords

All-ceramic; CAD/CAM; clinical performance; hypocalcified enamel; orthognathic surgery; zirconia.

Correspondence

Catherine Millet, Faculty of Dentistry—Prosthodontics, 11 Rue Guillaume Paradin, 69372 Lyon Cedex 08, France. E-mail: cathymillet@yahoo.fr

The authors deny any conflicts of interest.

Accepted July 30, 2014

Published in *Journal of Prosthodontics* July 2015; Vol. 24, Issue 5

doi: 10.1111/jopr.12242

ABSTRACT

This manuscript describes an interdisciplinary approach over a period of 8 years combining surgical and prosthodontic treatment of a young patient diagnosed with hypocalcified-type amelogenesis imperfecta and anterior open bite. The treatment procedures included transitional restorations, orthodontic treatment, and maxillofacial surgery with a one-piece Le Fort I osteotomy, bilateral mandibular osteotomy, and genioplasty. The definitive prosthetic rehabilitation consisted of 28 zirconia-based ceramic single crowns restoring both esthetics and function. Photographs and radiographs associated with clinical evaluation were used in the maintenance period. Two-year follow-up revealed satisfactory results and no deterioration in the restorations.

Amelogenesis imperfecta (AI) is the expression of a heterogeneous inherited enamel disorder, associated with mutations in many genes encoding enamel proteins such as amelogenin, enamelin, enamelysin, KLK4, WDR72, and FAM83H.[1,2] This genetic expression affects the quantity and quality of tooth enamel in both primary and permanent dentition, with variable prevalence from 1/700 to 1/14,000.[3] AI has been reported as an isolated or syndromic finding with an autosomal dominant, autosomal recessive, or X-linked inheritance.[4] The AI enamel defects are highly variable and may be classified as hypoplastic, hypomineralized (hypomaturation and hypocalcification), or both.[5] Major oral complications in patients with AI are rapid wear and compromised dental esthetics that may disrupt their social lives. Other associated clinical features include gingival hyperplasia, delayed dental eruption, tooth agenesis, pulp stones, progressive root and crown resorption, and short roots.[6,7] Craniofacial features may also be present, acting as constricted maxillary arch, reversed mandibular curve of Spee, and anterior and posterior open bite occlusions. In addition, these patients may face nutrition problems due to dental sensitivity and loss of occlusal vertical dimension caused by attrition.[8,9] The management of the most complex cases with severe malocclusion is a challenge for clinicians and usually requires an interdisciplinary approach.[10,11] The use of all-ceramic systems in such cases is considered, but some concerns regarding their durability have been reported.[12,13] The purpose of this clinical report is to describe the interdisciplinary management and fixed rehabilitation with computer-assisted design (CAD)/computer-aided manufacturing (CAM) zirconia-based ceramic crowns of a young girl suffering from AI, and the 2-year follow-up results.

CLINICAL REPORT

A 10-year-old girl and her parents presented to the Pediatric Dentistry Department of the Hospices Civils of Lyon, France, with the chief complaints of dental sensitivity to hot and cold food and discolored teeth. The patient reported difficulty with mastication and poor self-image due to teeth appearance. No remarkable findings were identified in her medical record. There was no evidence of systemic disease, nutritional deficiency, or drug treatments that may have affected dentition structure during development. According to her parents, none of her first-degree family members (mother, father, and sister) exhibited the same dental problems. The clinical examination showed a skeletal class II malocclusion with a severe mandibular retrognathism, a 5-mm anterior open bite, and incompetent lips at rest (Fig 15.1). Oral hygiene was poor, with evidence of gingivitis due to severe plaque accumulation, particularly around the existing composite resin restorations on the mandibular incisors. The patient had a mixed dentition. All erupted teeth had a yellowish discoloration, with rough surfaces and irregular defects (Fig 15.2). Enamel was softer than normal and showed some signs of detachment from the dentin. Intraoral periapical radiographs revealed no missing teeth, a reduced enamel thickness, a lack of distinction in density between enamel and dentin, and a carious lesion on the mandibular right first premolar (Fig 15.3). Pulp chambers had normal shape, and no calcification was noted. The clinical and radiographic appearance suggested a hypocalcified form of

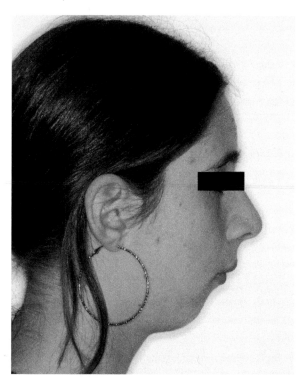

FIGURE 15.1 Initial presentation at age 10. Note the severe mandibular retrognathism and the convex profile.

AI. According to the Prosthodontic Diagnostic Index, the patient was classified as class IV.[14]

The treatment objectives were to reduce tooth sensitivity, attain ideal functional occlusion, and improve esthetic appearance. Because of the severity of the problem and the young age of the patient, an interdisciplinary consultation with a pediatric dentist, an orthodontist, and a prosthodontist was necessary. Specialists jointly evaluated the case and discussed treatment planning and the ultimate restorative requirements. Lateral cephalometric analysis showed a mandibular retrognathia (ANB 14°) and an accentuated inclination of the mandibular plane (FMA 35°). The diagnostic procedure on casts mounted in centric relation indicated that mandibular and maxillary surgery, after completion of facial growth, combined with orthodontic treatment, was needed to correct the skeletal imbalance. The proposed treatment was surgical-orthodontic management followed by complete mouth rehabilitation using all-ceramic crowns to stabilize the results and improve tooth form and color. Despite the length, cost, and difficulty, this option would provide an esthetic change and correct the patient's convex facial profile and the malocclusion. She and her parents were informed about the treatment plan with its objectives and possible complications. The importance of oral hygiene, caries control, and cooperation was emphasized. The patient and her parents gave their informed consent. The initial therapy consisted of dietary counseling and oral hygiene instructions

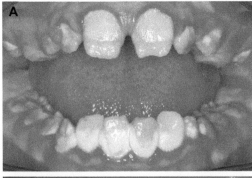

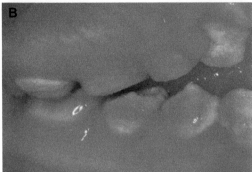

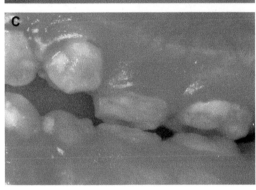

FIGURE 15.2 Initial presentation of the patient in mixed dentition with hypocalcified AI and anterior open bite. The photographs show extensive discoloration of the teeth, and teeth with a "moth-eaten appearance." (A) Anterior view; (B) right lateral view, maximum intercuspation; (C) left lateral view, maximum intercuspation.

emphasizing the use of tempered water to rinse the mouth. During the first sessions, preformed stainless steel crowns (Ion; 3M ESPE, St. Paul, MN) were placed subgingivally on the first permanent molars following minimal slice preparation of the teeth. The main goal of these crowns was to protect the dentin–pulp complex as well as to decrease the risk of loss of vertical dimension. Maxillary and mandibular incisors received preformed polycarbonate resin crowns (Ion). During this initial phase the child was monitored every 3 months to follow-up the eruption of all permanent teeth. Her cooperation and hygiene were good, confirmed by the improvement of her gingival health. After eruption, the premolars, canines, and second molars were fitted with preformed crowns cemented with glass ionomer cement (GIC; Fuji I;

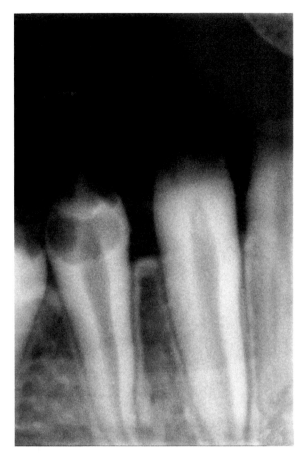

FIGURE 15.3 Initial periapical radiograph showing similar radio densities of enamel and dentin. Note the carious lesion of mandibular right first premolar.

GC Corporation, Tokyo, Japan; Fig 15.4). Pulp vitality was maintained for all the teeth except the mandibular right first premolar, which required endodontic treatment after caries excavation.

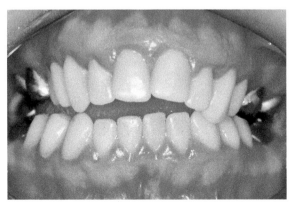

FIGURE 15.4 Appearance of the patient at age 13 with completed temporary preformed crowns in maximum intercuspation before orthodontic treatment. Note the periodontal inflammation.

When the patient was 14 years, 8 months old, fixed orthodontic appliances were placed on preformed crowns to align and level the dentition of both arches, to achieve better arch coordination prior to surgery. The presurgical operative orthodontic treatment was achieved within 21 months. After bone growth completion, preoperative planning of orthognathic surgery was realized through the use of 3-D computer-assisted simulation. Visual treatment objectives of the orthodontic treatment could achieve an angle class I profile by a posterior impaction of the maxilla and an 8 mm advance at the mandible. Orthognathic surgical splints were produced using the computerized digital model simulation. The patient underwent a midline segmental split Lefort I osteotomy in the upper jaw with impaction in the posterior region. In addition, a bilateral sagittal split osteotomy with genioplastic procedure was realized to advance the mandible and correct the mandibular retrognathism. After the consolidation period, postsurgical orthodontic treatment was processed on old preformed crowns for 11 months. Meanwhile, a preformed polycarbonate resin crown on the maxillary left lateral incisor crown was damaged and replaced by a new one. The retrusive chin and convex profile improved (Fig 15.5). A class I occlusion with both normal horizontal and vertical overlap was achieved (Fig 15.6). During the retention phase of treatment, a maxillary removable wraparound retainer was used, and a fixed wire retainer was bonded from canine to canine in the mandibular arch. The overall orthodontic treatment lasted 32 months.

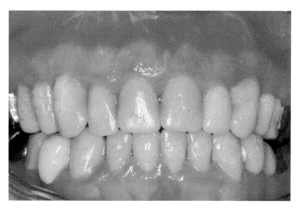

FIGURE 15.6 Postsurgical view of initial preformed crowns in maximum intercuspation after 5 to 7 years of clinical service.

Following orthodontic treatment completion, the prosthodontic treatment was initiated at the age of 18. First, diagnostic casts of the patient's jaws with the preformed crowns were obtained and mounted on a semiadjustable articulator SAM 2 (S.A.M. Praezisiontechnik; GmbH, Munich, Germany) using centric relation record. All posterior teeth had the necessary minimum clinical crown length. Therefore, no crown lengthening seemed necessary; however, the patient had an asymmetrical gingival level between the central and lateral incisors and canines of the maxillary dental arch. Periodontal surgery to correct the gingival level with a 3-month healing period was proposed, but the patient rejected this option. A wax-up was generated for the realization of interim prostheses with the purpose of serving as a blueprint for the definitive restorations. At this point, the patient requested that the definitive crowns on the anterior maxillary teeth be slightly less triangular than the preformed crowns. Furthermore, the patient's expectation was to achieve some resemblance to her sister who presented with a slight extruded and rotated maxillary left lateral incisor. Thus, the wax-up was modified according to the patient's demand (Fig 15.7). Central incisors were equal in

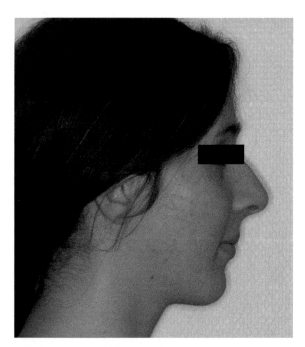

FIGURE 15.5 Lateral facial profiles at age 17 after maxillofacial surgery with a one-piece Le Fort I osteotomy, bilateral mandibular osteotomy, and genioplasty. Note the improvement in facial appearance.

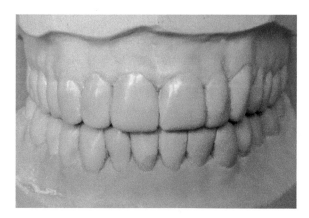

FIGURE 15.7 Mounted centric relation of diagnostic wax-up casts.

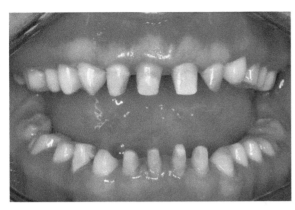

FIGURE 15.8   Frontal view of tooth preparations for all-ceramic crowns.

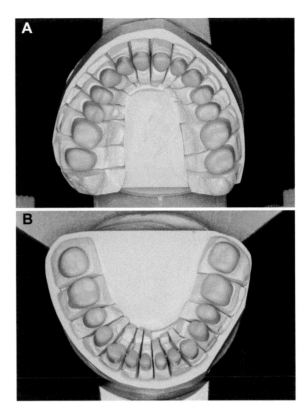

FIGURE 15.9   Master casts with CAD/CAM-manufactured zirconia copings. Note the anatomical shape: (A) maxillary master cast; (B) mandibular master cast.

width but not in height due to the asymmetric gingival heights. The wax-up was duplicated, and a vacuum-formed matrix was made. Preformed crowns were removed, and teeth were prepared under local anesthesia for all-ceramic single crowns. All teeth were prepared with an occlusal reduction of 1.5 to 2 mm, an axial reduction of 1 mm, and a finish line located below the cementoenamel junction to lower the risk of secondary caries due to altered enamel. Tooth preparations were finished by rounding sharp angles (Fig 15.8). Interim prostheses with a mutually protected occlusal scheme were made chairside using the matrix and autopolymerized acrylic resin (Unifast Trad; GC America, Alsip, IL). They were temporarily cemented using a zinc oxide-eugenol cement (TempBond; Kerr Italia, Scafati, Salerno, Italy). The patient wore her interim prostheses for 3 months, allowing sufficient time for adjustments to validate esthetics and function. Adjustments of the incisal edge position of the two maxillary central incisors were made both according to the patient's esthetic expectations, and to the fleshy and slightly asymmetrical lower lip (slightly higher on left side). The restorations were further adjusted to avoid any occlusal interference in protrusive and lateral excursions.

Poly(vinyl siloxane) material (Express; 3M ESPE) was used for the master impressions in custom impression trays. The maxillomandibular relationship was registered using wax wedges (Moyco Industries Inc, Philadelphia, PA). The maxillary and mandibular working casts (New Fujirock; GC) were mounted on a semi-adjustable articulator SAM 2. The dies were scanned using the CAD system (Cercon; DeguDent, Hanau, Germany) to acquire the data for a 3-D virtual model. All zirconia frameworks were designed using CAD software with anatomical shape to guarantee sufficient support for the veneering porcelain, and a thickness of 0.5 mm (Fig 15.9). Presintered zirconium oxide frameworks (Cercon HT; DeguDent) for each tooth were milled individually by CAM. The zirconia copings were sintered and then clinically fitted on the abutments with a film of silicone material (Fit Checker; GC). All copings showed a satisfactory marginal adaptation with a dental explorer (Fig 15.10). For the veneering process, the copings were covered with a manual layering technique using a ceramic material (Cercon Ceram-Kiss; DeguDent). The occlusion was constructed as mutually protected occlusion without eccentric contacts. Canines disengaged the posterior teeth during lateral movements. Protrusive guidance was evenly distributed across the maxillary and mandibular incisors. A trial evaluation of the ceramic before glazing enabled minor occlusal adjustments using a turbine and diamond burs with

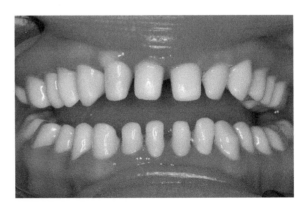

FIGURE 15.10   Clinical evaluation of CAD/CAM-manufactured zirconia copings.

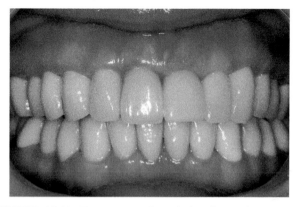

FIGURE 15.11 Posttreatment frontal view in centric occlusion position at age 18. Widespread recession was observed in interdental papillae.

30 to 40 μm grain size. No crowns were provisionally cemented before definitive cementation. The luting of the 28 single-tooth crowns was achieved with a resin-modified GIC (Fuji Cem 2; GC).

Both the patient and her parents were very satisfied with the esthetic and functional results despite the occurrence of interdental papillae recessions (Figs 15.11 and 15.12). In the follow-up, maintenance of oral hygiene was emphasized, and an occlusal night guard was prescribed to prevent the restorations from chipping; however, the patient declined to wear the occlusal guard at night. The patient was recalled for follow-up at 3, 6, 12, and 24 months. During follow-up appointments, the crowns were clinically evaluated for marginal adaptation, fracture, surface chipping, retention, color stability, and wear. The clinical evaluation was performed using tactile perception with a sharp explorer and visual inspection. Biological properties, such as tooth sensitivity, secondary caries, and periodontal response were also evaluated. Radiographic and photographic evaluations were made at 1- and 2-year recall visits. Intraoral digital photographic evaluation included frontal view of the anterior teeth and occlusal views of the full maxillary and mandibular

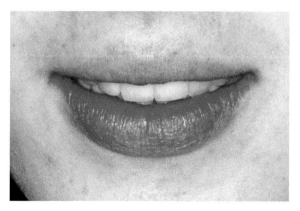

FIGURE 15.12 Posttreatment smile frontal view at age 18.

arches. Radiographic assessment included bitewing and periapical radiographs. Evaluation, 2 years after treatment, showed good stability of both orthodontic and prosthodontic results. This esthetic result has definitely affected the quality of life of the patient. Teeth showed no sensitivity, and the restorations exhibited no signs of complication. Marginal adaptations were good. No fracture of framework, chipping of veneered porcelain, or loss of retention was noted. There was no radiographic evidence of proximal caries (Fig 15.13). As for gingival response, an improvement of interdental papillae was observed (Fig 15.14), and no functional complaint was noted. The clinical evaluation according to a modified California Dental Association (CDA) ranking, as confirmed with high patient satisfaction, yielded an "excellent" ranking for the 28 zirconia-based ceramic single crowns.[13,15]

DISCUSSION

This clinical report demonstrates that timely diagnosis and individual approach is important for adequate treatment of patients with severe AI and anterior open bite. The interdisciplinary approach is essential for successful management of structural, esthetic, and functional issues. Numerous treatment modalities have been described for rehabilitation of AI patients: adhesive restorative techniques, overdentures, fixed dental prostheses, all-ceramic crowns, metal ceramic restorations, and inlay/onlay restorations.[16,17] Treatment modality includes consideration of a patient's age, severity of AI, orthodontic and maxillofacial needs, periodontal condition, financial implications for the patient's family, and long-term prognosis. In this young patient, preformed crowns were placed as transitional treatment prior to orthognathic surgery, which should be performed after the completion of growth to prevent recurrence and interference with craniofacial development. The management by direct interim bonding resin composite was not used due to poorly mineralized and friable enamel. In addition, interim prostheses should have been maintained in the mouth for several years (for 5–7 years) during the eruption of all permanent teeth and then throughout the orthodontic stage prior to surgery.[18,19] Furthermore, prefabricated stainless steel crowns are reported to be the most effective and efficient restorations in managing tooth sensitivity and restoring primary and permanent molars in children.[20]

The option of initially using interim prostheses based on wax-up was not considered in this case due to the patient's young age, the presence of mixed dentition, and insufficient space to correct tooth shape before the orthodontic treatment. In addition, tooth preparations had to be minimized due to large pulps. Here, orthodontic and maxillofacial procedures were realized prior to the wax-up, since a satisfactory occlusal relation could be established with the preformed

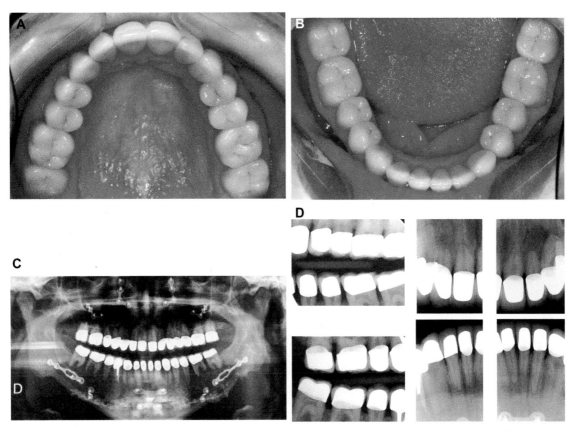

FIGURE 15.13 Treatment result 24 months after crowns insertion: (A) occlusal view, maxillary arch; (B) occlusal view, mandibular arch; (C) panoramic radiography; (D) bitewing and periapical radiographs.

crowns. Alternatively, in more complex occlusal conditions, the wax-up may be performed prior to orthognathic surgery. This enables the placement of interim prostheses in the desired occlusal final relationship, prior to surgery, thus guiding the surgeon for proper intraoperative jaw positioning.[18] In the present case, an alternative orthodontic treatment could have been proposed to the patient to avoid maxillofacial surgery. It consisted of intruding the posterior teeth in both arches and extruding the maxillary anterior teeth to close the open bite; however, the potential change was not considered sufficient with this option. In case of denial of orthodontic and surgical treatments, periodontal surgical procedures with bone reduction on molars would have been needed for improving the occlusal plane and the anterior open bite. This option would not allow maintaining posterior tooth vitality and correction of skeletal discrepancy to achieve a normal profile. For the above reasons, orthodontic and surgical corrections were accomplished for a better esthetic and functional result.

Complete crown coverage is commonly recommended for the definitive restorative procedure in most severe hypocalcified AI cases.[21,22] Even though significant reduction of tooth structure is required, such restorations protect the dental tissues from further destruction due to brittle enamel structure. Adequate tooth preparation and appropriate choice of restorative materials are essential to limit biological complications like loss of pulp vitality and to ensure long-term success. All-ceramic zirconia-based restorations were selected because all-ceramic restorations show good success rates with better esthetics compared to metal ceramic restorations. Besides, all-ceramic materials hold other advantages including low plaque retention and optimum biocompatibility inducing favorable biological responses in the soft tissues. In particular, zirconia demonstrated the possibility of inducing an epithelial attachment to its surface.[23] Recent improvements in CAD/CAM technology enable shaping the zirconium dioxide framework with anatomic form. Thus a layer of uniform veneering porcelain can be created throughout the framework, substantially reducing the risk of chipping, especially in the posterior area.[24–28] In addition, chipping may be reduced by using a coefficient of thermal expansion of veneering porcelain similar to zirconia.[28] For this patient, these recommendations were followed, and the complete mouth rehabilitation provided a mutually protected occlusion to prevent structural alteration of the ceramic in the posterior area during excursions. At the 24-month clinical short-term examination, no fracture or

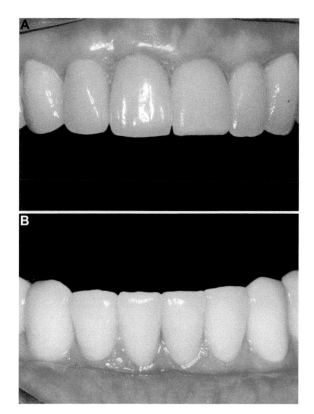

FIGURE 15.14 Definitive single crowns after 24 months. Note good gingival response with improving recession of interdental papillae. (A) Maxillary anterior teeth; (B) mandibular anterior teeth.

chipping problems were recorded in the 28 single crowns. This observation was in agreement with data from recent published studies on the clinical short/medium-term performance of zirconia-based ceramic single crowns.[29–31] Besides the ceramic system selected, the choice of the luting agent is important because the ceramic fracture strength decreases as the restoration ages and the bond strength degrades in the oral cavity.[32] Because of its high flexural strength, zirconia can be conventionally cemented just like metal ceramic crowns, without the need for any pretreatment, or bonded with adhesive resin cements.[33] For this young patient with vital teeth and retentive preparations, resin-modified GIC was chosen due to its lower technique sensitivity, its good long-term results, and its potential for fluoride release. Although this luting agent provides inferior bond strength compared with resin cements, in vitro studies have demonstrated an improved retention strength for zirconia crowns compared to zinc phosphate and GIC cements.[32,34]

CONCLUSION

Management of AI patients is a long and complex process requiring a carefully established protocol, generally extending over several years. Coordinated interdisciplinary procedures are critical for a successful outcome and patient satisfaction. Prosthodontic rehabilitation with zirconia-based restorations represents a promising alternative, especially in the posterior area, to preserve and stabilize weakened tooth substance; however, longer observation periods and randomized controlled trials with a large number of treatments are necessary to assess the long-term success of such restorations.

REFERENCES

1. Chan HC, Estrella NM, Milkovich RN, et al: Target gene analyses of 39 amelogenesis imperfecta kindreds. *Eur J Oral Sci* 2011;119:311–323.
2. Wright JT, Torain M, Long K, et al: Amelogenesis imperfecta: genotype–phenotype studies in 71 families. *Cells Tissues Organs* 2011;194:279–283.
3. Sundell S: Hereditary amelogenesis imperfecta: an epidemiological, genetic and clinical study in a Swedish child population. *Swed Dental J Suppl* 1986;31:4–38.
4. CAU American Academy of Pediatric Dentistry Council on Clinical Affairs: Guideline on oral health care/dental management of heritable dental development anomalies. *Pediatr Dent* 2008–2009;30(7 Suppl):196–201.
5. Witkop CJ: Amelogenesis imperfecta, dentinogenesis imperfecta and dentin dysplasia revisited: problems in classification. *J Oral Pathol* 1988;17:547–553.
6. Gadhia K, McDonald S, Arkutu N, et al: Amelogenesis imperfecta: an introduction. *Br Dent J* 2012;212:377–379.
7. Poulsen S, Gjørup H, Haubek D, et al: Amelogenesis imperfect—a systematic literature review of associated dental and oro-facial abnormalities and their impact on patients. *Acta Odontol Scand* 2008;66:193–199.
8. Hoppenreijs TJ, Freihofer HP, Stoelinga PJ, et al: Skeletal and dento-alveolar stability of Le Fort I intrusion osteotomies and bimaxillary osteotomies in anterior open bite deformities. A retrospective three-centre study. *Int J Oral Maxillofac Surg* 1997;26:161–175.
9. Persson M, Sundell S: Facial morphology and open bite deformity in amelogenesis imperfecta. A roentgenocephalometric study. *Acta Odontol Scand* 1982;40:135–144.
10. Gisler V, Enkling N, Zix J, et al: A multidisciplinary approach to the functional and esthetic rehabilitation of amelogenesis imperfecta and open bite deformity: a case report. *J Esthet Restor Dent* 2010;22:282–293.
11. Wright J, Waite P, Mueninghoff L, et al: The multidisciplinary approach managing enamel defects. *J Am Dent Assoc* 1991;122:62–65.
12. Siadat H, Alikhasi M, Mirfazaelian A: Rehabilitation of a patient with amelogenesis imperfecta using all-ceramic crowns: a clinical report. *J Prosthet Dent* 2007;98:85–88.
13. Groten M: Complex all-ceramic rehabilitation of a young patient with a severely compromised dentition: a case report. *Quintessence Int* 2009;40:19–27.

14. McGarry TJ, Nimmo A, Skiba JF, et al: Classification system for completely dentate patient. *J Prosthodont* 2004;13: 73–82.

15. California Dental Association: *Quality Evaluation for Dental Care: Guidelines for The Assessment of Clinical Quality and Professional Performance.* Los Angeles, CDA, 1977.

16. Malik K, Gadhia K, Arkutu N, et al: The interdisciplinary management of patients with amelogenesis imperfecta—restorative dentistry. *Br Dent J* 2012;212:537–542.

17. Patil PG, Patil SP: Amelogenesis imperfecta with multiple impacted teeth and skeletal class III malocclusion: complete mouth rehabilitation of a young adult. *J Prosthet Dent* 2014;111:11–15.

18. Kinzer GA: Commentary. A multidisciplinary approach to the functional and esthetic rehabilitation of amelogenesis imperfecta and open bite deformity: a case report. *J Esthet Restor Dent* 2010;22:294–296.

19. Millet C, Duprez JP: Multidisciplinary management of a child with severe open bite and amelogenesis imperfecta. *J Contemp Dent Pract* 2013;14:320–326.

20. Seow WK: Clinical diagnosis and management strategies of amelogenesis imperfecta variants. *Pediatr Dent* 1993;15:384–393.

21. Chen CF, Hu JCC, Bresciani E, et al: Treatment considerations for patient with amelogenesis imperfecta: a review. *Braz Dent Sci* 2013;16:7–18.

22. Urzúa B, Ortega-Pinto A, Farias DA, et al: A multidisciplinary approach for the diagnosis of hypocalcified amelogenesis imperfecta in two Chilean families. *Acta Odontol Scand* 2012;70:7–14.

23. Tetè S, Zizzari VL, Borelli B, et al: Proliferation and adhesion capability of human gingival fibroblasts onto zirconia, lithium disilicate and feldspathic veneering ceramic in vitro. *Dent Mater J* 2014;33:7–15.

24. Land MF, Hopp CD: Survival rates of all-ceramic systems differ by clinical indication and fabrication method. *J Evid Based Dent Pract* 2010;10:37–38.

25. Swain M: Unstable cracking (chipping) of veneering porcelain on all ceramic dental crowns and fixed partial dentures. *Acta Biomaterials* 2009;5:1668–1677.

26. Rosentritt M, Steiger D, Behr M, et al: Influence of substructure design and spacer settings on the in vitro performance of molar zirconia crowns. *J Dent* 2009;37:978–983.

27. Vavřičková L, Dostálová T, Charvát J, et al: Evaluation of the 3-year experience with all-ceramic crowns with polycrystalline ceramic cores. *Prague Med Rep* 2013;114:22–34.

28. Raigrodski AJ, Hillstead MB, Meng GK, et al: Survival and complications of zirconia-based fixed dental prostheses: a systematic review. *J Prosthet Dent* 2012;107:170–177.

29. Ortorp A, Kihl ML, Carlsson GE: A 5-year retrospective study of survival of zirconia single crowns fitted in a private clinical setting. *J Dent* 2012;40:527–530.

30. Rinke S, Schäfer S, Lange K, et al: Practice-based clinical evaluation of metal-ceramic and zirconia molar crowns: 3-year results. *J Oral Rehabil* 2013;40:228–237.

31. Monaco C, Caldari M, Scotti R: Clinical evaluation of 1132 zirconia-based single crowns: a retrospective cohort study from the AIOP Clinical Research Group. *Int J Prosthodont* 2013;26: 435–442.

32. Dhima M, Paulosova V, Carr AB, et al: Practice-based clinical evaluation of ceramic single crowns after at least 5 years. *J Prosthet Dent* 2014;111:124–130.

33. Al-Amleh B, Lyons K, Swain M: Clinical trials in zirconia: a systematic review. *J Oral Rehabil* 2010;37:641–652.

34. Ernst CP, Cohnen U, Stender E, et al: In vitro retentive strength of zirconium oxide ceramic crowns using different luting agents. *J Prosthet Dent* 2005;93:551–558.

16

MAXILLARY REHABILITATION USING A REMOVABLE PARTIAL DENTURE WITH ATTACHMENTS IN A CLEFT LIP AND PALATE PATIENT: A CLINICAL REPORT

MARINA RECHDEN LOBATO PALMEIRO, DDS, MS, PHD, CAROLINE SCHEEREN PIFFER, DDS, MS, VIVIAN MARTINS BRUNETTO, DDS, PAULO CÉSAR MACCARI, DDS, MS, PHD, AND ROSEMARY SADAMI ARAI SHINKAI, DDS, MS, PHD

Department of Prosthodontics, Pontifical Catholic University of Rio Grande do Sul, Porto Alegre, Brazil

Keywords

Telescopic crowns; dental prosthesis; birth defects; quality of life; cleft lip; cleft palate; removable partial denture; removable prosthesis; telescopic retainers.

Correspondence

Marina Rechden Lobato Palmeiro, Pontifical Catholic University of Rio Grande do Sul – School of Dentistry, Av. Ipiranga, 6681 Pré dio 6, Porto Alegre, RS 90619-900, Brazil. E-mail: marina.lobato@pucrs.br

This research was partially supported by the Brazilian Ministry of Education and Culture/CAPES (BEX: 12312-12-6 and CAPES I scholarship for M.R.L. Palmeiro).

The authors deny any conflicts of interest.

Accepted January 22, 2014

Published in *Journal of Prosthodontics* April 2015; Vol. 24, Issue 3

doi: 10.1111/jopr.12188

ABSTRACT

Clefts of the lip and/or palate (CLP) are oral-facial defects that affect health and overall quality of life. CLP patients often need multidisciplinary treatment to restore oral function and esthetics. This paper describes the oral rehabilitation of a CLP adult patient who had maxillary bone and tooth loss, resulting in decreased occlusal vertical dimension. Functional and cosmetic rehabilitation was achieved using a maxillary removable partial denture (RPD) attached to telescopic crowns. Attachment-retained RPDs may be a cost-effective alternative for oral rehabilitation in challenging cases with substantial loss of oral tissues, especially when treatment with fixed dental prostheses and/or dental implants is not possible.

Clefts of the lip and/or palate (CLP) are oral-facial defects that affect the health, quality of life, and socioeconomic well-being of both the affected individuals and their families.[1–3] Clefts are associated with cosmetic deformities and dental abnormalities; difficulties with speaking, chewing, and swallowing; and psychological problems.[4–6] Treatment of CLP patients spans from birth to adulthood and often requires a multidisciplinary team of nurses, plastic surgeons, oral and maxillofacial surgeons, otolaryngologists, speech therapists, psychologists, orthodontists, and prosthodontists.[7–10]

In the older generation of CLP patients (those born in the 20th century) there are some problems with residual fistulae (scarring), and surgery and orthodontics cannot achieve a complete oral rehabilitation without a complementary prosthodontic approach. Restorative dentistry offers several options for prosthetic rehabilitation in patients with clefts. These options include fixed partial dentures (FPDs), removable partial dentures (RPDs), adhesive FPDs, and implant-supported dentures.[2,11–13]

Because many types of surgery performed in cleft patients result in anatomical and functional complications, some modifications from conventional prosthetic treatment may be necessary to achieve satisfactory functional and esthetic results. This study presents a case involving the oral rehabilitation of one adult CLP patient using an RPD connected with telescopic crowns.

CLINICAL REPORT

A 54-year-old woman with a unilateral cleft lip and hard palate on the left side was referred to the Prosthodontics Clinic Unit of the PUCRS School of Dentistry. She stated that she avoided social contact because of her physical appearance. Another complaint was difficulty in chewing due to missing and incorrectly positioned teeth, as well as temporomandibular joint discomfort. An initial X-ray, before the treatment, revealed the absence of bone in the cleft region, periapical lesion on tooth #11, periodontal lesion on teeth #14 and #27, impaction of tooth #18, and misalignment of tooth #23 (Fig 16.1A). Nonsurgical periodontal therapy, root canal treatment of tooth #11, and extraction of teeth #14 and #27 were performed. After the initial therapy, clinical reevaluation showed teeth #14–17, #21, #22, and #27 were missing, and tooth #23 was misaligned (Fig 16.1B). Abnormal tooth color was associated with external factors (staining from intake of dark colored foods and smoking). Furthermore, a scar from correction of the left unilateral CLP was observed (Fig 16.1C).

Diagnostic models were mounted on a semi-adjustable articulator to plan treatment. The patient was missing bone tissue in the maxilla, but bone grafts and dental implants were not a primary option because she was an active heavy smoker and asked for a nonsurgical treatment. The absence of teeth

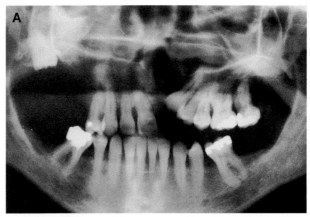

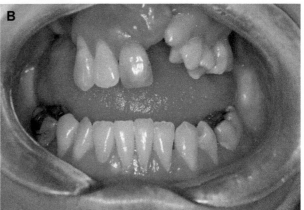

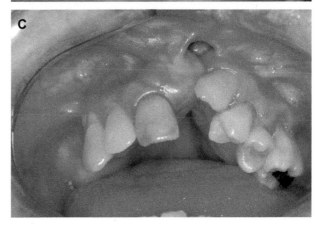

FIGURE 16.1 Initial appearance before prosthetic treatment. (A) Panoramic X-ray: area with bone defect between teeth #21 and #22. (B) Front view, missing teeth in the maxillary arch, and misaligned teeth #23 to #25. (C) Occlusal view, surgical scar from surgery procedures for correction of the oral-facial defect.

#14–17, resulting in a large prosthetic space (free end), excluded the possibility of an FPD in the right hemi-arch. A conventional RPD would neither seal the oronasal communication nor support the upper lip. Thus, the chosen treatment plan consisted of an association of RPD, attachments, and telescopic crowns to seal the oronasal communication and restore function and esthetics.

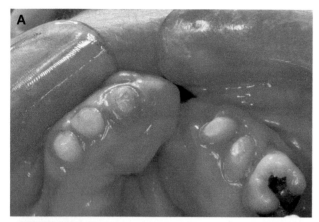

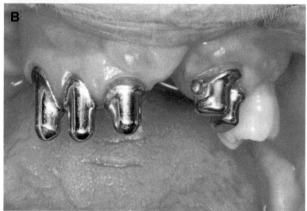

FIGURE 16.2   Tooth preparations for fabrication of telescopic crowns. (A) Occlusal view. (B) Inner telescopic copings, supragingival location of the crown edge.

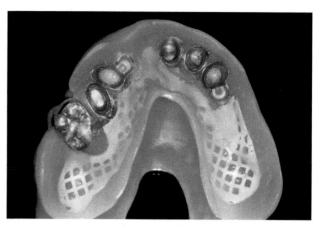

FIGURE 16.3   Internal view of the removable partial prosthesis with the matrix connectors on the telescopic crowns. An extracoronal retaining element (SD-attachment; Servo-Dental GmbH & Co. KG, Hagen, Germany) was added to copings of teeth #24 and #13 to improve retention.

Extraction of tooth #23 was indicated and performed to facilitate the path of insertion of the RPD. Teeth #11–13, #24, and #25 were prepared for telescopic crown fabrication (Fig 16.2A). According to the Glossary of Prosthodontic Terms, a telescopic crown is "an artificial crown constructed to fit over a coping (framework). The coping can be another crown, a bar, or any suitable rigid support for the dental prosthesis."[14] Some authors describe the telescopic retainer as an inner telescopic coping, or sleeve coping, cemented to the dental abutment that telescopes within an outer telescopic coping, or secondary crown, connected to a detachable prosthesis.[9,15–17]

After tooth preparation, a full-arch impression was obtained with an acrylic custom tray and addition silicone (Express™; 3M ESPE, Seefeld, Germany). The casts were mounted on the semi-adjustable articulator in centric relation for the fabrication of the inner telescopic copings. On teeth #13 and #24, an extracoronal retaining attachment (SD attachment; Servo-dental, Hagen, Germany) was added for extra retention. Telescopic crowns were custom made with patrix connectors to support the RPD with matrix connectors and to splint the remaining teeth. The metal copings cast in

nickel–chromium alloy (Dan Ceramalloy, Osaka, Japan) were tried in, and fit accuracy was verified (Fig 16.2B).

A second full-arch impression with silicone was made to transfer the position of the inner telescopic copings in relation to the maxilla. A new cast was remounted for laboratory fabrication of the outer telescopic copings and RPD framework. Both metal structures were tested clinically to check fit and occlusion. A bite record was made using a wax baseplate attached to the RPD saddle. Facial parameters such as lip support, smile line, and upper lip length were evaluated, and vertical dimension was reestablished before selection of artificial tooth size and color. After a wax-up trial with the patient's approval, the RPD was finished in the laboratory (Fig 16.3).

In the following clinical session, the crowns and RPD were adjusted and installed. The inner telescopic copings were cemented with resin-modified glass ionomer cement (RelyX Luting Plus; 3M ESPE, St. Paul, MN). The RPD was immediately positioned over the dental abutments, providing a splint to form a stabilized polygon (Fig 16.4). The patient was instructed on how to wear the RPD. Oral hygiene instructions were also given, such as removing the prosthesis for cleaning after meals and brushing teeth at least three times a day. Recalls were completed weekly for 1 month, then every 6 months. The procedures described in this article were successful, and the results surpassed the patient's cosmetic and functional needs.

DISCUSSION

Oral rehabilitation in CLP patients requires an interdisciplinary view to make the prosthesis capable of blocking oronasal communication, restoring masticatory and phonetic

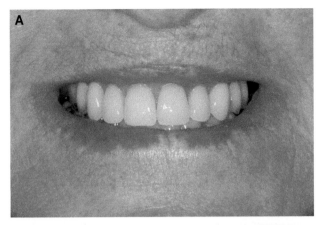

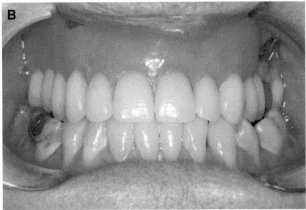

FIGURE 16.4 Final appearance after prosthetic treatment. (A) Front extraoral view. (B) Intraoral view.

functions, and improving cosmetics considering the overall cost/benefit analysis and gain in quality of life.[8,9,12,13] Choosing between the many prosthetic rehabilitation options is based on the specific clinical situation of the patient and his/her main complaints and wishes. Clinical examination should evaluate not only the dental conditions but also the presence and extension of alveolar ridge defects, scar tissue, and oronasal communication.[7–9] It is the responsibility of the prosthodontist to provide a prosthesis that should be simple to handle and easy to maintain.

The treatment plan presented here consisted of a maxillary rehabilitation using an association of RPD, attachments, and telescopic crowns to seal the oronasal communication and restore dental occlusion and lip support.[9,15] The patient chose this treatment option because the procedures were less complex, less invasive, less expensive, and less time consuming than alternatives involving bone grafts and dental implants. A systematic review demonstrated that complications occur early in most cases of implant-supported prostheses in patients with clefts.[12] The fact that the patient can remove the prosthesis also facilitates the hygiene of dental abutments and residual cleft under the RPD.

If the implant placement conditions are not ideal, and adjacent teeth need cosmetic corrections, conventional prostheses may be the best treatment option; however, adhesive fixed prostheses with minimally invasive preparations are not indicated for definitive treatment of patients with clefts because small premaxillary movements or mobility of the dental abutments can cause cement failure.[11] Another common problem in CLP patients is deficient lip support. Removable prostheses are indicated in cases with severe bone loss that affects the lip position or when the cleft needs to be blocked.[9,13] The major resistance to using RPDs for partially edentulous patients is due to cosmetic reasons, such as the visibility of metallic clamps, as well as functional concerns during speech and chewing because the prostheses are not fixed.[11]

The principles involved in the use of telescopic crowns and RPDs have been well described in the literature as a valuable therapy option.[15–17] Yalisove and Dietz[16] reported the following advantages of this treatment modality: accessibility to oral hygiene maintenance by the patient; reduction of lateral stress on abutment teeth; independence of the individual abutments; use of weak abutments with questionable prognosis that should not be used in an FPD; bilateral splinting; and esthetic replacement of extensive alveolar bone loss.[15,16]

In this clinical case, the prosthetic rehabilitation using an RPD connected to telescopic crowns successfully splinted and corrected the position of the remaining teeth. When connected to the RPD, telescopic crowns increase the prosthetic stability and retention, optimize favorable force transmission to the long dental axis, and improve esthetics.[9,14] The present findings using telescopic crowns are in line with Yalisove's[15,16] reports, which suggested that, apart from the benefits mentioned above, other benefits include maintenance of centric relation and occlusal vertical dimension, preservation of the ridges, minimal number of adjustments, and improvement in patient acceptance, from the standpoint of function and psychological impact.[15,16] A positive impact on daily living and quality of life has been reported following restoration with an RPD retained by telescopic crowns, particularly for patients with few remaining teeth.[17,18]

CONCLUSION

There are several treatment options for patients with CLP; however, in patients missing several dental elements (making dental treatment difficult) and/or those who have experienced bone loss, a good option may be removable partial prostheses connected to telescopic crowns. This article shows that this alternative is effective for patients missing various dental elements and who lack osseous tissue and lip support as it corrects dental misalignment, restoring oral function, esthetics, and overall satisfaction.

ACKNOWLEDGMENTS

The authors thank the patient who participated in this study, as well as all the staff at PUCRS School of Dentistry.

REFERENCES

1. Hunt O, Burden D, Hepper P, et al: The psychosocial effects of cleft lip and palate: a systematic review. *Eur J Orthod* 2005;27:274–285.

2. Foo P, Sampson W, Roberts R, et al: General health-related quality of life and oral health impact among Australians with cleft compared with population norms; age and gender differences. *Clef Palate Craniofac J* 2012;49:406–413.

3. Oosterkamp BCM, Dijkstra PU, Remmelink HJ, et al: Satisfaction with treatment outcome in bilateral cleft lip and palate patients. *Int J Oral Maxillofac Surg* 2007;36:890–895.

4. Mossey PA, Litle J, Munger RG, et al: Cleft lip and palate. *Lancet* 2009;374:1773–1785.

5. Krieger O, Matuliene G, Hüsler J, et al: Failures and complications in patients with birth defects restored with fixed dental prostheses and single crowns on teeth and/or implants. *Clin Oral Implants Res* 2009;20:809–816.

6. Moore D, McCord JF: Prosthetic dentistry and the unilateral cleft lip and palate patient. The last 30 years. A review of the prosthodontic literature in respect of treatment options. *Eur J Prosthodont Restor Dent* 2004;12:70–74.

7. Kramer FJ, Baethge C, Swennen G, et al: Dental implants in patients with orofacial clefts: a long-term follow-up study. *Int J Oral Maxillofac Surg* 2005;34:715–721.

8. Cune MS, Meijer GJ, Koole R: Anterior tooth replacement with implants in grafted alveolar cleft sites: a case series. *Clin Oral Implants Res* 2004;15:616–624.

9. Mañes Ferrer JFM, González AM, Galdón BO, et al: Telescopic crowns in adult case with lip and palate cleft. Update on etiology and management. *Med Oral Patol Oral Cir Bucal* 2006;11:e358–e362.

10. Vargervik K, Oberoi S, Hoffman WY: Care for the patient with cleft: UCSF protocols and outcomes. *J Craniofac Surg* 2009;20Suppl 2:1668–1671.

11. Reisberg DJ: Dental and prosthodontic care for patients with cleft or craniofacial conditions. *Cleft Palate Craniofac J* 2000;37:534–537.

12. Krieger O, Matuliene G, Hüsler J, et al: Failures and complications in patients with birth defects restored with fixed dental prostheses and single crowns on teeth and/or implants. *Clin Oral Implants Res* 2009;20:809–816.

13. Landes CA, Ghanaati S, Ballon A, et al: Severely scarred oronasal cleft defects in edentulous adults: initial data on the long-term outcome of telescoped obturator prostheses supported by zygomatic implants. *Cleft Palate Craniofac J* 2013;50:e74–e83.

14. The glossary of prosthodontic terms. *J Prosthet Dent* 2005;94:10–92.

15. Yalisove IL: Crown and sleeve-coping retainers for removable partial prosthesis. *J Prosthet Dent* 1966;16:1069–1085.

16. Yalisove IL, Dietz JR: *Telescopic Prosthetic Therapy.* Philadelphia, George F Stickley Co., 1977, p 11.

17. Breitman JB, Nakamura S, Freedman AL, et al: Telescopic retainers: an old or new solution? A second chance to have normal dental function. *J Prosthodont* 2012;21:79–83.

18. Preshaw PM, Walls AW, Jakubovics NS, et al: Association of removable partial denture use with oral and systemic health. *J Dent* 2011;39:711–719.

17

TREATMENT OF A PATIENT WITH CLEIDOCRANIAL DYSPLASIA USING A SINGLE-STAGE IMPLANT PROTOCOL

Vicki C. Petropoulos, DMD, MS,[1] Thomas J. Balshi, DDS, PHD, FACP,[2] Glenn J. Wolfinger, DMD, FACP,[3] and Stephen F. Balshi, MBE[4]

[1]Prosthodontist and Associate Professor, Department of Preventive and Restorative Sciences, School of Dental Medicine, University of Pennsylvania, Philadelphia, PA

[2]Founder and Prosthodontist, PI Dental Center, Institute for Facial Esthetics, Fort Washington, PA

[3]Prosthodontist, PI Dental Center, Institute for Facial Esthetics, Fort Washington, PA

[4]President, CM Prosthetics, Inc., Fort Washington, PA; Director of Research, PI Dental Center, Institute for Facial Esthetics, Fort Washington, PA

Keywords

Cleidocranial dysplasia; dental implants; edentulism; immediate loading; conversion prosthesis; osseointegration.

Correspondence

Vicki C. Petropoulos, Department of Restorative and Preventive Sciences, School of Dental Medicine, University of Pennsylvania, 4001 Spruce St., Philadelphia, PA 19147. E-mail: vp718@comcast.net

The Teeth in a Day Protocol described in this report is trademarked by Prosthodontics Intermedica (PI Dental Center). Dr. T Balshi is the founder of Prosthodontics Intermedica; Dr. Wolfinger is an employee of Prosthodontics Intermedica; Dr. S. Balshi is the Director of Research of Prosthodontics Intermedica.

Accepted August 14, 2011

Published in *Journal of Prosthodontics* October 2011; Vol. 20, Suppl 2

doi: 10.1111/j.1532-849X.2011.00781.x

ABSTRACT

This patient report describes the treatment of a 45-year-old Caucasian woman with cleidocranial dysplasia who had significant dental problems that greatly affected her quality of life. The patient had orthodontic treatment in her earlier years along with surgical removal of supernumerary teeth. Using implants, the maxillary and mandibular arches were restored with fixed screw-retained prostheses. Eight and six implants were placed in the maxilla and mandible, respectively. Both arches were immediately loaded following the Teeth in a Day™ protocol using an all-acrylic resin provisional prosthesis. Five months later, definitive maxillary and mandibular prostheses were fabricated. The patient has been followed for a period of 5 years, and all postoperative evaluations have been uneventful.

In 2005, the patient described in this article had just seen her local dentist in Sydney, OH. Her dentist recommended extracting all her teeth and placing maxillary and mandibular complete dentures. The patient had reviewed the dental literature and come across a case study the authors of this article had published where a patient with her similar congenital condition was successfully treated using dental implants. She immediately contacted the treatment center asking if there was any hope for her. In response, she was told not to have any of her teeth removed and that she could be helped if she could travel to Pennsylvania. This article describes the treatment that significantly enhanced her quality of life.

In 1897, Marie and Sainton[1] first described cleidocranial dystosis, a rare inherited skeletal dysplasia. It has since been known as cleidocranial dysplasia. Its underlying pathology is a generalized skeletal dysplastic condition.[2] It is an autosomal dominant pattern of inheritance; however, it has been suggested that between 20% and 40% of cases represent new mutations.[3] It is best known for its dental and clavicular abnormalities, and it is a disorder of bone caused by a defect in the CBFA 1 gene of chromosome 6p21. This gene guides osteoblastic differentiation and appropriate bone formation when expressed under normal conditions.

Individuals with cleidocranial dysplasia tend to be of short stature and have proportionally large heads with pronounced parietal and frontal bossing. A broad base of the nose with a depressed nasal bridge as well as ocular hypertelorism can be observed. The most dramatic finding, odontologically, is the presence of numerous unerupted permanent and supernumerary teeth.

The dental abnormalities associated with cleidocranial dysplasia represent a remarkable dental challenge.[4] Treatment of the dental problems associated with cleidocranial dysplasia may be difficult.[4] These treatments are difficult due to the supernumerary teeth, malformed and shortened roots, delayed eruption of permanent teeth, and underdeveloped maxilla and mandible. The treatment often involves multidisciplinary approaches with a combination of orthodontics, orthognathic surgical interventions, and interim prostheses. This process of involving all these disciplines can take several years until patients can receive their definitive prostheses.

Therapeutic dental options include a crown sleeve coping overdenture,[5] full-mouth extractions followed by denture fabrication, autotransplantation of selected impacted teeth followed by prosthetic restoration, or removal of primary and supernumerary teeth followed by exposure of permanent teeth subsequently extruded orthodontically. The use of implants in a patient with cleidocranial dysplasia has been documented to support a removable implant-retained overdenture.[6] Petropoulos et al[7] documented a treatment using implants to support an implant-supported fixed prosthesis. To date, there is a limited amount of documented cleidocranial

dysplasia treatments using an implant-supported fixed prosthesis with immediate loading. Using implants in such situations seems logical, since there have been documented cases of bone formation around teeth that have been orthodontically erupted in patients with cleidocranial dysplasia.

CLINICAL REPORT

Patient History

The patient was a 45-year-old woman (Figs 17.1A–17.1C) born with cleidocranial dysplasia. She was missing a piece of her clavicle (Fig 17.1D) and had other facial anomalies common with this condition. Her father, middle sister, daughter, and son also carry this genetic defect. The patient was in excellent general health, with allergy to codeine, when presenting for treatment related to reconstruction of her dentition (Fig 17.1E). Her past dental history revealed that at age 12, she had undergone multiple tooth extractions (about 30 teeth), which took 6 hours (according to her recollection), where all her deciduous teeth and supernumerary teeth were removed (Figs 17.2A–17.2C). Subsequently, she underwent orthodontic treatment for 7 years. Following these treatments, she was strongly dissatisfied with her appearance. This strong discontent continued throughout her life. Her teeth were misaligned and did not show when she spoke and smiled. In addition, some of her teeth were loose. Her dentist told her to be satisfied with what she had, as she would "never have that Colgate smile." She was advised to have all her teeth extracted; however, she was afraid and concerned about not being able to function properly with removable dentures. She was also told that due to excessive bone loss she was not a candidate for dental implants. Her chief complaints were, "I have some missing teeth," "I am unable to chew properly," "my teeth do not show when I speak," and "I am very ashamed of my appearance and extremely dissatisfied" (Fig 17.1B).

Clinical Evaluation and Diagnosis

At the initial visit, the patient presented with the following teeth in the maxillary arch: #s 1–6, 8, 9, and 11–16 (Fig 17.2C); and in the mandibular arch: teeth #s 18–20, 22–25, and 27–31. Teeth #17 and 32 were unerupted and had two supernumerary teeth in the posterior maxilla and one in the mandible.

Clinical examination revealed that the patient was in a dental class I relationship with an anterior cross bite and malaligned teeth. She showed severe occlusal wear on her posterior teeth, loss of occlusal vertical dimension (OVD, Fig 17.1C), and severe horizontal and vertical bone loss. She had generalized chronic advanced periodontitis. Tooth #6 was abscessed and extremely loose and was

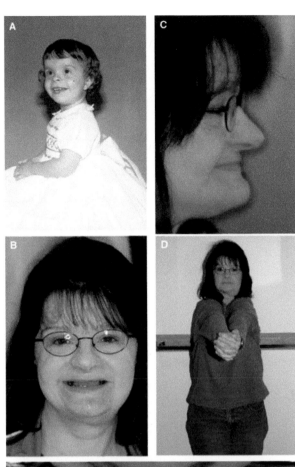

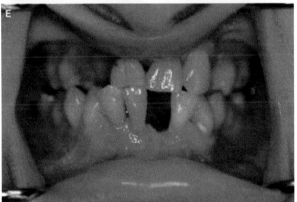

FIGURE 17.1 (A) Patient at 2 years old. (B) Preoperative full face showing a broad base of the nose with a depressed nasal bridge. (C) Concave preoperative profile view of patient showing loss of vertical dimension. (D) Approximation of clavicles; characteristic of cleidocranial dysplasia. (E) Preoperative intraoral photograph of maxillary and mandibular teeth in occlusion.

extracted prior to fabricating diagnostic casts. In addition, the patient had periodontal abscesses around #8 and 13. She was classified according to the ACP Prosthodontic Diagnostic Index classification for partial edentulism as class IV.[8]

Diagnostic casts were made and articulated at her existing OVD (Fig 17.2D). Intraoral and extraoral visual examination

determined that the patient had an existing interocclusal rest space of 7 mm (Fig 17.1C). A second set of diagnostic casts were made and articulated at a newly reestablished OVD, giving the patient 3 mm of freeway space. The reestablished vertical dimension was recorded with an interocclusal bite registration (Regisil, Denstsply York, PA). Diagnostic casts were articulated at this improved and increased OVD, which was later used to fabricate transitional immediate dentures for the maxillary and mandibular arches.

The patient had short conical roots along with generalized chronic advanced periodontitis, which did not make her a good candidate for orthodontic intervention. Her remaining dentition had a poor prognosis to serve as abutments for fixed restorations. Other options included complete maxillary and mandibular dentures, or implant-retained overdentures. A complete maxillary denture would have presented retention challenges for the patient due to her maxillary palate being extremely shallow; she also had a severe gag reflex. Not replacing the teeth with implants would also have allowed continued ridge resorption in both arches.[9] The patient expressed her desire for something not removable and desired fixed prostheses. She was presented with the fixed implant reconstruction and accepted this treatment approach.

Clinical Treatment

Local anesthesia was administered using Marcaine (Abbott Laboratories, Abbott Park, IL) 1:200 × 5 carpules and Ligno-span (Septodent, New Castle, DE) 1:50 × 5 carpules. All maxillary and mandibular teeth were extracted. Crestal incisions were made, along with flap elevation for both arches. The necessary anatomic landmarks in both arches were identified prior to making any preparations in the bone. In the mandibular arch, the critical anatomic landmarks are the mental foramina, positioning of the inferior alveolar canal, and positioning of the anterior loop; these are identified visually. The anterior loop was carefully probed to determine the extent of the anterior extension. In the maxilla, the floor of the nose could be visualized from a labial flap elevation. In addition, the floor and the walls of the sinuses could be visualized through the thin lateral walls.

Prior to surgery, the determination on the position of the implants and the decision of whether to bone graft were made from panoramic radiographic analysis. The patient and the clinicians were ready to revert to a two-stage procedure if an adequate bone was available for implant placement following the removal and debridement of the alveolar bone. This would obligate the patient to wear interim complete removable dentures during the time of bone healing. Fortunately for this patient, following the removal of all her teeth, adequate bone remained for implant placement.

The implants were placed without a surgical guide. Freehand surgery was done with fully elevated mucosal flaps to allow optimal visibility of the bone. Saline

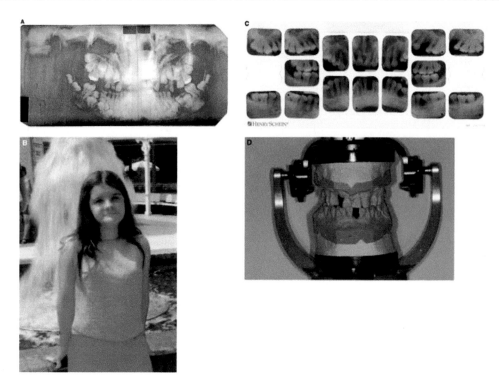

FIGURE 17.2   (A) Panoramic radiograph showing numerous supernumerary and deciduous teeth taken in 1971 when patient was 11 years old. (B) Photograph of patient at 13 years old. (C) Full-mouth series radiographs taken in 2005 when patient was 45 years old. (D) Pretreatment articulated mounted diagnostic cast.

irrigation was used throughout the implant drilling and placement procedure. Table 17.1 shows distribution of the 14 implants used to support this patient's prostheses. The implants were coated with autogenous platelet-rich plasma (PRP)[10] and placed using a torque-controlled machine (45 N cm) and checked manually. Primary closure of the incisions was made with interrupted Vicryl 4.0 sutures (Ethicon Inc., Somerville, NJ).

The Teeth in a Day™ protocol[11] was followed by placing transmucosal abutments (Estheticone and Standard, Nobel Biocare, Yorba Linda, CA) on all the Brånemark System implants. A rubber dam was then used to isolate the abutments from the mucosa and underlying bone. The prosthetic components were installed on the abutments with

TABLE 17.1   **Location of Implant (Tooth #), Implant Size, and Type**

Location of Implant (Tooth #)	Implant Size and Type
3,4,7	13 × 4 mm MKIV
6	15 × 4 mm MKII
9,11	13 × 3.75 mm MKIII
13,14	13 × 4 mm MKIII
20	13 × 3.75 mm MKIII
22,24,25,27	15 × 3.75 mm MKIII
29	15 × 4 mm MKIV

moderate length guide pins. All the maxillary and mandibular implants were immediately loaded using the interim complete denture prostheses made from the diagnostic casts, which were previously articulated at the newly reestablished OVD, and were converted to all-acrylic resin conversion prostheses by connecting the interim complete denture prostheses with the prosthetic cylinders using autopolymerizing resin (Jet; Lang Dental Manufacturers, Wheeling, IL). The conversion prosthesis[12],[13] was first described at the 1986 International Congress on Tissue Integration in Oral and Maxillofacial Reconstruction in Brussels, Belgium. The implant-supported all-acrylic resin conversion prostheses were delivered (Fig 17.3). The newly established OVD was checked using phonetic tests, checking the lip support, and extraoral measurements. The patient had 3 mm of interocclusal rest space.

Postsurgical Patient Management

Following the mandibular and maxillary implant surgeries, the patient was provided with postsurgical instructions, including cold therapy, standard medications of Pen VK 500 mg (SmithKline Beecham Corp., King of Prussia, PA), Peridex (Dentsply Caulk, Milford, DE), and Decadron 0.75 mg (Merck and Co., Inc., Whitehouse Station, NJ), and a soft diet for 8 weeks.

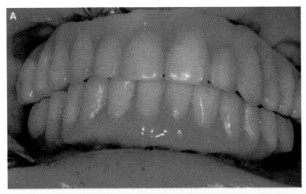

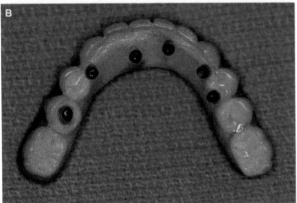

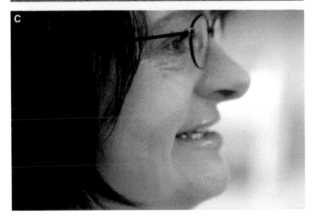

FIGURE 17.3   (A) Maxillary and mandibular conversion prostheses. (B) Mandibular conversion prosthesis. (C) Profile view of maxillary and mandibular conversion prostheses in place.

Definitive Prostheses for Maxillary and Mandibular Arches

Five months following surgical and provisional restorative procedures, the patient presented for fabrication of the definitive prostheses for the maxillary and mandibular arches. An interocclusal registration was made using Regisil. The final impressions were made using the existing maxillary and mandibular fixed all-acrylic resin conversion prostheses as an impression splint. Heavy body Reprosil (Dentsply) impression material was syringed beneath the

prostheses, and pick-up impressions were made using long guide pins (Nobel Biocare). The master casts were created by placing abutment analogs into the temporary cylinders within the all-acrylic resin prostheses. In addition, maxillomandibular relation records were made using the conversion prostheses at the tested OVD. Using the immediately loaded conversion prosthesis as an impression splint has been shown to create an exceptionally accurate master cast. The laboratory then began fabrication of the definitive metal-reinforced implant-supported prostheses. The patient was appointed for a variety of tryins, including functional and esthetic assessments as well as verification of the recorded OVD.

A metal ceramic prosthesis was planned for the maxilla, and a gold framework wrapped with acrylic was planned for the mandible. The gold casting frameworks were tried in 2 weeks following the final impressions. The fit was verified clinically using the single-screw test and also reconfirmed radiographically.[14] At final delivery, the occlusion was adjusted so that all the contacts were even. The access holes were sealed using cotton and Fermit (Ivoclar Vivadent, Buffalo, NY). The patient was extremely pleased with the results (Fig 17.4). A maxillary occlusal guard was made to be worn at night. The patient has been followed on a yearly basis for maintenance visits (Fig 17.5) for the past 5 years. She resides in Sydney, OH, and is being seen by a local dentist.

DISCUSSION

Brånemark System implants were used successfully in treating a 45-year-old woman with cleidocranial dysplasia. The patient had struggled odontologically from a combination of delayed eruption, malformation, and the absence of many of her permanent teeth. The patient had undergone years of orthodontic treatment along with the extraction of her supernumerary and deciduous teeth. Due to her current state of generalized chronic advanced periodontitis, along with short conical roots, her remaining teeth were unable to serve as useful abutments for a fixed reconstruction, and it was necessary to edentulate the patient, followed by immediate implant reconstruction. The removal of all her teeth without this immediate reconstruction would most likely have left the patient with an edentulous state that would continue to deteriorate due to ongoing alveolar atrophy. The treatment described in this report provided the patient with an excellent long-term prognosis and had a huge positive emotional impact. Following her treatment, she stated that her "impossible dream of having teeth became possible." Moreover, her self-confidence grew to the point that she became an enthusiast for fellow patients with similar afflictions, starting a blog and a support group.

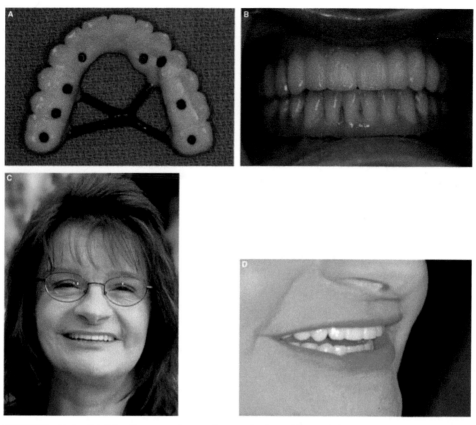

FIGURE 17.4   (A) Maxillary metal-ceramic prosthesis at bisque bake stage. (B) Postoperative esthetics of final prostheses. (C) Postoperative esthetics. (D) Profile view esthetics.

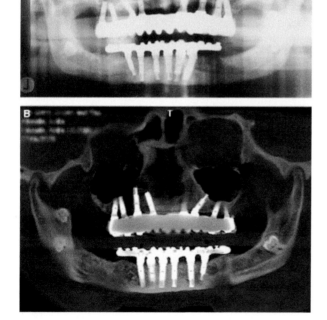

FIGURE 17.5   (A) Panoramic radiograph following definitive prosthesis delivery. (B) Follow-up panoramic radiograph 5 years postoperatively.

SUMMARY

Using implants to support fixed prostheses is an effective treatment option for patients with cleidocranial dysplasia and eliminates the long-standing struggle with ill-fitting, uncomfortable, or unsightly removable prostheses. The Teeth in a Day™ protocol far exceeded the patient's expectations for clinical rehabilitation. The patient's care was executed by a team consisting of surgical prosthodontists, a biomedical engineer, laboratory technicians, and support staff focusing on the patient's emotional well-being. Her dental makeover took only 1 day. This aspect of her treatment cannot be overstated. Final prosthesis delivery occurred in less than 5 months. This treatment protocol is an improved standard of care for patients suffering from cleidocranial dysplasia.

ACKNOWLEDGMENTS

The authors acknowledge the kind and gentle treatment of the patient by the staff at PI Dental Center; and the laboratory support from Fort Washington Dental Laboratory.

REFERENCES

1. Marie P, Sainton P: Observation d'hydrocephailie hereditaire (pere et fils) par vice de development du crane et du cerveux. *Bull Soc Med Hop Pairs* 1897;14:706–712.

2. Butterworth C: Cleidocranial dysplasia: modern concepts of treatment and a report of an orthodontic resistant case requiring a restorative solution. *Dental Update* 1999;12:458–463.

3. Fitchet SM: Cleidocranial dysostosis: hereditary and familial. *J Bone Joint Surg* 1929;11:8383–8866.

4. Shafer WG, Hine MK, Levy BM: Diseases of the bone and joints. In: Shafer WG, Hine MK, Levy BM (eds): *A Textbook of Oral Pathology*. Philadelphia, Saunders, 1974, pp. 622–664.

5. Weintraub GS, Yalisove IL: Prosthodontic therapy for clidocranial dysostosis: report of a case. *J Am Dent Assoc* 1978;96: 301–305.

6. Lombardas P, Toothaker RW: Bone grafting and osseointegrated implants in the treatment of cleidocranial dysplasia. *Compend Contin Educ Dent* 1997;18:509–514.

7. Petropoulos VC, Balshi TJ, Balshi SF, et al: Treatment of a patient with cleidocranial dysplasia using osseointegrated implants: a patient report. *Int J Oral Maxillofac Implants* 2004;19:282–287.

8. McGarry TJ, Nimmo A, Skiba JF, et al: Classification system for partial edentulism. *J Prosthodont* 2002;11:181–193.

9. Jahangiri L, Derlin H, Ting H, et al: Current perspectives in residual ridge remodeling and its clinical implications. *J Prosthet Dent* 1998;80:224–237.

10. Anitua E: Enhancement of osseointegration by generating a dynamic implant surface. *J Oral Implantol* 2006;32:72–76.

11. Balshi T, Wolfinger G: Teeth in a day for the maxilla and mandible: case report. *Clin Impl Dent Relat Res* 2003;5: 11–16.

12. Balshi TJ: The conversion prosthesis: a provisional fixed prosthesis supported by osseointegrated titanium fixtures. In: Albrektsson T, Branemark PI, Holt R, et al (eds): *Tissue Integration in Oral and Maxillofacial Reconstruction: Proceedings of an International Congress, May 1985*, Excerpta Medica Brussels. Amsterdam 1986, pp. 354–365.

13. Balshi TJ: The biotes conversion prosthesis: a provisional fixed prosthesis supported by osseointegrated titanium implants for restoration of the edentulous jaw. *Quintessence Int* 1985;16: 667–677.

14. Branemark PI, Zarb GA, Albreksston T: *Tissue-Integrated Prostheses: Osseointegration in Clinical Dentistry*. Chicago, Quintessence, 1985.

18

FULL-MOUTH REHABILITATION OF AN EDENTULOUS PATIENT WITH PAPILLON–LEFÈVRE SYNDROME USING DENTAL IMPLANTS: A CLINICAL REPORT

LEILA AHMADIAN, DDS, MSC,[1] ABBAS MONZAVI, DDS, MSC,[2] RASOUL ARBABI, DDS, MSC,[1] AND HAMID MAHMOOD HASHEMI, DDS, MSC[3]

[1]Private Practice, Department of Prosthodontics, School of Dentistry, Zahedan, Iran
[2]Department of Prosthodontics and Dental Implants, School of Dentistry, Tehran University of Medical Sciences, Tehran, Iran
[3]Department of Maxillofacial Surgery and Dental Implants, School of Dentistry, Tehran University of Medical Sciences, Tehran, Iran

Keywords
Papillon–Lefèvre syndrome; dental implants; mouth rehabilitation; treatment plan; atrophic jaw.

Correspondence
Leila Ahmadian, Department of Prosthodontics, School of Dentistry, Azadegan St., Zahedan, Iran. E-mail: leilaahmadian@yahoo.co.in

Accepted January 24, 2011

Published in *Journal of Prosthodontics* December 2011; Vol. 20, Issue 8

doi: 10.1111/j.1532-849X.2011.00768.x

ABSTRACT

Papillon–Lefèvre syndrome (PLS) is a rare autosomal recessive disorder. The oral manifestations of the syndrome include rapidly progressive periodontal disease resulting in premature exfoliation of primary and permanent dentitions. Patients are often edentulous at an early age and require prosthodontic treatment. This report is the oral rehabilitation of an edentulous 21-year-old woman with PLS. Treatment included maxillary and mandibular fixed prostheses supported by osseointegrated dental implants. At the 4-year follow-up, the patient presented significant improvements in oral function and psychosocial activities and no prosthetic complications.

Papillon–Lefèvre syndrome (PLS) is a rare autosomal recessive disorder occurring approximately in one to four cases per million.[1] The syndrome is characterized by diffused or localized hyperkeratoses of the palms and soles. Cutaneous lesions of PLS, referred to as keratoderma, may appear at birth[2] or 1 to 2 months after birth,[1,3] but are most commonly manifested between 6 months and 4 years of age.[4,5] Males and females are equally affected, and no racial predilection seems to exist. Life expectancy in these patients is in the normal range.[3] The etiology and pathogenesis of PLS are not fully understood; however, PLS is associated with cathepsin-C gene mutations, located on chromosome 11q14. Cathepsin

C is a lysosomal enzyme expressed in the epithelial regions such as palms, soles, and knees.[6] Oral manifestations of PLS appear approximately when palmar-plantar hyperkratoses present (Table 18.1). These manifestations include rapidly progressive periodontal disease, resulting in premature exfoliation of primary and permanent dentitions. Patients are often edentulous at an early age and require prosthodontic treatment. In PLS patients both dentitions erupt at the expected age and in normal sequence, and they usually have normal form and structure.[7] The pathognomonic dental features of PLS are hypermobility, drifting, migration, and exfoliation of teeth without any signs of root resorption. Therefore, these patients are usually edentulous in their teens.

The oral bacterial flora in afflicted individuals is similar to those found in adult periodontitis, including gram-negative cocci, rods, and spirochetes.[8] Other findings reported in PLS cases include marked chronic inflammation with predominant plasma-cell infiltration, osteoclastic activity, and lack of osteoblastic activity.[9] Rapid progression of periodontitis is not arrested by conventional periodontal treatments; therefore, generalized, severe, and rapid destruction of alveolar bone around the primary and permanent teeth leaves atrophic jaws.[10,11] Due to the lack of improvement in the patients' periodontal condition, treatment has focused on elimination of pockets by extractions of all permanent teeth. Some clinicians believe that alveolar bone is preserved in this manner.

Oral rehabilitation of PLS patients consists of various combinations of conventional complete dentures and overdentures. In recent years, endosseous dental implants have been considered important alternatives. Implant-supported prostheses enhance the support, stability, and retention of prostheses. The use of implants in patients with PLS has been reported in limited cases, and the results indicate that PLS patients can be successfully treated with implants.[12,13] Available bone is an important factor for the successful placement of endosseous dental implants in an edentulous case.[14] As mentioned earlier, available bone in these patients is jeopardized; therefore, the treatment of choice in reported cases is an implant-supported overdenture. Fixed implant-supported prostheses in these patients necessitate a variety of reconstructive procedures, such as sinus floor elevation in the posterior maxilla and nerve repositioning in the posterior mandible for compensation of severe alveolar resorption.

TABLE 18.1   **Diagnostic Features of PLS**

Diffuse or localized hyperkeratoses of the palms and soles
Rapidly progressive periodontal disease not arrested by conventional periodontal treatments
Hypermobility, drifting, migration, and exfoliation of teeth without any signs of root resorption
Premature exfoliation of primary and permanent dentitions

This report details the oral rehabilitation of an edentulous 21-year-old woman with PLS. Treatment included maxillary and mandibular fixed prostheses supported by osseointegrated dental implants. At the 4-year follow-up, the patient exhibited significant improvements in oral function and psychosocial activities without any prosthetic complications.

CLINICAL REPORT

A 21-year-old woman with PLS was referred to the Postgraduate Prosthodontics Clinic at Tehran University of Medical Sciences, Iran. The patient presented with a chief complaint of "I don't like my appearance. I want dental implants and fixed prostheses." The patient's medical history was unremarkable. The patient was only under medical care for hyperkeratosis of palms and soles. There were no abnormal findings or contraindications to dental treatment.

Extraoral examination revealed decreased lower facial height, a prominent chin, mandibular prognathism, and resultant concave facial profile. Premature loss of teeth and resorption of alveolar bone had resulted in decreased facial height (Fig 18.1). Intraoral examination revealed partial edentulism of the upper and lower arches with only third molars present. All the third molars were partially erupted and malformed (Fig 18.2). Periodontal examination of teeth

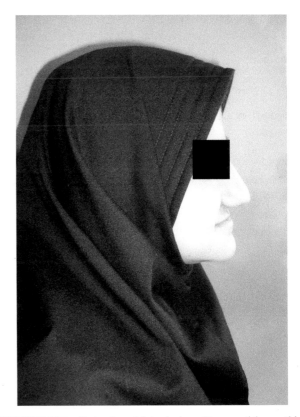

FIGURE 18.1   Pretreatment lateral view. Decreased lower third face height.

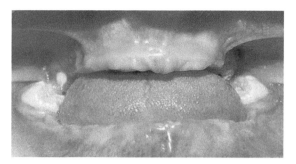

FIGURE 18.2 Pretreatment intraoral condition.

revealed probing depths of 4 to 5 mm. Abnormal tooth mobility was noted. The mucosa appeared to be generally smooth and shiny, with loss of stippling. The maxillary and mandibular residual ridge appeared narrow and demonstrated severe resorption.

Panoramic radiographic examination revealed severe bone loss of the jaw and pneumatized sinuses that would require sinus augmentation before implant placement. The posterior mandibular ridge was resorbed, and the mandibular nerve canal was near the crest of the ridge. The alveolar bone appeared to have normal density and trabeculation. The third molars were judged to have a poor prognosis due to severe alveolar bone loss (Fig 18.3). According to the American College of Prosthodontists Prosthodontic Diagnostic Index (ACP PDI), this patient was categorized as class IV for partially edentulous patients.[15] She had upper and lower acrylic transitional prostheses with poor esthetics and function, and therefore did not wear them.

Diagnostic impressions and record bases were used to mount the casts. It was determined that an Angle's class III relationship was present. Diagnostic wax dentures were fabricated at an optimal occlusal vertical dimension (OVD) with esthetics approved by the patient. The treatment plan was then established after consultation with a surgeon. Several treatment alternatives were reviewed and discussed with the patient. Treatment options included conventional complete dentures, implant-supported overdentures, implant-supported fixed prostheses, and combinations of these. Based on the patient's expectations and her chief complaint, fixed prostheses for both arches were selected. Complications and

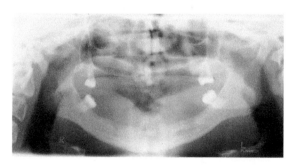

FIGURE 18.3 Preoperative panoramic radiograph.

limitations of the treatment plan such as extrasurgical steps, high cost, time considerations, and unpredictable failure of implants were explained. The patient and her parents appeared to understand the complications and limitations of the treatment plan and signed a consent form. The sequence of the selected treatment plan is summarized in Table 18.2.

In the initial step, the conventional complete dentures were fabricated as an interim prosthesis. Model surgery was carried out on duplicated casts, revealing that a mandibular osteotomy could create a more favorable arch alignment and improve the appearance. The mandible was set back by sagittal split ramus osteotomy. One month after osteotomy, another mandibular complete denture with a new centric relation record was fabricated.

Nine months later, transitional complete dentures were duplicated to fabricate radiographic templates with radiopaque markers to determine proper implant locations. The surgical procedure was performed in the operating room under general anesthesia. Eight ITI SLA implants (Institute Straumann AG, Waldenburg, Switzerland) with regular platforms were placed in the mandibular arch according to the predetermined positions. In the posterior segments of the mandible, the mandibular nerve was repositioned, and longer implants were placed. During the same surgical session, bilateral sinus grafts along with window technique were performed to idealize implant placement in the maxilla. The tibia was chosen as the donor site due to the fact that a high volume of bone marrow could be harvested. One month following the surgical procedure, the interim complete dentures were relined with a soft liner (UFI Gel P, Voco, Cuxhaven, Germany). The postsurgical recovery period was unremarkable with no chief complaint or complications.

Nine months subsequent to sinus augmentation, the same number of implants were placed in the maxillary arch in the predetermined locations. Six months later, clinical and radiographic examinations confirmed the osseointegration of all 16 implants. The criteria for success were the absence of mobility, the absence of radiographic gap in the bone/implant interface, and the absence of pain or infection at the periimplant area.[16] Then, a vestibuloplasty procedure was performed as the final step of surgical treatment. This procedure created adequate attached gingiva necessary for a successful fixed prosthesis. In this step, the soft tissue around the implants was corrected as needed.

After the healing period, preliminary impressions for implant-supported restorations were made. Custom open trays (SR Ivolen, Ivoclar, Vivadent, Schaan, Liechtenstein) were fabricated on these casts for final impressions. Screw-retained impression copings (Institute Straumann AG) were placed into implant bodies, and final impressions were made with polyether (Impregum Penta; 3M ESPE, St. Paul, MN) using an open-tray technique. Each impression was poured

TABLE 18.2   **Selected Treatment Plan**

Correction the current functional status	● Placement of an interim complete denture
Correction of jaw relationship	● Model surgeries on the mounted casts to choose the surgical technique
	● Surgical stent fabrication in corrected relationship as the surgical guide
	● Orthognathic surgery with set-back of mandible
Correction of current functional status	● Placement of a new set of provisional complete dentures
Idealization of maxillary and mandibular anatomy	● Bone grafting at posterior segment of maxilla with the open window technique
	● Nerve repositioning at posterior segment of mandible
Implant placement	● Radiographic guide fabrication
	● Surgical guide fabrication
	● Implant placement
	● Vestibuloplasty procedure to create adequate attached gingiva
	● Extraction of remaining hopeless teeth
Fabrication of the definitive prostheses	● Fabrication of interim prostheses
	● Fabrication of definitive prostheses

with type IV dental stone (Prima-Rock, Whip Mix Corp., Louisville, KY). Then the master casts were mounted on the articulator using the facebow and centric relation records. To obtain an accurate centric relation record, screw-retained record bases were also used.[17]

The initial step in the fabrication of the definitive prostheses required determining the position of the artificial teeth and supporting structure in relation to the final casts. New flangeless wax trial dentures were fabricated on the screw-retained record bases, which were used to improve esthetics and phonetics intraorally. The trial dentures were then used to determine the position of the final prostheses in relation to the implants on the final casts through the use of putty matrices (Lab-Putty; Coltene/Whaledent, Cuyahoga Falls, OH).

Premounted transfer portions of the implants were retained after the surgical procedure to serve as temporary screw-retained abutments. Temporary abutments were placed on the final casts, and autopolymerizing acrylic resin (permanent reline and repair resin; The Hygienic Co., Akron, OH) was bead-brushed and poured around them. An acrylic resin framework outline was then created. In the next step, the fit of these acrylic frames was evaluated by the alternate pressure technique[18] and the screw resistance test.[19] The acrylic frameworks assembled on the articulator and matrices made from the trial denture were used to position the artificial teeth over it. This finished diagnostic setup was examined and tried in, and the occlusion was adjusted. A mutually protected occlusion was achieved and verified intraorally.[20,21]

In this step, the wax used to attach the artificial teeth to the acrylic frame was eliminated and replaced by the same acryl. Then the screw-retained interim acrylic prostheses were polished and delivered. A mutually protected occlusion was verified intraorally using articulating paper (AccuFilm II, Parkell, Farmingdale, NY) and 12-μm thick shimstock (Almore, Darby Spencer Mead, Westbury, NY) (Fig 18.4).

Vinyl polysiloxane material (Reprosilputty; Dentsply Intl, York, PA) was placed into the occlusal access openings. A panoramic radiograph was taken as a baseline for future follow-up. The patient functioned with the interim prostheses for 12 weeks to further assess the adaptation of the proposed OVD for the definitive restorations. The patient was instructed regarding posttreatment care. This included

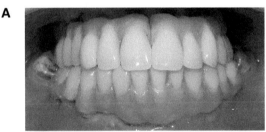

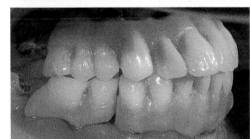

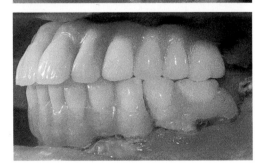

FIGURE 18.4   Acrylic screw-retained interim prostheses in place; (A) frontal view; (B) right lateral view; (C) left lateral view.

home-care instructions of twice-per-day brushing with an electric toothbrush (Sonicare; Philips Electronics, Stamford, CT) and use of an oral irrigator (Waterpik Ultra Dental Water Jet, WP-100W; Water Pik Inc., Newport Beach, CA) once daily. The patient was placed on 1-week recall appointments. She was referred to the surgeon for the extraction of remaining teeth including teeth #1, #16, #17, and #32.

The interim prostheses were retrieved after 12 weeks of comfortable function and were assembled on the master casts. Maxillary and mandibular polystyrene templates (Coping Material, National Keystone Products Co., Cherry Hill, NJ) were fabricated from the patient's interim prostheses for use as a guide in the full-contour waxing of the definitive prostheses.[22] The final implant-supported fixed partial dentures were fabricated by developing a full-contour waxing based on the templates. The waxing was then cut back and separated into several pieces (two pieces in the maxilla and four pieces in the mandible) for the fabrication of the cast framework. The several-piece design was used to decrease laboratory complexity and to allow for easy retrieval for maintenance and repair, if necessary. The completed wax patterns were cast in a gold–palladium alloy (Olympia, Heraeus Kulzer Inc., Armonk, NY). The castings were evaluated under a microscope, and the fit was verified on the master cast. The metal frameworks were clinically and radiographically evaluated in the mouth. The left side of the maxilla had a misfit, and was therefore cut and indexed using autopolymerizing PMMA resin (GC Pattern Resin; GC America Inc., Alsip, IL). The framework was preporcelain soldered (Jelenko Olympia Pre Solder, Heraeus Kulzer Inc.) using a torch. After being soldered, the framework was evaluated again to ensure proper marginal fit and absence of any "rocking" movement.

Following framework preparation, dental porcelain was applied, using feldspathic porcelain (Vita Omega Metal Ceramics, Vita Zahnfabrik, Bad Sackingen, Germany) fired according to the manufacturer's instructions. Gingival-tone porcelain was added to the soft tissue area of the framework. A mutually protected occlusion was developed again. The restorations were returned to the patient for a bisque bake try-in. Contour, occlusion, and shade were modified and verified. The metal ceramic restorations were characterized, and finally glazed.

At delivery, abutment screws and superstructure screws were tightened, as suggested by the manufacturer. Guttapercha was placed over the fastening screws, and the access holes were covered with light-cured composite resin (Z250, 3M ESPE). Postoperative instructions were given to the patient again, and a panoramic radiograph was taken (Fig 18.5). The patient was placed on 6-month recall appointments. Figure 18.6 illustrates the patient's presentation to the clinic at a recall appointment of 6 months posttreatment. No prosthetic complications were reported by the patient at the 4-year follow-up appointment.

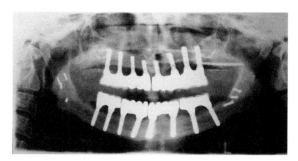

FIGURE 18.5   Posttreatment panoramic radiograph.

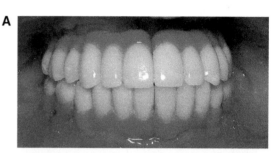

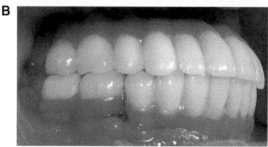

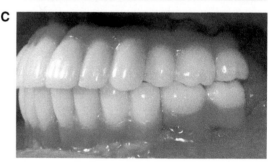

FIGURE 18.6   Definitive screw-retained restorations in place; (A) frontal view; (B) right lateral view; (C) left lateral view.

DISCUSSION

PLS is a devastating disease process characterized by rapid destruction of the dental alveolar complex. It affects both the deciduous and permanent dentitions and leads to edentulism in the teens; therefore, the affected individuals are socially, psychologically, and physically debilitated. Conventional treatment plans for oral rehabilitation of these patients consist of removable partial or complete dentures.

During the last three decades, implant dentistry has enabled clinicians to treat edentulous and partially edentulous patients predictably with fixed restorations. Osseointegrated implants offer an alternative that will provide major improvements in the long-term prognosis for oral rehabilitation.[23,24]

Dental implants are used to retain, support, and stabilize prostheses. Implant placement is not contraindicated in these patients, and the outcome of the implant treatment in our subject was successful and similar to healthy individuals.

Available bone in an edentulous site is a determining factor in treatment planning, implant design, surgical approach, healing time, and initial progressive bone loading during prosthetic reconstruction.[25,26] Because of the severe alveolar bone loss in these patients, this factor is more critical. One of the reasons for short-term implant failure is lack of primary stability. Impaired bone height, especially in the posterior segments of the maxilla and mandible, contribute significantly to such diminished implant longevity.[27] To decrease stress, the clinician may elect to increase the number of implants or use different preprosthetic surgeries for correction of anatomic variations.[28–31] In our case a combination of these modalities was used.

This report illustrates the importance of proper and logical treatment planning as well as clear communication between the dental team and the patient regarding the outcomes of the planned dental treatment. An esthetic and functional result can only be achieved if the clinician communicates well with the patient and plans a logical treatment sequence. On the other hand, the complexity of a case can be simplified if it is broken down into separate parts that can be addressed sensibly. In our patient, the treatment outcome exceeded her expectations. Certainly, her quality of life has greatly improved, and she is very happy with the function, fit, and appearance of the prostheses.

SUMMARY

The case we presented suggests that the use of dental implants in the rehabilitation of PLS patients provides excellent support for functional and esthetic dental rehabilitation.

ACKNOWLEDGMENTS

The authors would like to thank all the professors in the Prosthodontic Department of Tehran University of Medical Sciences who have shared their knowledge in the pursuit of excellence, and would also like to thank Mr. Hasan Zade and Mr. Khodadad for laboratory support of this case.

REFERENCES

1. Gorlin RJ, Sedano H, Anderson VE: The syndrome of palmar-plantar hyperkratosis and premature periodontal destruction of the teeth. *J Pediatr* 1964;65:895–898.

2. Galanter DR, Bradford S: Case report. Hyperkeratosis palmoplantaris and periodontosis: the Papillon–Lefèvre syndrome. *J Periodontol* 1969;40:40–47.

3. Haneke E: The Papillon–Lefèvre syndrome: keratosis palmoplantaris with periodontopathy. Report of a case and review of the cases in the literature. *Hum Genet* 1979;51:1–35.

4. Hattab FN, Rawashdeh MA, Yassin OM, et al: Papillon–Lefèvre syndrome: a review of the literature and report of 4 cases. *J Periodontol* 1995;66:413–420.

5. Wiebe CB, Hakkinen L, Putnins EE, et al: Successful periodontal maintenance of a case with Papillon–Lefèvre syndrome: 12-year follow-up and review of the literature. *J Periodontol* 2001;72:824–830.

6. Canger EM, Celenk P, Devrim I, et al: Intraoral findings of Papillon–Lefèvre syndrome. *J Dent Child* 2008;75:99–103.

7. Baghdady VS: Papillon–Lefèvre syndrome: report of four cases. *ASDC J Dent Child* 1982;49:147–150.

8. Newman M, Angel I, Karge H, et al: Bacterial studies of the Papillon–Lefèvre syndrome. *J Dent Res* 1977;56:545.

9. Martinez Lalis RR, Lopez Otero R, Carranza FA Jr: A case of Papillon–Lefèvre syndrome. *Periodontics* 1965;3:292–295.

10. Rateitschak-Pluss EM, Schroeder HE: History of periodontitis in a child with Papillon–Lefèvre syndrome. A case report. *J Periodontol* 1984;55:35–46.

11. Shapira J, Eidelman E, Fuks A, et al: Treatment of Papillon–Lefèvre syndrome with chemotherapy: report of cases. *Spec Care Dentist* 1985;5:71–74.

12. Ullbro C, Crossner CG, Lundgren T, et al: Osseointegrated implants in a patient with Papillon–Lefèvre syndrome. A 4 1/2-year follow up. *J Clin Periodontol* 2000;27:951–954.

13. Woo I, Brunner DP, Yamashita DD, et al: Dental implants in a young patient with Papillon–Lefèvre syndrome: a case report. *Implant Dent* 2003;12:140–144.

14. Orsini G, Bianchi AE, Vinci R, et al: Histologic evaluation of autogenous calvarial bone in maxillary onlay bone grafts: a report of 2 cases. *Int J Oral Maxillofac Implants* 2003;18:594–598.

15. McGarry TJ, Nimmo A, Skiba JF, et al: Classification system for partial edentulism. *J Prosthodont* 2002;11:181–193.

16. Buser D, Weber HP, Lang NP: Tissue integration of non-submerged implants. 1-year results of a prospective study with 100 ITI hollow-cylinder and hollow-screw implants. *Clin Oral Implants Res* 1990;1:33–40.

17. Hobo S, Ichida E, Garcia LT: *Osseointegration and Occlusal Rehabilitation* (ed 1) Tokyo, Quintessence, 1991.

18. Henry PJ: An alternative method for the production of accurate casts and occlusal records in osseointegrated implant rehabilitation. *J Prosthet Dent* 1987;58:694–697.

19. Jemt T: Failures and complications in 391 consecutively inserted fixed prostheses supported by Branemark implants in edentulous jaws: a study of treatment from the time of prosthesis placement to the first annual checkup. *Int J Oral Maxillofac Implants* 1991;6:270–276.

20. Kim Y, Oh TJ, Misch CE, et al: Occlusal considerations in implant therapy: clinical guidelines with biomechanical rationale. *Clin Oral Implants Res* 2005;16:26–35.

21. Misch CE, Bidez MW: Occlusal considerations for implant-supported prostheses. In Misch CE (ed): *Dental Implant Prosthetics* (ed 1) St. Louis, Mosby, 1999, pp. 629–645.

22. Sotera AJ: A direct technique for fabricating acrylic resin temporary crowns using the Omnivac. *J Prosthet Dent* 1973;29:577–580.

23. Adell R, Eriksson B, Lekholm U, et al: Long-term follow-up study of osseointegrated implants in the treatment of totally edentulous jaws. *Int J Oral Maxillofac Implants* 1990;5:347–359.

24. Adell R, Lekholm U, Rockler B, et al: A 15-year study of osseointegrated implants in the treatment of the edentulous jaw. *Int J Oral Surg* 1981;10:387–416.

25. Brunski JB: In vivo bone response to biomechanical loading at the bone/dental-implant interface. *Adv Dent Res* 1999;13:99–119.

26. Geng JP, Tan KB, Liu GR: Application of finite element analysis in implant dentistry: a review of the literature. *J Prosthet Dent* 2001;85:585–598.

27. Rieger MR, Adams WK, Kinzel GL: A finite element survey of eleven endosseous implants. *J Prosthet Dent* 1990;63:457–465.

28. Misch CE: Density of bone: effect on treatment plans, surgical approach, healing, and progressive bone loading. *Int J Oral Implantol* 1990;6:23–31.

29. Sahin S, Cehreli MC, Yalcin E: The influence of functional forces on the biomechanics of implant-supported prostheses—a review. *J Dent* 2002;30:271–282.

30. Siegele D, Soltesz U: Numerical investigations of the influence of implant shape on stress distribution in the jaw bone. *Int J Oral Maxillofac Implants* 1989;4:333–340.

31. Papavasiliou G, Kamposiora P, Bayne SC, et al: Three-dimensional finite element analysis of stress-distribution around single tooth implants as a function of bony support, prosthesis type, and loading during function. *J Prosthet Dent* 1996;76:633–640.

PART IV

MANAGEMENT OF ORTHODONTIC/PROSTHODONTIC PATIENTS

19

ASPECTS OF ORTHODONTIC-PROSTHETIC REHABILITATION OF DENTOFACIAL ANOMALIES

Zorica Ajdukovic, dds, phd,[1] Mirjana Janosevic, dds, phd,[2] Gordana Filipovic, dds, phd,[2] Stojanka Arsic, md, phd,[3] Predrag Janosevic, dds,[2] and Nenad Petrovic, dds[1]

[1]Department of Prosthodontics, University of Nis, Faculty of Medicine in Nis, Clinic of Stomatology, Nis, Serbia
[2]Department of Orthodontics, University of Nis, Faculty of Medicine in Nis, Clinic of Stomatology, Nis, Serbia
[3]University of Nis, Faculty of Medicine in Nis, Institute of Anatomy, Nis, Serbia

Keywords
Class III malocclusion; orthodontic–prosthetic rehabilitation.

Correspondence
Zorica Ajdukovic, Department of Prosthodontics, Faculty of Medicine in Nis, Clinic of Stomatology, University of Nis, Bul. Dr. Zorana Djindjica 52, 18000 Nis, Serbia. E-mail: ajdukoviczorica@yahoo.com

This research was financed by funds from the project of the Ministry of Education and Science of Serbia No III41018 and No III45004.

The authors deny any conflicts of interest.

Accepted April 2014

Published in *Journal of Prosthodontics* April 2014; Vol. 23, Issue 3

doi: 10.1111/jopr.12091

ABSTRACT

Skeletal class III malocclusion is one of the most difficult dentofacial anomalies, characterized by deviation in the development of the mandible and maxilla in the sagittal plane, where the mandible is dominant in relation to the maxilla. In patients with class III malocclusion, anomalies in the dentoalveolar level and esthetic discrepancies are also frequent. The etiology of class III malocclusion is multifactorial due to the interaction of hereditary and environmental factors. Rehabilitation and treatment of malocclusion is one of the major goals of modern dentistry. This article presents the orthodontic-prosthetic therapy and rehabilitation of a 45-year-old patient with an abnormal occlusal vertical dimension and a skeletal class III malocclusion. The patient came to the clinic complaining about degraded esthetics and disordered functions of the orofacial region (functions of eating, swallowing, speech) and also pain in the temporomandibular joint. After the diagnosis was made, the patient was first referred to orthodontic treatment with fixed orthodontic appliances (self-ligating brackets system Rot 0.22). Upon completion of the orthodontic treatment, the patient was sent for further prosthetic treatment. Fixed prosthetic restorations were made in the upper and lower jaw, thus achieving a satisfactory result in terms of esthetics and function of the stomatognathic system.

Class III malocclusion is a craniofacial anomaly and belongs to the group of most severe deformities. Class III malocclusions are characterized by the overgrowth of the lower jaw in relation to the overdeveloped, normal, or underdeveloped upper jaw.[1,2] In addition to changes in the mandible and/or maxilla, anomalies in the dentoalveolar level and esthetic discrepancies, such as facial asymmetry, are also frequent in this type of patient. For example, the angle of the cranial base is often decreased in these patients, making the problem more severe and visible on the face. Dentoalveolar disorders arise as a consequence of nature striving to balance the existing skeletal problems.[3] The etiology of class III malocclusion is multifactorial, due to the interaction of hereditary and environmental factors.[4]

The diagnostic approach to class III malocclusion is reflected in the identification and assessment of morphological and functional differences and variations in growth and development of the craniofacial complex. The initial criterion in the prosthetic-orthodontic diagnostics of dentofacial anomalies is the eugnathic relationship (i.e., the proper relationship of the upper and lower jaw to the skull).[5]

Treatment, rehabilitation, and esthetics represent the main tasks of modern dentistry. Class III malocclusion is one of the most severe dentofacial anomalies that threatens esthetics and requires very complex treatment and rehabilitation. Adequate treatment and rehabilitation are determined by various factors. Class III malocclusion requires early orthodontic treatment in the period of deciduous and early mixed dentition; however, the outcome is difficult to predict while the patient is still growing.[6,7]

Orthodontic-prosthetic treatment presents itself as an option in adult patients with class III malocclusion where the skeletal discrepancy is relatively low. Given that the modification of the growth of craniofacial structures cannot be effected in these patients, therapeutic procedures are limited to the dentoalveolar level. Orthodontic and prosthetic rehabilitation of these patients represents a so-called camouflage therapy.[8]

Temporomandibular disorders (TMD) are often present inpatients with class III malocclusion. They may be a consequence of occlusal interferences, loss of occlusal vertical dimension (OVD), or the psychological state of the patient.[9] Pronunciation difficulties, as well as masticatory problems, are also reported in this type of patient.[10–21]

Esthetics and impaired function are the main reasons an adult patient comes to a dental office. Our goals in this case were to achieve functional occlusion and to improve facial esthetics, phonetics, and masticatory function in a patient with class III malocclusion by using orthodontic and prosthetic treatment.

CLINICAL REPORT

After a detailed clinical examination, the male patient, age 45, underwent orthodontic-prosthetic treatment for reasons of disturbed esthetics, lack of a normal diet, disordered speech, and pain in the temporomandibular joint. After a thorough clinical and functional examination, X-ray diagnostics were performed (teleroentgen and digital orthopantomography).

Clinical and Functional Findings

Intraorally: Posterior teeth in class III, a narrow upper jaw with crowding in the front, an anterior crossbite and crossbite of the left canine, missing first and second right premolars, missing second left premolar and first left permanent molar in the upper jaw and two first permanent molars in the lower jaw, as well as missing third molars, a deep bite, and a positive overjet of 3.2 mm (Fig 19.1) were found.

Analysis of the face (profile): In the biometric field, the upper lip is positioned behind the nasal vertical, while the lower lip and the chin are positioned in front of the nasal vertical, which corresponds to a progenic profile.

Analysis of the face (en face): Shortened lower third of the face, with no visible asymmetry (Fig 19.2) was found.

OVD: OVD decreased by 3 mm as determined clinically, pronounced nasolabial and mentolabial sulcus, and lowered mouth corners.

Functional findings: These included disturbed functions of the orofacial region and pain in TMJ.

Pronunciation disorders: These included slightly noticeable difficulties in pronunciation of labio-dental voices "f"/f/and,"v"/v/, a mild lisp and difficulties in pronunciation of dental voices "d"/d/, "t"/t/, "z"/z/, "s"/s/, "c"/ts/, as well as a mild distortion of voices "č"/tʃ/, "ć"/tɕ/,"ž"/ʒ/, "š"/ʃ/(/ʃ*/International Phonetic Alphabet—IPA).

Radiographic Findings

Teleroentgenogram analysis showed a class III relationship by Steiner (ANB 1°), a combination of real and pseudo progenia. Cephalometric analysis also showed normognathism of the maxilla relative to the cranial base (SNA 83°), while at the same time the body length of the maxilla was 5.6 mm shorter in relation to the anterior part of the cranial base. There was also a mandibular prognathism SNB 84o, while the corpus of the mandible was 6.1 mm longer in relation to the anterior part of the cranial base. An anterior (hypodivergent) type of growth was found in this patient. Bjork polygon angles sum was 390.5o, causing an increase in the bite depth (Tables 19.1, 19.2).

Course of Treatment

Based on the diagnosis, the patient was first referred to orthodontic treatment with fixed orthodontic appliances

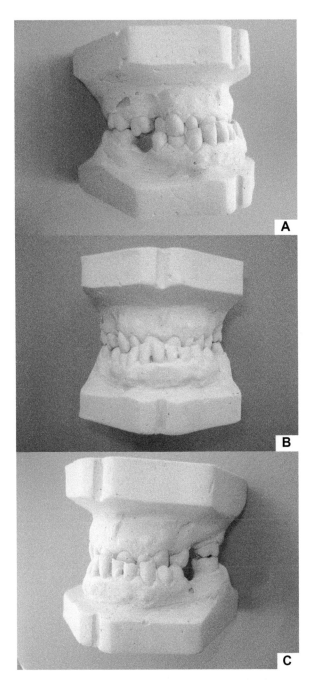

FIGURE 19.1   A, B, C initial dental casts before therapy.

(Damon self-ligating system Rot 0.22) (Fig 19.3). The goal of this therapy was the leveling of the maxillary dental arch and the mesial movement of the upper left first premolar as well as protrusion of the upper front teeth to establish a better sagittal relationship with the lower anterior teeth. Since the majority of the space for the upper left first molar was closed by the mesial movement of the upper left second molar, the orthodontic decision was not to distalize the upper left second molar to make that space. Due to the existence of a reverse overlap of incisors and a deep bite that would have caused the

overthrow of the orthodontic brackets during treatment, disarticulation was done with glass ionomer cement (Fuji; GC America, Alsip, IL) applied on the occlusal surfaces of the lower molars before the fixed appliance was placed.

Orthodontic therapy lasted 12 months. After final leveling of the dental arches and achieving all the above-mentioned goals of orthodontic treatment, the patient was immediately referred for further prosthetic treatment. The retention splint was not used (Fig 19.4).

Analysis of the study casts made after orthodontic therapy provided the data necessary for further prosthetic treatment: occlusal relation of the upper and lower jaw, sagittal and vertical relation of the anterior teeth, and the position of the edentulous ridge compared to the antagonist. Orthodontic treatment brought the front teeth in an edge-to-edge articulation. Although two teeth were missing on each side of the upper arch, the edentulous space could only accommodate one restoration on each side. The final prosthodontic plan was to do a semicircular, fixed, nine-unit metal-ceramic prosthesis consisting of seven crowns on abutment teeth and two cantilevered crowns in the upper jaw, and to do two lateral, four-unit, metal-ceramic fixed partial dentures (FPDs) in the lower jaw. The restorations were made to permanently fix the changed relations between the upper and lower teeth achieved by orthodontic treatment (i.e., to bring the teeth from edge-to-edge to a proper correlation and to reconstruct the bite).

The teeth were prepared using a standard high-powered hand-piece with water cooling and a standard set of diamond burs. In the upper jaw, teeth 11 to 13 and 22 to 24 were prepared, and impressions were taken with a plane to add two cantilevers to the semicircular construction, replacing teeth 14 and 25. In the lower jaw, two lateral four-crown FPDs were made. On the left side teeth 34, 35, and 37 were prepared, and impressions were taken with planes to add a pontic replacing tooth 36. On the right side, teeth 44, 45, and 47 were prepared, and impressions were taken with a plan to add a pontic crown replacing missing tooth 46. The impressions were taken using a standard tray and elastomers (Zeta Plus; Zhermack, Rovigo, Italy). Working casts were made following standard procedures (Fig 19.5). Proper OVD vas determined using esthetic and phonetic signs—determining vertical dimension of rest (VDR) position by establishing ordinary configuration of the patient's nose, lips, and chin, and through pronunciation of sibilant and fricative sounds, as well as the word "Emma" commonly used for this purpose.[22] The value of VDR was reduced by 3 mm, and thus the appropriate OVD was obtained.

Wax paterns of the FPD were modeled on the working cast and then invested and cast from base metal alloys. Metal suprastructures were tried on in the mouth to check the sealing of the abutment teeth, as well as the relations to the antagonists and mucosa. Metal casts were then brought back to the laboratory and ceramics applied and fired.

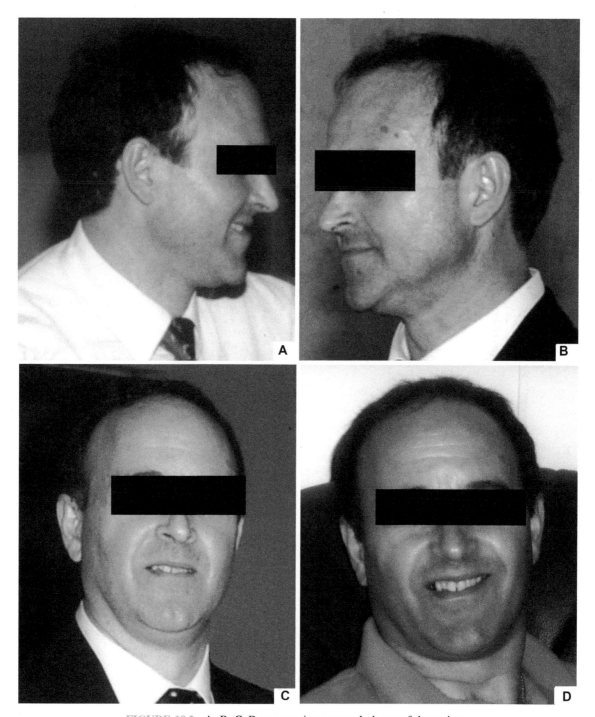

FIGURE 19.2 A, B, C, D preoperative extraoral photos of the patient.

Another try-in in the mouth was made before glazing of the ceramics. After the glazing, metal-ceramic FPDs were temporarily cemented using RelyX Temp NE (3M ESPE, Seefeld, Germany), and after 4 months, permanently cemented with glass-ionomer cement (Aqua Meron; VOCO, Cuxhaven, Germany).

The global articulation test (GAT) was used for assessing articulation of voices of Serbian language. The test consists of 30 words. Observed voice is marked by the corresponding letter in front of the word. If there are two of the same voices in the word, only the first is assessed. The word is repeated three times, and only the most appropriate response is recorded. Marks 1, 2, and 3 represent good voices, mark 4 represents borderline distorted voices, mark 5 represents distorted voices, mark 6 represents voices difficult to understand out of context, mark 7 represents voices the patient

TABLE 19.1   **Angular Parameter Values for Cephalometric Teleroentgen Analysis**

Parameters	Measured values	Required values	Results
SNA	83°	82°	Maxillary normognathism
SNB	84°	80°	Mandibular prognathism
ANB	−1°	2° to 4°	Mesial jaw relationship
NS/SpP	3°	8 ± 3°	Anteinclination of the maxilla
NS/MP	29°	33 ± 6°	Anteinclination of the mandible
J/SpP	67°	70°	Mild protrusion of upper incisors
i/MP	93°	80°	Retrusion of lower incisors
Bjorksum	390.5°	396°	Anterior growth type

TABLE 19.2   **Linear Parameter Values for Cephalometric Teleroentgen Analysis**

Parameters	Measured values (mm)	Required values (mm)	Results
Cor. max	49	54.6	Reduced maxillary body length—5.6 mm
Cor. mand	88	81.9	Increased mandibular body length + 6.1 mm

cannot pronounce. The sum of good, marginal, damaged, or missing voices is scored. The test was applied by an experienced clinician before the start of orthodontic treatment, and 6 months after completion of prosthetic treatment.[23]

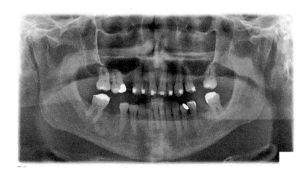

FIGURE 19.3   Orthopantomography during the course of treatment.

A questionnaire was used to evaluate the patient's perceived masticatory ability. Five questions were asked to evaluate the patient's ability to chew foods of different hardness:

1. Are you ordinarily, or would you be, able to chew or bite fresh carrot?
2. Are you ordinarily, or would you be, able to chew or bite fresh lettuce or spinach?
3. Are you ordinarily, or would you be, able to chew or bite steak, chops, or firm meat?
4. Are you ordinarily, or would you be, able to chew or bite boiled peas, carrots, or yellow beans?
5. Are you ordinarily, or would you be, able to chew or bite a whole fresh apple without cutting?

After having read the questions, the patient was asked to indicate his response on a visual analog scale (VAS) 150 mm long (limited by "not" and "very") located below each question. The scale provided a means of assigning a metric value to each

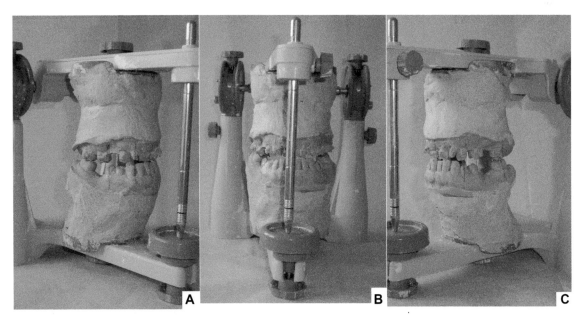

FIGURE 19.4   A, B, C dental casts postorthodontic treatment.

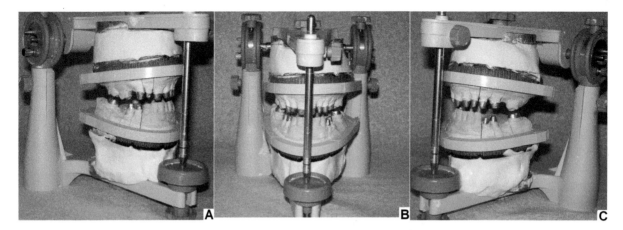

FIGURE 19.5   A, B, C dental casts after tooth preparation at a proper OVD (as determined clinically).

response, based on the distance of the marked response from the ends of the line.[20] The patient filled in the first questionnaire just before the start of orthodontic treatment, and the second questionnaire 6 months after the end of prosthetic treatment.

OUTCOME

Upon completion of treatment, the esthetic success was apparent, achieved by combining the orthodontic and prosthetic rehabilitation of the patient with class III malocclusion (Figs 19.6 and 19.7). The lower third of the face is now within normal proportions. The upper lip is supported by the upper anterior teeth and moved slightly in the anterior direction. Although the changes in the patient's profile were not dramatic, the progenic facial appearance was no longer the main characteristic of the patient's facial esthetic. The success of the therapy was confirmed by a teleroentgen analysis (Fig 19.8, Table 19.3).

The functions of the orofacial region have returned to normal (pronunciation and mastication), while the pain in the TMJ partially decreased during orthodontic treatment. Complete disappearance of the TMJ problem came several months after final prosthetic rehabilitation of the patient, at which time the prosthesis was permanently cemented.

The patient's pronunciation of voices in Serbian before orthodontic-prosthetic therapy was: "f"/f/, "v"/v/, "d"/d/, "t"/t/, "z"/z/, "s"/s/, "c"/ts/—borderline distorted voices (mark 4 on GAT); "ć"/tɕ/—distorted voice (mark 5 on GAT); "č"/tʃ/, "ž"/ʒ/, "š"/ʃ/—voices difficult to understand out of context (mark 6 on GAT); Remaining voices were marked as "good voices" with marks 1, 2, or 3 on GAT. After 6 months, the patient's pronunciation was within acceptable boundaries. Voices "f"/f/, "v"/v/, "d"/d/, "t"/t/, "z"/z/, "s"/s/, "c"/ts/, "ć"/tɕ/, "č"/tʃ/were marked as "good voices" with marks 1, 2, or 3 on GAT, while voices "ž"/ʒ/and "š"/ʃ/remained in the category borderline distorted voices (mark 4 on GAT).

Also, the patient stated that his mastication significantly improved. Before therapy, the patient's response to question 1 from the questionnaire was within the 61 to 75 range on the VAS. The answer to question 2 was within the 106 to 120 range on the VAS. Answers to questions 3 and 5 were within the 31 to 45 range on the VAS. The answer to question 4 was within the 121 to 135 range on the VAS. After the end of prosthetic treatment, his answers to the questions from the questionnaire were as follows:

1. Question 1: within the 121 to 135 range on the VAS
2. Question 2: within the 136 to 150 range on the VAS
3. Question 3: within the 106 to 120 range on the VAS
4. Question 4: within the 136 to 150 range on the VAS
5. Question 5: within the 121 to 135 range on the VAS

DISCUSSION

To achieve good results in the treatment of class III malocclusion in adult patients, a combination of orthodontic-surgical or orthodontic-prosthetic therapy is often needed.[24] Treatment of class III malocclusion represents a great challenge, but fortunately the incidence of this anomaly is not large (2% to 10%, depending on the population). The clinical picture is easily recognized, ranging from the mildest form, where the only disturbance is in the position of the front teeth, to the worst forms, where there is a significant disorder in skeletal relations.[25,26]

Woodside classified adult patients with class III malocclusion according to the dento-skeletal characteristics into three main categories. The first type is dentoalveolar or pseudo-class III. Each part of the face is well related with good prognosis after treatment. The second type is related to skeletal variation, which could result from the combination of retrognatic or orthognathic maxilla, with prognathic or

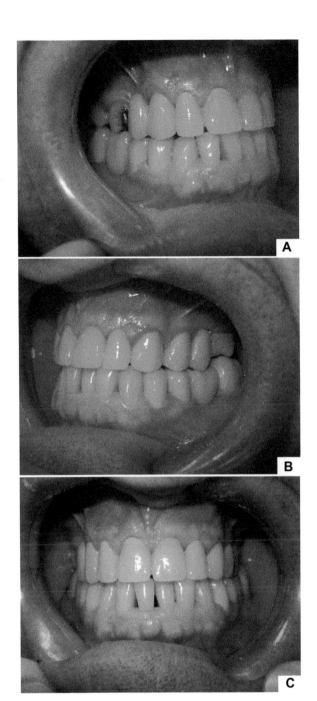

FIGURE 19.6 A, B, C intraoral finding after completion of therapy.

orthognathic mandible causing a skeletal class III pattern. Dental compensations for skeletal class III are commonly found in this group. The third type is related to neuromuscular adaptation, such as opening rotation of the previously prognathic mandible resulting in more harmonious facial profile, or overclosure of the orthognathic mandible through a large freeway space, resulting in a more severe class III profile.[27]

Skeletal jaw relations can be disrupted in the sagittal as well as in the transverse and vertical planes, and abnormal relations between the upper and lower teeth are always present in these cases. A higher degree of mandibular prognathism may be due to changes in the lower jaw, and it can be conditioned by its length, mesial position, or by a combination of its abnormal size and position.[28] As part of the abovementioned anomalies in the lower jaw, disrupted morphometric characteristics of the upper jaw can also be present. These skeletal and dental irregularities disturb the harmony of the soft-tissue profile of the patient, forming craniofacial-dental abnormalities, which many authors, because of their complexity, define as a syndrome.[24–32] Despite the fact that class III malocclusions are anomalies that require prompt treatment, numerous studies have shown that the use of an appropriate orthodontic-prosthetic procedure can lead to good results in the treatment of malocclusion even in elderly patients.[33–35]

In this patient, the undertaken orthodontic treatment was critical in terms of bringing his occlusion to the stage when it was possible to do a successful prosthetic camouflage therapy. An alternative to this approach in the treatment might have been a bilateral mandibular split osteotomy combined with prosthetic rehabilitation.[36] Given that surgical therapy is still a drastic procedure that entails a long postoperative recovery and the potential complications, orthodontic-prosthetic treatment in this case proved to be a safer solution for this patient, presenting excellent posttreatment results.

Patients with class III malocclusion often report a history of TMD problems. In a study of 44 patients in the year 2000, it was stated that TMD is much more likely to occur when a class III malocclusion is associated with asymmetry. Recent studies reported the influences of psychological stress on the occurrence of TMJ dysfunction.[37] In this case, the patient came to our clinic complaining, among other things, of pain in the TMJ. After the fixed prosthesis was completed and ready for cementation, TMJ problems, even though decreased, were still present. For that reason, FPDs were temporarily cemented at the first phase of therapy. The pain in the TMJ subsided, most likely due to the establishment of functional occlusion, bite-raising to the proper, clinically determined level of OVD, and the patient's accommodation to the new situation. After complete disappearance of TMJ problems, the prosthesis was permanently cemented.

Six months and 1 and 2 years after definite cementation of the prosthesis, the patient did not show any TMD symptoms.

Studies done on the subject of speech disorders related to malocclusions suggest that the risk ratio for producing consonants too far anteriorly was greater by 4.5 times for individuals with mesial occlusion, 3.7 times for those with mandibular overjet, 3.4 times for those with incisal open bite, and 1.7 for those with lateral cross-bite compared to individuals without those occlusal anomalies. This study suggests that mesial occlusion is related to more severe misarticulations of consonants.[10] Chinese individuals with a class III relationship may distort the consonants

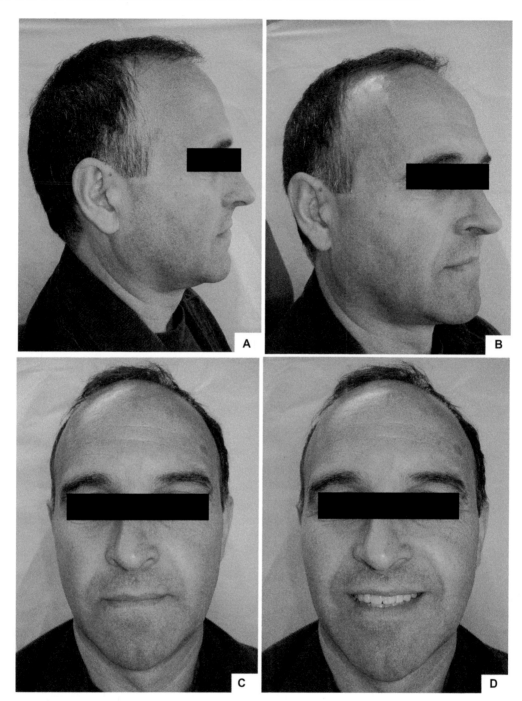

FIGURE 19.7 A, B, C, D facial appearance of the patient after the completion of treatment (extraoral findings).

/zh/, /ch/, /sh/, and/z/.[11] Several studies have suggested that combined surgical and orthodontic treatment can result in positive changes in articulation for most patients.[12,13] It is difficult to draw firm conclusions on the correlation between malocclusion and speech disorder, since speech is a complex process for putting thought into words involving several organs, such as the brain, teeth, lips, tongue, and muscles. These organs can compensate mutually to ensure that pronunciation is correct.[14] In our case, the GAT, commonly used in this region, was used to express the number and type of voices damaged and the extent of their damage. The GAT includes good voices, marginal voices, distorted voices, difficult-to-understand voices, and voices the patient cannot pronounce. At the individual level, the GAT tells us what voices deviate from desired pronunciation. In our case, the majority of speech difficulties significantly improved, and

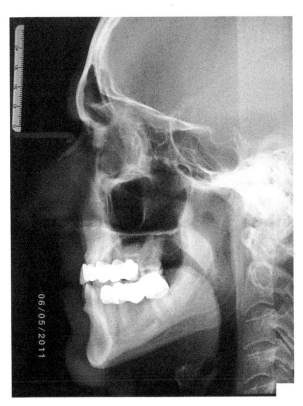

FIGURE 19.8 Lateral cephalograph of the patient upon completion of treatment.

after a 6-month follow-up, the patient's pronunciation was within acceptable boundaries.

Mastication can be measured by several means, including masticatory ability, efficiency, and performance. Masticatory ability is a subjective measure, a perception of how well individuals think they break down foods.[15] Several factors influence masticatory performance, including body size, bite force, number of functional tooth units, occlusal contact area, and malocclusions.[16–19] Although not as potent a factor as the mutilated dentition, malocclusions

can negatively affect individuals' ability to process and break down foods.[20] Malocclusions cause decreased masticatory performance, especially as it relates to a reduced occlusal contact area.[21] In this case, when the patient first came to our clinic, he reported a history of disturbed function of mastication as well as a history of TMJ pain. In more detail, he stated that he could only eat soft and pureed food because of unfavorable tooth relations, and because of the pain in the TMJ, which amplified when chewing tough foods. We decided to quantify this problem, by asking the patient to complete a questionnaire about his ability to chew different foods. He reported significant improvement in his ability to chew fresh carrots, steak, and other firm meats, on the VAS, after orthodontic-prosthetic therapy. He has also reported an improvement in his ability to chew or bite a whole fresh apple without cutting. This corresponds with the previously reported results.[20,38] This improvement is most likely caused by the establishment of functional occlusion, with a higher number and greater size of occlusal contacts.[39] The improvement was apparent 6 months after orthodontic-prosthetic treatment, which is significantly sooner than surgically treated malocclusion patients in which masticatory performance significantly increased only after a period of 5 years, as suggested in previous studies.[40,41]

CONCLUSION

On the basis of the presented clinical report, it can be concluded that class III malocclusion in an adult patient can be successfully resolved using a combination of orthodontic and prosthetic treatment in a relatively short time interval, even though the growth of facial and jaw bones ended long ago. It is necessary to comply with all phases of orthodontic and prosthetic treatment for the rehabilitation therapy to be a complete success. The presented patient suggests that patient age does not limit the success of therapy if he/she is diagnosed correctly and if an appropriate therapeutic approach is selected in the rehabilitation of complex dentofacial anomalies. Application of combined orthodontic-prosthetic rehabilitation procedures in a patient with a dentofacial anomaly restored his lost esthetics, phonetics, and masticatory function.

TABLE 19.3 **Angular Parameters for Cephalometric Teleroentgen Analysis Before and After Therapy**

Cephalometric measurements	Norms	Pretreatment	Posttreatment	Pre- & posttherapy changes
SNA	82°	83°	83°	0°
SNB	80°	84°	83°	1°
ANB	2° to 4°	−1°	0°	1°
NS/SpP	8 ± 3°	3°	3°	0°
NS/MP	33 ± 6°	29°	33°	4°
J/SpP	70°	67°	62°	5°
i/MP	80°	93°	93°	0°
Björk sum	396°	390.5°	394.5°	4°

REFERENCES

1. Kuntza TR, Staleyb RN, Bigelowc HF, et al: Arch widths in adults with class I crowded and class III malocclusions compared with normal occlusions. *Angle Orthod* 2008;78:597–603.
2. Bukhary MT: Comparative cephalometric study of class III malocclusion in Saudi and Japanese adult females. *J Oral Sci* 2005;47:83–90.

3. Anwar N, Fida M: Evaluation of dentoalveolar compensation in skeletal class II malocclusion in a Pakistani university hospital setting. *J Coll Physicians Surg Pak* 2009;19:11–16.

4. Hickey AJ, Salter M: Prosthodontic and psychological factors in treating patients with congenital and craniofacial defects. *J Prosthet Dent* 2006;95:392–396.

5. Uysal T, Usumez S, Memili B, et al: Dental and alveolar arch widths in normal occlusion and class III malocclusion. *Angle Orthod* 2005;75:809–813.

6. Jefferson Y: Orthodontic diagnosis in young children: beyond dental malocclusions. *Gen Dent* 2003;51:104–111.

7. Lin J, Yan Gu: Preliminary investigation of nonsurgical treatment of severe skeletal class III malocclusion in the permanent dentition. *Angle Orthod* 2003;173:401–410.

8. Doshi SS, Jayarama M, Gaikwad S, et al: Nonsurgical treatment of patient with class III malocclusion and missing maxillary lateral incisors: a combined orthodontic-prosthodontic approach. *J Contemp Dent* 2012;2:57–63.

9. Ueki K, Nakagawa K, Takatsuka S, et al: Temporomandibular joint morphology and disc position in skeletal class III patients. *J Craniomaxillofac Surg* 2000;28:362–368.

10. Laine T: Malocclusion traits and articulatory components of speech. *Eur J Orthod* 1992;14:302–309.

11. Hu W, Zhou Y, Fu M: Effect of skeletal class III malocclusion on speech articulation. *Chin J Stomatol* 1997;32:344–346.

12. Lee AS, Whitehill TL, Ciocca V, et al: Acoustic and perceptual analysis of the sibilant sound/s/before and after orthognatic surgery. *J Oral Maxillofacial Surg* 2002;60:364–372.

13. Ruscello DM, Tekieli ME, Van Sickels JE: Speech production before and after orthognathic surgery: a review. *Oral Surg Oral Med Oral Pathol Oral Radiol Endod* 1985;59:10–29.

14. Johnson NC, Sandy JR: Tooth position and speech—is there a relationship? *Angle Orthod* 1999;69:306–310.

15. Carlsson GE: Masticatory efficiency: the effect of age, the loss of teeth and prosthetic rehabilitation. *J Int Dent* 1984;34:93–97.

16. Fontijn-Tekamp FA, Slagter AP, van der Bilt A, et al: Biting and chewing in overdentures, full dentures, and natural dentitions. *J Dent Res* 2000;79:1519–1524.

17. Hatch JP, Shinkai RS, Sakai S, et al: Determinants of masticatory performance in dentate adults. *Arch Oral Biol* 2001;46:641–648.

18. Owens S, Buschang PH, Throckmorton GS, et al: Masticatory performance and areas of occlusal contact and near contact in subjects with normal occlusion and malocclusion. *Am J Orthod Dentofacial Orthop* 2002;12:602–609.

19. Buschang Peter H: Masticatory ability and performance: the effects of mutilated and maloccluded dentitions. *Semin Orthod* 2006;12:92–101.

20. English JD, Buschang PH, Throckmorton GS: Does malocclusion affect masticatory performance? *Angle Orthod* 2002;72:21–27.

21. Magalhaes IB, Pereira JP, Marques LS, et al: The influence of malocclusion on masticatory performance: a systematic review. *Angle Orthod* 2010;80:981–987.

22. Bhat VS, Gopinathan M: Reliability of determining vertical dimension of occlusion in complete dentures: a clinical study. *J Indian Prosthodont Soc* 2006;6:38–42.

23. Vesela M, Mikov A: Risk factors for development speaking disorders at praematurus. *Medicina Danas* 2009;8:330–339.

24. Ostyn JM, Maltha JC, van't Hof MA, et al: The role of interdigitation in sagittal growth of the maxillomandibular complex in *Macaca fascicularis*. *Am J Orthod Dentofacial Orthop* 1996;109:71–78.

25. Abdelnaby YL, Nassar EA: Chin cup effects using two different force magnitudes in the management of class III malocclusions. *Angle Orthod* 2010;80:957–962.

26. Yamada K, Hanada K, Sultana MH, et al: The relationship between frontal facial morphology and occlusal force in orthodontic patients with temporomandibular disorder. *J Oral Rehabil* 2000;27:413–421.

27. Sirabanchongkran S, Nimitpornsuko C, Pornthongprasert C, et al: Surgical treatment in skeletal class III malocclusion: a case report. *Kerala Dent J* 2002;5:45–54.

28. Singh GD: Morphologic determinants in the etiology of class III malocclusions: a review. *Clin Anat* 1999;12:382–405.

29. Goto TK, Yamada T, Yoshiura K: Occlusal pressure, contact area, force and the correlation with the morphology of the jaw-closing muscles in patients with skeletal mandibular asymmetry. *J Oral Rehabil* 2008;35:594–603.

30. Hashim HA, Sarhan OA: Dento-skeletal components of class III malocclusions for children with normal and protruded mandibles. *J Clin Pediatr Dent* 1993;18:12–16.

31. Uysal T, Sari Z, Basciftci FA, et al: Intermaxillary tooth size discrepancy and malocclusion: is there a relation? *Angle Orthod* 2005;75:208–213.

32. Tollaro I, Baccetti T, Bassarelli V, et al: Class III malocclusion in the deciduous dentition: a morphological and correlation study. *Eur J Orthod* 1994;16:401–408.

33. Ditschi D: Indication and potential of bonded metal-ceramic fixied partial dentures. *Pract Periodont Aesthet Dent* 2000;12:51–58.

34. Tahmina K, Tanaka E, Tanne K: Craniofacial morphology in orthodontically treated patients of class III malocclusion with stable and unstable treatment outcomes. *Am J Orthod Dentofacial Orthop* 2000;117:681–690.

35. In-Phill P, Seong-Joo H, Jai-Young K, et al: Post traumatic malocclusion and its prosthetic treatment. *J Adv Prosthodont* 2010;2:88–91.

36. Proffit WR: Combined surgical and orthodontic treatment. In Profit WR, Fields HW (eds): *Contemporary Orthodontics* (ed 3). St. Louis, Mosby, 2000, pp 674–709.

37. Slade GD, Diatchenko L, Bhalang K, et al: Influence of psychological factors on risk of temporomandibular disorders. *J Dent Res* 2007;86:1120–1125.

38. Henrikson T, Ekberg E, Nilner M: Can orthodontic treatment improve mastication? A controlled, prospective and longitudinal study. *Swed Dent J* 2009;33:59–65.

39. Fontijn-Tekamp FA, van der Bilt A, Abbink JH, et al: Swallowing threshold and masticatory performance in dentate adults. *Physiol Behav* 2004;432:431–436.

40. van den Braber W, van der Glas H, van der Bilt A, et al: Masticatory function in retrognathic patients, before and after mandibular advancement surgery. *J Oral Maxillofac Surg* 2004;62:549–554.

41. van den Braber W, van der Bilt A, van der Glas H, et al: The influence of mandibular advancement surgery on oral function in retrognathic patients: a 5-year follow-up study. *J Oral Maxillofac Surg* 2006;64:1237–1240.

20

ORTHODONTIC TREATMENT AND IMPLANT-PROSTHETIC REHABILITATION OF A PARTIALLY EDENTULOUS PATIENT

MILTON M.B. FARRET, DDS, MSD, PHD,[1] MARCEL MARCHIORI FARRET, DDS, MSD, PHD,[2] JHOSUÉ CARLESSO, DDS,[2] AND OSCAR CARLESSO, DDS[2]

[1]Department of Orthodontics, Federal University of Santa Maria, Santa Maria, Brazil
[2]Private Practice, Santa Maria, Brazil

Keywords
Orthodontics; implant-prosthetic rehabilitation; partial edentulism.

Correspondence
Marcel Marchiori Farret, 1000/113 Floriano Peixoto St., Santa Maria, RS 97015370, Brazil. E-mail: marcelfarret@yahoo.com.br

The authors deny any conflicts of interest.

Accepted November 19, 2012

Published in *Journal of Prosthodontics* October 2013; Vol. 22, Issue 7

doi: 10.1111/jopr.12033

ABSTRACT

This article describes the treatment of a 61-year-old man who had a completely edentulous maxillary arch and partially edentulous mandibular arch. The patient was orthodontically treated to correct an anterior crossbite by distalization of the mandibular teeth using a removable prosthesis serving as an anchorage unit. Subsequently, the patient received two zygomatic implants, five conventional implants in the maxillary arch, and six conventional implants in the mandibular arch. By the end of treatment, the convexity of the facial profile improved, and esthetic and functional occlusion was established.

Orthodontic treatment is restricted or sometimes even impossible in the case of partially edentulous patients due to difficulty in obtaining anchorage for tooth movements,[1] reduced periodontal support,[1] and presence of a prosthesis, which can interfere or prevent tooth movements.[2] Dental implants, which can be inserted and serve as anchorage units after osseointegration, can be used as an alternative treatment for such patients.[1–4] However, the site of insertion of the implant should be precisely defined, but it becomes difficult for patients to be treated orthodontically based on the necessity of dental movement during treatment.[2]

Early loss of the entire maxillary dentition results in loss of height and width of the alveolar bone,[5–8] thereby preventing the use of conventional implants for supporting the prosthesis. Zygomatic implants can be used as an alternative to ordinary implants when the bone area available for implantation is not sufficient to provide support for implants.[9,10] Currently, the use of zygomatic implants together with conventional implants is one of the best options for replacing maxillary teeth in patients with completely edentulous maxillae.[9,10]

This study presents the case of a 61-year-old patient who wore a total prosthesis in the maxillary arch and partial prosthesis in the mandibular arch, and who was orthodontically treated using implants and a prosthesis to achieve adequate posterior rehabilitation.

CLINICAL REPORT

Facial analysis showed that the patient had a straight-to-concave facial profile while wearing the maxillary prosthesis due to the presence of an anterior crossbite and accentuated projection of the mandibular incisors. The patient wore a complete denture in the maxillary arch and a partial prosthesis in the mandibular arch. All the anterior teeth (maxillary canines of the prosthesis) were in a crossbite with a class III canine relationship (Figs 20.1–20.3). Radiographic examination showed high resorption in the maxillary and mandibular alveolar bones from the natural teeth (Fig 20.4). The chief complaints of the patient were prosthetic instability and poor facial and dental esthetics.

The treatment was aimed at retracting the mandibular anterior teeth to correct the anterior crossbite to allow rehabilitation with implants and prostheses without the formation of a crossbite, thereby improving the facial profile of the patient. Furthermore, the molars were to be made upright to allow the insertion of mandibular implants at an adequate inclination and position. The option for bone grafting and conventional implants in the maxilla was disregarded due to extensive bone loss and need for large amount of graft, which would have a lower probability of success compared to the zygomatic implants.

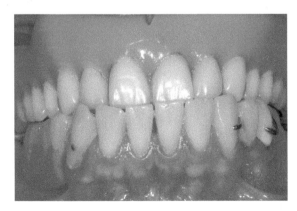

FIGURE 20.1   Initial intraoral frontal view.

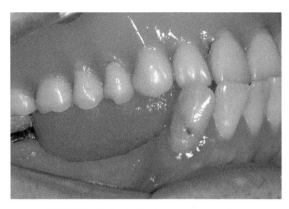

FIGURE 20.2   Initial intraoral right view.

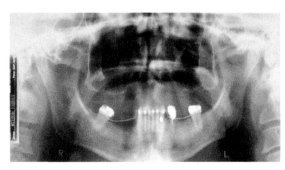

FIGURE 20.3   Initial intraoral left view.

First, orthodontic alignment and leveling were performed using 0.012-inch to 0.020-inch stainless steel archwires. Subsequently, the mandibular removable prosthesis was cut in the anterior region to allow distal movement of the anterior teeth. The posterior part of the prosthesis was used as an anchorage unit for keeping the molars in position. Initially, the canines were distalized using elastic chains connected to the molars. Subsequently, the incisors were retracted. After total distalization of the anterior teeth, the molars were made upright. The first step of the rehabilitation procedure was the insertion of six mandibular conventional implants (Straumann, Basel, Switzerland) measuring 4 × 18 mm (2 implants), 4 × 9 mm

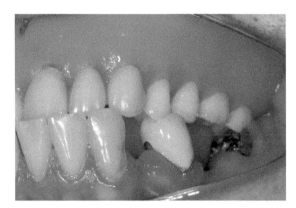

FIGURE 20.4   Initial panoramic radiography.

(2 implants), 3.75 × 11 mm (1 implant), and 4 × 11 mm (1 implant). Of the six implants, two were inserted close to the canines because of the availability of a large amount of bone area, another two were inserted between the molars and canines, and the remaining two were inserted closer to the molars. After 6 months, maxillary implants were surgically inserted using the original Brånemark technique for zygomatic implants. In this procedure, two implants (Straumann) measuring 4.0 × 5.0 × 50.0 mm were inserted in the zygoma, together with five conventional implants (Straumann) inserted anteriorly and measuring 3.75 × 13 mm (two implants), 3.75 × 13 mm (one implant), 4 × 18 mm (one implant), and 5 × 13 mm (one implant). After the surgery, a metalloplastic implant-supported temporary prosthesis was inserted and was worn until the metal-ceramic definitive prosthesis was delivered 6 months later. Occlusal contacts in maximum intercuspation matching the posterior centric occlusion were established in the temporary and definitive prostheses. Lateral canine guidance and incisal guidance were also established.

At the end of the treatment, the convexity of the facial profile improved, as shown in the lateral view (Figs 20.5 and 20.6) as a result of the lower anterior teeth retraction and new upper prosthesis with incisors positioned anteriorly and due to the correction of the habitual protrusive position and

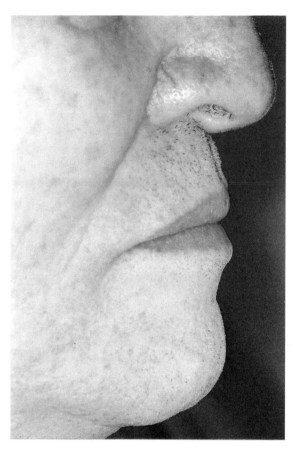

FIGURE 20.6   Posttreatment facial profile.

restoration of the occlusal vertical dimension. Functional occlusion was established with ideal intercuspation, good vertical and horizontal overlap, coincident midlines, and well-distributed posterior contacts (Fig 20.7). A fixed retainer made with 0.0195″ twist-flex stainless steel wire was bonded on the lower six anterior teeth. The posttreatment panoramic radiograph showed good parallelism among teeth and implants and good tissue health (Fig 20.8). The analysis 8 years posttreatment revealed excellent stability of the results and optimal periodontal tissue health (Figs 20.9–20.11).

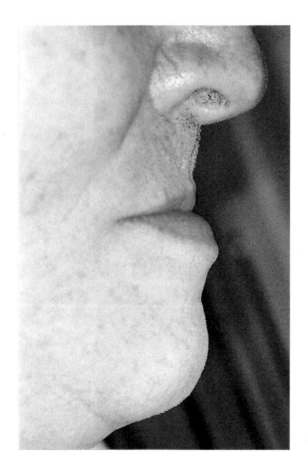

FIGURE 20.5   Initial facial profile.

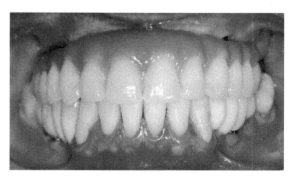

FIGURE 20.7   Posttreatment intraoral frontal photograph.

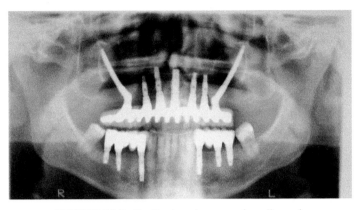

FIGURE 20.8   Posttreatment panoramic radiograph.

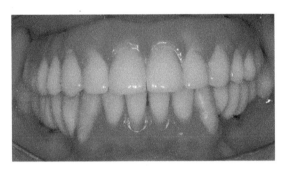

FIGURE 20.9   Intraoral frontal view 8 years after treatment.

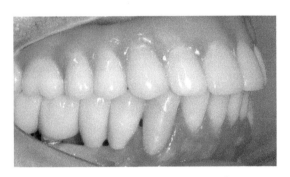

FIGURE 20.10   Intraoral right side 8 years after treatment.

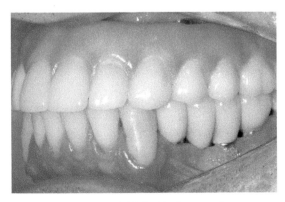

FIGURE 20.11   Intraoral left side 8 years after treatment.

DISCUSSION

Partially edentulous patients present a great challenge to orthodontists because anchorage is reduced or sometimes even absent in these patients.[2,7,11] Furthermore, loss of some teeth may cause inclination, rotation, and extrusion of the remaining teeth, thereby possibly jeopardizing the treatment and the reference for movements.[3] Moreover, the presence of a fixed and removable prosthesis might limit movements.[4] However, as in the present patient, the prosthesis may be used as an anchorage unit, thus facilitating the treatment.

For rehabilitation, mandibular implants were first inserted. Four of these implants were inserted near the canines and molars to take advantage of the larger amount of bone area available in these regions. After uprighting the molars, an osseous neoformation area was created because of the stretching of the fibers in the mesial region of these teeth.[12] This neoformation allowed the surrounding bone area to be used as an implantation site.[8,12] The mandibular right molar showed a slight inclination even after implant insertion. This was corrected using a combination of provisional crowns and by using the implants as anchorage units.[3] The region distal to the canines was another good site for implantation because the decrease in bone width and height was less in this region. Consequently, this region was also used as an implantation site. In the present patient, the implants were inserted very close to the canines. This implantation had to be performed very carefully to prevent contact with the canine roots.

Zygomatic implants are an alternative for patients with accentuated bone loss in the posterior region of the maxilla.[10,13] Normally, such patients are treated by reconstructing the large bones in the extraoral donor areas. This procedure always involves a certain degree of morbidity, high cost, and various biological risks beyond the control of the professional, which may lead to failure.[10] In contrast, zygomatic implants have a high success rate (approximately 97%).[9] Furthermore, using the zygoma as an implantation site reduces the need for conventional implants in the anterior region of the maxilla.

Correction of the crossbite and rehabilitation in the maxillary anterior region improved the convexity of the facial profile. The nasogenian sulcus, which was deep at the beginning of the treatment, flattened as a result of the rehabilitation. The upper lip was projected and vermilion border was more displayed. In contrast, the lower lip was retracted as a result of the retraction of the mandibular anterior teeth, thereby reducing the lower lip vermilion border displayed.

REFERENCES

1. Gallas MM, Abeleira MT, Fernandez JR, et al: Three-dimensional numerical simulation of dental implants as orthodontic anchorage. *Eur J Orthod* 2005;27:12–16.

2. Maruo H, Maruo IT, Saga AY, et al: Orthodontic prosthetic treatment of an adult with a severe Class III malocclusion. *Am J Orthod Dentofacial Orthop* 2010;138:820–828.

3. Drago CJ: Use of osseointegrated implants in adult orthodontic treatment: a clinical report. *J Prosthet Dent* 1999;82:504–509.

4. Moslehifard E, Nikzad S, Geraminpanah F, et al: Full-mouth rehabilitation of a patient with severely worn dentition and uneven occlusal plane: a clinical report. *J Prosthodont* 2011;21:56–64.

5. Salinas TJ, Sheridan PJ, Castellon P, et al: Treatment planning for multiunit restorations—the use of diagnostic planning to predict implant and esthetic results in patients with congenitally missing teeth. *J Oral Maxillofac Surg* 2005;63:45–58.

6. Vitral RWF, da Silva Campos MJ, de Andrade Vitral JC, et al: Orthodontic distalization with rigid plate fixation for anchorage after bone grafting and maxillary sinus lifting. *Am J Orthod Dentofacial Orthop* 2009;136:109–114.

7. Geckili O, Sakar O, Yurdakuloglu T, et al: Multidisciplinary management of limited interocclusal space: a clinical report. *J Prosthodont* 2011;20:329–332.

8. Capri D: Augmentation of an anterior edentulous ridge for fixed prosthodontics with combined use of orthodontics and surgery: a clinical report. *J Prosthet Dent* 2003;90:111–115.

9. Bedrossian E: Rehabilitation of the edentulous maxilla with the zygoma concept: a 7-year prospective study. *Int J Oral Maxillofac Implants* 2010;25:1213–1221.

10. Sherry JS, Balshi TJ, Sims LO, et al: Treatment of a severely atrophic maxilla using an immediately loaded, implant-supported fixed prosthesis without the use of bone grafts: a clinical report. *J Prosthet Dent* 2010;103:133–138.

11. Rose TP, Jivraj S, Chee W: The role of orthodontics in implant dentistry. *Br Dent J* 2006;201:753–764.

12. Mantzikos T, Shamus I: Forced eruption and implant site development: soft tissue response. *Am J Orthod Dentofacial Orthop* 1997;112:596–606.

13. Ferreira EJ, Kuabara MR, Gulinelli JL: "All-on-four" concept and immediate loading for simultaneous rehabilitation of the atrophic maxilla and mandible with conventional and zygomatic implants. *Br J Oral Maxillofac Surg* 2010;48:218–220.

21

PROSTHETIC REHABILITATION OF A CLEIDOCRANIAL DYSPLASIA PATIENT WITH VERTICAL MAXILLOFACIAL DEFICIENCY: A CLINICAL REPORT

KWANTAE NOH, DMD, MSD, PHD,[1] KUNG-ROCK KWON, DMD, MSD, PHD,[2] HYOWON AHN, DMD, MSD, PHD,[3] JANGHYUN PAEK, DMD, MS, PHD,[1] AND AHRAN PAE, DMD, MSD, PHD[4]

[1]Clinical Instructor, Department of Prosthodontics, School of Dentistry, Kyung Hee University, Seoul, South Korea
[2]Professor and Chairman, Department of Prosthodontics, School of Dentistry, Kyung Hee University, Seoul, South Korea
[3]Assistant Professor, Department of Orthodontics, School of Dentistry, Kyung Hee University, Seoul, South Korea
[4]Assistant Professor, Department of Prosthodontics, School of Dentistry, Kyung Hee University, Seoul, South Korea

Keywords
Telescopic detachable prosthesis; cleidocranial dysplasia; occlusal vertical dimension; maxillary hypoplasia.

Correspondence
Ahran Pae, Department of Prosthodontics, School of Dentistry, KHU, 1 Hoegi-Dong, Dongdaemun-Gu, Seoul, 130-701, South Korea. E-mail: ahranp@khu.ac.kr

The authors deny any conflicts of interest.

Accepted February 11, 2013

Published in *Journal of Prosthodontics* January 2014; Vol. 23, Issue 1

doi: 10.1111/jopr.12056

ABSTRACT

Cleidocranial dysplasia (CCD) is a rare congenital disorder characterized by skeletal and dental anomalies. This clinical report describes the prosthodontic approach to treating a CCD patient who presented with decreased facial height and relative mandibular protrusion due to maxillary hypoplasia after orthodontic treatment. Functional and esthetic rehabilitation was achieved using telescopic detachable prostheses in the maxilla and osseointegrated implants and metal-ceramic fixed dental prostheses in the mandible. These treatment approaches precluded the need for orthognathic surgical correction and presented a favorable prognosis during the 5-year observation period.

Cleidocranial dysplasia (CCD) is a rare autosomal-dominant skeletal dysplasia best known for its dental and clavicular abnormalities.[1] The most characteristic feature of CCD is hypoplasia or aplasia of the clavicles, resulting in hypermobility of the shoulders.[2] Patients with CCD tend to be of moderately short stature and have proportionally large heads with pronounced frontal and parietal bossing. A broad base of the nose with a depressed nasal bridge as well as ocular hypertelorism may also be observed. The face appears small in relation to the cranium due to the presence of hypoplastic maxillary, lacrimal, nasal, and zygomatic bones.[3]

Dental problems are a significant manifestation of CCD. Retained deciduous dentition, delayed eruption or retention of the permanent dentition, and multiple supernumerary teeth are common findings in CCD patients.[4] The maxilla is under-developed, while the growth of the mandible is normal, which results in decreased facial height and relative mandibular prognathism.[5] Growth variation of the stomatognathic system may influence the occlusal vertical dimension (OVD) in CCD patients.[6,7] Therefore, the treatment objectives of these patients must include restoring the OVD, establishing masticatory function, improving the patient's facial appearance, and improving the patient's psychological well-being.[8,9]

Regarding the dental treatment of CCD, different approaches have been reported over the decades. Treatment options are prosthetic replacement by complete dentures after extraction of the remaining teeth, overdentures that cover the remaining teeth, and surgical repositioning or transplantation of selected impacted teeth followed by prosthetic rehabilitation.[4,10–12] In recent years, the use of implants to support a removable overdenture or an implant-supported fixed prosthesis has also been reported in CCD patients.[13,14]

At a young age, treatment options involving combinations of surgical and orthodontic treatment are usually indicated.[2,8] Despite orthodontic treatment, decreased lower-third facial height and relative mandibular prognathism may often be present due to the underdeveloped maxilla.[3,5] Therefore, LeFort I orthognathic surgery is often needed to correct underlying skeletal discrepancies and to establish appropriate OVD after the alignment of all permanent teeth.[5,8,15] However, orthognathic surgery is not always feasible for patients with CCD, in which case the prosthodontic approach is the treatment of choice.

Although some cases of maxillary overdentures have been reported, no published reports use tooth-supported telescopic detachable prostheses on the maxilla to increase the OVD and to improve facial esthetics. In selected complex patients, telescopic detachable prostheses may be effective for cleaning or repairing localized failures without reconstruction. The purpose of this clinical report is to present an alternative treatment approach using a telescopic prosthesis for a cleidocranial dysplasia patient with vertical maxillofacial deficiency.

CLINICAL REPORT

Patient History and Chief Complaint

In 2005, a 27-year-old woman was referred from the Department of Orthodontics, Kyung Hee University for prosthetic consultation. The chief complaint was that her maxillary teeth were not visible during speaking and smiling.

The patient was first diagnosed with cleidocranial dysplasia, based on bilateral hypoplasia of the clavicles, the presence of an enlarged cranium, frontal bossing, failed eruption of permanent teeth, and presence of supernumerary teeth. She had previously undergone orthodontic treatment starting in 1993 for 8 years due to the complaint of mandibular prognathism. Rapid maxillary expansion with a hyrax and facemask was performed for 1 year to resolve the maxillary hypoplasia. The patient had undergone surgeries to remove all deciduous and supernumerary teeth and to expose the unerupted permanent teeth. The forced eruption of impacted teeth and leveling and alignment of both arches were completed by 2000; however, when she revisited the clinic after 5 years, an edge-to-edge state with posterior open occlusal relationship due to delayed mandibular growth was observed. She was interested in retreatment due to her esthetic and masticatory functional problems.

Diagnosis and Complaints

The intraoral examination presented class III malocclusion with an anterior edge-to-edge relationship (Fig 21.1). Occlusal contacts were present on the maxillary anterior teeth only. The maxillary central incisors displayed some gingival recession and grade 1 mobility. The maxillary right posterior teeth, mandibular right canine, and first and second premolars had been prepared, but not restored. The mandibular right first molar was missing. Brackets had been prepared on the left mandibular first and second premolars for vertical control. At clinical examination, the patient showed a severely decreased lower facial height and mandibular prognathism with significant overclosure in maximal intercuspal position (Fig 21.1). The maxillary teeth were not exposed when the patient attempted to smile. The interocclusal distance at rest position was 13 mm, and the general facial appearance improved with the mandible in the physiological rest position.

Cephalometric evaluation demonstrated decreased lower facial height, decreased mandibular plane angle, and sagittal and vertical deficiency of the maxilla with relative mandibular protrusion. The panoramic radiograph showed distinct features of CCD: the parallel-sided ascending ramus of the mandible, the upward-pointed coronoid process, and the downward-tilting zygomatic arch (Fig 21.2).

The goal of treatment was to improve facial esthetics by increasing the OVD in order to obtain an esthetic upper tooth/lip relationship and to achieve satisfactory masticatory function. To obtain these ends, LeFort I osteotomy followed by prosthetic rehabilitation was presented as a treatment option; however, the patient refused orthognathic surgery because of fear of extensive surgery. Therefore, the alternative treatment option was limited to prosthetic rehabilitation.

Treatment Plan

The treatment plan for the patient was divided into two phases. The first phase was the fabrication of the maxillary and mandibular interim prostheses to evaluate facial esthetics

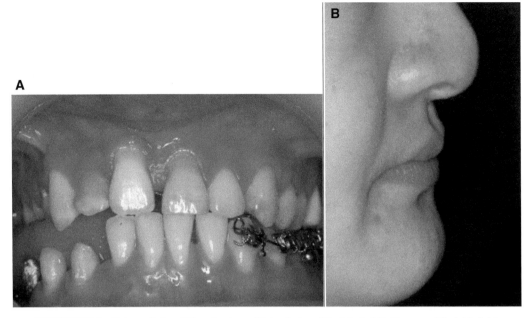

FIGURE 21.1   Intraoral view (A) and extraoral lateral view (B) at first visit. Decreased facial height, anterior edge-to-edge articulation, and posterior open occlusal relationship were present.

and function. Adequate OVD was to be verified after trials with interim prostheses. The second phase consisted of the fabrication of definitive prostheses. The prosthetic options considered for the mandible were implant-supported fixed dental prostheses (FDPs) for the missing teeth and metal ceramic restorations. The advantages and disadvantages of maxillary overdenture and FDPs as prosthetic options for the maxilla were considered. Facial parameters, such as lip support, smile line, and upper lip length, were evaluated with interim prostheses for decision making. The decision was to be finalized after evaluation of the interim prostheses.

Interim Prostheses Phase

To evaluate the appropriate OVD and masticatory function, a maxillary interim overdenture was designed to cover all the maxillary teeth. An impression of the maxilla was made using vinylpolysiloxane (VPS) (Silagum DMG; Chemisch-Pharmazeutische Fabrik GmbH, Hamburg, Germany) with a custom-made acrylic impression tray (OSTRON100; GC Co., Tokyo, Japan) and poured with type IV gypsum material (Fujirock EP; GC America, Alsip, IL). After the maxillary cast was trimmed, a record base and wax occlusion rim were fabricated. The optimal OVD was established with wax rim by evaluating the height of the upper lip, swallowing, and phonetics.[17-21] The wax rim was inserted intraorally, and an adequate OVD as well as the centric relationship and upper tooth/lip relationship were verified. As a result, the OVD was increased by 11 mm, measured from nose tip to mentum. The maxillary and mandibular casts were articulated on a semi-adjustable articulator (Hanau Modular Articulator System; Whip Mix Corp., Louisville, KY) (Fig 21.3), and denture teeth (Endura, Shofu, San Marcos, CA) were arranged.

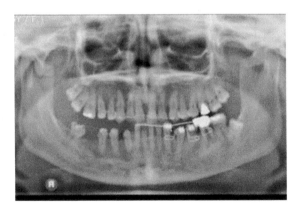

FIGURE 21.2   Panoramic view after orthodontic treatment.

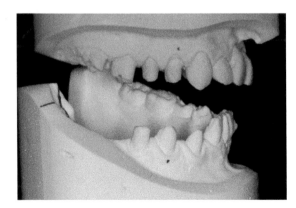

FIGURE 21.3   Increased OVD.

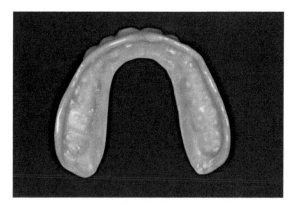

FIGURE 21.4   Intaglio surface of maxillary interim overdenture.

The mandibular left premolars were only partially erupted and presented spacing. The mandibular left first molar presented with an ill-fitting restoration and incomplete root canal treatment. Therefore, the incomplete root canal treatment was redone; these teeth also needed prosthetic restorations. The hopelessly compromised mandibular right second molar needed to be extracted, and implant prostheses were planned. Fixed interim restorations were fabricated for the mandibular teeth, and provisional cementation was done (Tempbond; Kerr; Orange, CA). Labial undercuts and the gingival region of the maxillary cast were relieved, and a maxillary interim overdenture was fabricated (Fig 21.4).

After insertion of the mandibular fixed interim prostheses and the maxillary interim overdenture, the patient adapted well to the increased OVD and experienced no functional problems. She was also satisfied with the esthetics of the interim prostheses while smiling, and her profile improved (Fig 21.5); however, she wanted an FDP as a definitive prosthesis.

For fixed interim prostheses, preparation was completed on the maxillary teeth via a 360° deep chamfer margin. Intentional endodontic treatment was done on the maxillary right and left central incisors. The maxillary interim

overdenture was relined intraorally with acrylic resin (Jet Acrylic; Lang Dental Manufacturing Co. Inc., Wheeling, IL) and trimmed (Figs 21.6 and 21.7). The interim prostheses were cemented with provisional cement (Tempbond). The patient was satisfied with the masticatory function and facial esthetics of the fixed interim prostheses. The decision to fabricate the definitive prosthesis was made based on these observations.

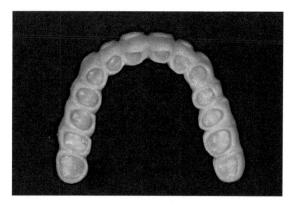

FIGURE 21.6   Intaglio surface of fixed interim prosthesis.

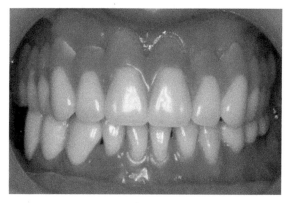

FIGURE 21.7   Frontal view of fixed interim prostheses.

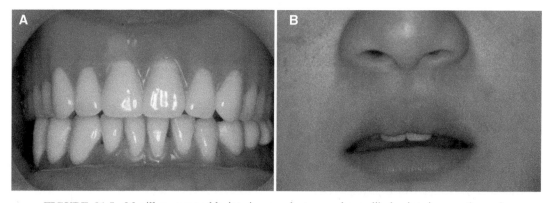

FIGURE 21.5   Maxillary removable interim overdenture and mandibular interim prostheses in place, intraoral (A) and extraoral (B) views.

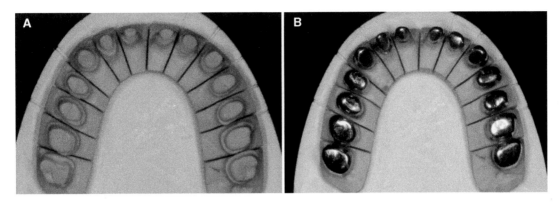

FIGURE 21.8 Definitive cast of maxillary arch. (A) Preparation for inner and outer telescopic crowns; (B) inner telescopic crowns.

Because the OVD was increased substantially to compensate the underdeveloped maxilla, the crown-to-root ratio of the maxillary teeth was increased as well. The crown-to-root ratio was increased to a maximum 2:1, and splinting of the maxillary teeth was considered to achieve stabilization against occlusal forces.

Stabilization of the maxillary teeth with fixed splinted restorations was considered inappropriate because of possible risk factors such as localized abutment failure. Splinting of telescopic restorations was considered to be as effective as that of FDPs. These restorations can be retrieved for repair and oral hygiene maintenance during long-term follow-up. Thus, a telescopic prosthesis was considered a better treatment option with promising results.

Definitive Restoration Phase

For implant placement, the patient was referred to the Department of Oral and Maxillofacial Surgery. Two dental implants (SLA® implants, Standard RN ø4.8 mm, 8 mm, and 10 mm; Straumann, Basel, Switzerland) were placed in the region of the mandibular right first and second molar, using a surgical guide. All implants had adequate primary stability at the time of placement.

Three months after implant placement, impressions of the implants and the prepared maxillary and mandibular teeth were made using a VPS impression material. A facebow transfer (Hanau Spring-Bows) and maxillomandibular relationship was recorded. The OVD of the interim prosthesis was transferred to the definitive restoration. The casts were articulated to a semiadjustable articulator.

The inner telescopic copings of the maxillary telescopic prosthesis were cast and milled to an average wall taper of 6° (Fig 21.8). After adaptation was confirmed intraorally, inner telescopic copings were cemented to the maxillary teeth with provisional cement (TempBond). A transfer impression of the telescopic crowns was then made using polyether (Impregum; 3M ESPE, Seefeld, Germany) in a custom-made acrylic impression tray.

An irreversible hydrocolloid impression (COE Alginate; GC America) of the interim FDP was also made and poured in type III dental stone (New Plastone; GC Co.), to be used as a guide to fabricate the definitive restorations. The abutments for the mandibular implants were selected (synOctaR Cementable Abutment; Straumann). Wax-ups for the maxillary telescopic prosthesis and mandibular metal ceramic restorations were done. The incisal length and position of the maxillary anterior teeth were determined from the interim prostheses. Full contoured wax-up was then cut back for the porcelain veneer and cast with a noble metal alloy (V-Supragold, Cendres + Metaux, Binne, Switzerland). After confirming the fit of the metal framework intraorally, a veneering porcelain material (VM-13, VITA Zahnfabrik, Bad Sackingen, Germany) was built up (Fig 21.9).

The final fit, esthetics, and lip support of the definitive prosthesis were verified. The inner telescopic crowns of the maxilla were cemented with resin-modified glass ionomer cement (GC FujiCEM; GC Co.). The superstructure was cemented with provisional cement (Tempbond). Abutments were placed on the implants in the mandibular right first and second molars and tightened with 35 N torque. Metal ceramic restorations for the mandible were delivered with resin-modified glass ionomer cement (GC FujiCEM). The occlusion was adjusted to present solid interdigitation, canine guidance, and consistent and regular occlusal contacts.

After delivery of the definitive restorations, harmonious vertical facial relations were achieved with a satisfactory nose/lip/chin relationship (Fig 21.10). A class I relationship was obtained. The patient was extremely satisfied with the treatment outcome. The patient received instructions on meticulous oral hygiene care. A strict 6-month recall regimen was maintained. To date, the patient has worn the prosthesis for 5 years and reported no complications (Figs 21.11 and 21.12).

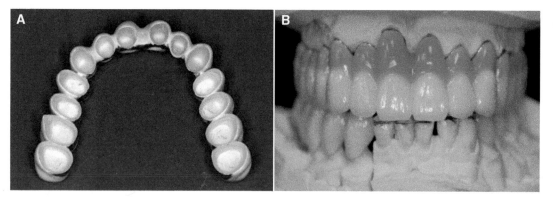

FIGURE 21.9   Definitive maxillary telescopic prosthesis; (A) intaglio surface; (B) frontal view.

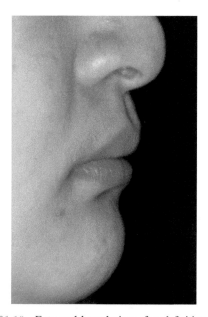

FIGURE 21.10   Extraoral lateral view after definitive prosthesis.

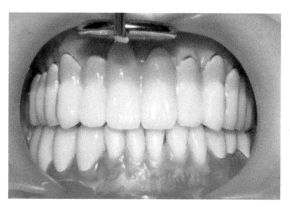

FIGURE 21.11   Intraoral view 5 years after placing definitive prosthesis.

DISCUSSION

This clinical report presents the prosthetic rehabilitation of a patient with CCD after orthodontic treatment. The treatment of dental abnormalities associated with CCD often requires multidisciplinary approaches with a combination of

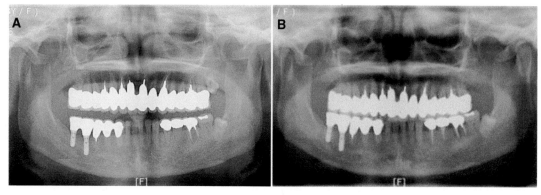

FIGURE 21.12   Panoramic radiograph; (A) after delivery of the definitive prosthesis; (B) 5 years after definitive prosthesis.

orthodontics, prosthodontics, and orthognathic surgical interventions. Despite orthodontic treatment, this patient presented a deficient lower facial height and unsatisfactory facial appearance because the underlying skeletal deformity had not been solved.

In treating this patient with decreased OVD, standard phonetic and esthetic criteria were evaluated to determine the appropriate OVD.[7,17–21] The patient's ability to adapt to the increased OVD was verified by an interim overdenture. The patient did not show any negative consequences to the increased OVD.

A maxillary overdenture covering the natural teeth could be a treatment option in this case. The advantages of overdentures compared with fixed prostheses include preservation of tooth structure and relatively low cost; however, there are disadvantages of overdentures as well. Caries tend to frequently occur because supporting teeth are isolated from normal salivary contact by the overdenture.[16] Occlusal wear of the overdenture can be a problem after long-term use. Here, the patient preferred an FDP to an overdenture. Facial esthetics and lip support were satisfactory with the fixed interim prosthesis.

Due to the increased OVD, the crown-to-root ratio was compromised for the fixed prosthesis. No objective criteria are yet identified to define the need for splinting in relation to violating the crown-to-root ratio.[22] However, splinting the maxillary teeth was considered to achieve stabilization against occlusal force. Splinting abutments may enhance stability and may significantly distribute horizontal forces.[23] A telescopic prosthesis was determined to be the treatment option. Inner telescopic copings were permanently cemented individually to the maxillary teeth, and then a detachable telescopic prosthesis (the superstructure) was cemented with provisional cement. Although this prosthesis requires complex laboratory procedures, there are many advantages.[24–27] The primary advantage of a telescopic prosthesis is retrievability. In patients whose remaining dentition is in a state of transition, the superstructure can be retrieved and repaired without reconstruction of the entire prosthesis. Also a telescopic prosthesis prevents cement leakage between the natural abutment and inner telescopic coping, because weaker provisional cement between inner coping and outer coping will fail prior to leakage. Satisfactory facial esthetics and function were achieved by the definitive telescopic prosthesis. At the labial surface of the telescopic prosthesis, a gingival portion was designed and added to provide lip and soft-tissue support, although the patient's smile line was low.

Throughout the follow-up period of 5 years, the patient maintained good periodontal health (Fig 21.11). The widened periodontal space on the mandibular left first molar that was initially successfully treated needs to be closely examined (Fig 21.12). Despite a poor crown-to-root ratio, mobility of the maxillary teeth did not increase. TMJ-related symptoms or mechanical complications were not noted, although the OVD was intentionally increased.

Mandibular right first and second molars and endosseous implants were placed for the missing teeth. Although CCD is a bone disorder caused by a defect in the gene that guides osteoblastic differentiation and bone formation, it has been reported that bone remodeling and osseointegration normally occur.[13,14] Stable osseointegration of the dental implants has been obtained in this patient, and no biologic complications were observed 5 years after implant placement (Fig 21.12).

SUMMARY

This clinical report describes an alternative prosthetic treatment option for a cleidocranial dysplasia patient with vertical max-illofacial deficiency. A telescopic detachable prosthesis with individual inner telescopic copings in the maxilla established masticatory function and improved facial esthetics. During 5 years of follow-up, there were no biological or technical complications. Telescopic detachable prostheses in patients with CCD can be considered as an alternative treatment option to orthognathic surgery or overdenture.

REFERENCES

1. Nebgen D, Wood RS, Shapiro RD: Management of a mandibular fracture in a patient with cleidocranial dysplasia: report of a case and review of the literature. *J Oral Maxillofac Surg* 1991;49:405–409.

2. Farronato G, Maspero C, Farronato D, et al: Orthodontic treatment in a patient with cleidocranial dysostosis. *Angle Orthod* 2009;79:178–185.

3. Jensen BL, Kreiborg S: Craniofacial abnormalities in 52 school age and adult patients with cleidocranial dysplasia. *J Craniofac Genet Dev Biol* 1993;13:98–108.

4. Winter GR: Dental conditions in cleidocranial dysplasia. *Am J Orthod Oral Surg* 1943;29:61–89.

5. Dann JJ 3rd, Crump P, Ringenberg QM: Vertical maxillary deficiency with cleidocranial dysplasia: diagnostic findings and surgical-orthodontic correction. *Am J Orthod* 1980;78:564–574.

6. Lux CJ, Conradt C, Burden D, et al: Three dimensional analysis of maxillary and mandibular growth increments. *Cleft Palate Craniofac J* 2004;41:304–314.

7. Pokorny PH, Wiens JP, Litvak H: Occlusion for fixed prosthodontics: a histological perspective of the gnathological influence. *J Prosthet Dent* 2008;99:299–313.

8. Becker A, Lustmann J, Shteyer A: Cleidocranial dysplasia. Part 1: general principles of the orthodontic and surgical treatment modality. *Am J Orthod Dentofac Orthop* 1997;111:28–33.

9. Berg RW, Kurtz KS, Watanabe I, et al: Interim prosthetic phase of multidisciplinary management of cleidocranial dysplasia: "the Bronx Approach." *J Prosthodont* 2011;20:S20–S25.

10. Weintraub GS, Yalisove IL: Prosthodontic therapy for cleidocranial dysostosis: report of case. *J Am Dent Assoc* 1978;96:301–305.

11. Kelly E, Nakamoto RY: Cleidocranial dysostosis—a prosthodontics problem. *J Prosthet Dent* 1974;31:518–526.

12. Jensen BL, Kreiborg S: Dental treatment strategies in cleidocranial dysplasia. *Br Dent J* 1992;172:243–247.

13. Lombardas P, Toothaker RW: Bone grafting and osseointegrated implants in the treatment of cleidocranial dysplasia. *Compend Contin Educ Dent* 1997;18:509–514.

14. Petropoulos VS, Balshi TJ, Balshi SF, et al: Treatment of a patient with cleidocranial dysplasia using osseointegrated implants: a patient report. *Int J Oral Maxillofac Implants* 2004;19:282–287.

15. Daskalogiannakis J, Piedade L, Lindholm TC, et al: Cleidocranial dysplasia: 2 generations of management. *J Can Dent Assoc* 2006;72:337–342.

16. Vertigo TJ: Prosthodontics for pediatric patients with congenital/developmental orofacial anomalies: a long-term follow-up. *J Prosthet Dent* 2001;86:342–347.

17. Willis FM: Features of the face involved in full denture prosthesis. *Dent Cosmos* 1935;77:851–854.

18. Turner KA, Missirlian DM: Restoration of the extremely worn dentition. *J Prosthet Dent* 1984;52:467–474.

19. Shanahan TE: Physiologic jaw relations and occlusion of complete dentures. *J Prosthet Dent* 1955;5:319–324.

20. Pound E: Let/S/be your guide. *J Prosthet Dent* 1977;38:482–489.

21. Silverman MM: Determination of vertical dimension by phonetics. *J Prosthet Dent* 1956;6:465–471.

22. Grossman Y, Sadan A: The prosthodontic concept of crown-to-root ratio: a review of the literature. *J Prosthet Dent* 2005;93:559–562.

23. Faucher RR, Bryant RA: Bilateral fixed splints. *Int J Periodontics Restorative Dent* 1983;3:8–37.

24. Langer A: Telescope retainers and their clinical application. *J Prosthet Dent* 1980;44:516–522.

25. Langer Y, Langer A: Tooth-supported telescopic prostheses in the compromised dentitions: a clinical report. *J Prosthet Dent* 2000;84:129–132.

26. Weaver JD: Telescopic copings in restorative dentistry. *J Prosthet Dent* 1989;61:429–433.

27. Breitman JB, Nakamura S, Freedman AL, et al: Telescopic retainers: an old or new solution? A second chance to have normal dental function. *J Prosthodont* 2012;21:79–83.

22

OCCLUSAL REHABILITATION OF PSEUDO-CLASS III PATIENT

Antônio Carlos Cardoso, dds, msc, phd,[1] Cimara Fortes Ferreira, dds, msc, phd,[2] Elisa Oderich, dds, msc, phd,[3] Moira Leão Pedroso, dds, msc, phd,[4] and Russell Wicks, dds, ms[5]

[1]Professor and Chairman, Department of Prosthodontics, Federal University of Santa Catarina, Florianópolis, Brazil

[2]Assistant Professor, Department of Periodontology, University of Tennessee Health Sciences College of Dentistry, Memphis, TN

[3]Assistant Professor, Department of Prosthodontics, Federal University of Santa Catarina, Florianópolis, Brazil

[4]Assistant Professor, Department of Prosthodontics, University Positivo, Curitiba, Paraná, Brazil

[5]Professor and Chairman, Department of Prosthodontics, University of Tennessee Health Sciences College of Dentistry Memphis, TN

Keywords
Occlusal adjustment; pseudo-class III; dental implant rehabilitation.

Correspondence
Cimara Fortes Ferreira, Department of Periodontology, University of Tennessee School of Dentistry, Dunn Dental Bldg, 875 Union Ave, Memphis, TN 38163. E-mail: cimarafortes@hotmail.com

The authors deny any conflicts of interest.

Accepted December 3, 2013

Published in *Journal of Prosthodontics* January 2015; Vol. 24, Issue 1

doi: 10.1111/jopr.12158

ABSTRACT

To treat a patient with anterior crossbite, the clinician should first assess if it is a genuine class III or a pseudo-class III malocclusion. Cephalometric analysis is important; however, registering a patient's centric relation (CR) is simple, quick, and costless and can play a decisive role in a differential diagnosis for this type of patient profile. This clinical report depicts a patient clinically diagnosed as class III. After mandible manipulation in CR, it was noted that the patient in question was a pseudo-class III. The treatment was based on the pseudo-class III diagnosis. Therefore, the patient was rehabilitated by occlusal adjustments and conventional and implant-supported prostheses and without the need for invasive orthognathic surgery.

The intermaxillary relation in Angle's class III malocclusion presents a diagnostic challenge. The causes of this type of malocclusion can be hereditary,[1,2] congenital,[3] or acquired.[4] Class III position is diagnosed through clinical, radiographic, and cephalometric analyses.[5]

Moyers suggested that pseudo-class III malocclusion was a positional malrelationship related to an acquired neuromuscular reflex.[6] In these cases, the occlusal analysis within the clinical exam becomes the key factor for diagnosis. Pseudo-class III malocclusion can be diagnosed by means

Journal of Prosthodontics on Complex Restorations, First Edition. Edited by Nadim Z. Baba and David L. Guichet.
© 2016 American College of Prosthodontists. Published 2016 by John Wiley & Sons, Inc.

of a cephalogram analysis, family history, molar and canine relationships at habitual occlusion and centric relation (CR), and dentoskeletal morphology.[7]

CR is recognized worldwide[6] and has been subject to broad discussions. The literature is vast on dental rehabilitations using CR as a starting point.[8–21] The use of CR as a diagnostic tool in full occlusal rehabilitation cases should be incorporated as part of a routine clinical exam practice.

There are two types of joint manipulation techniques: the chin point guidance[22] and the bilateral mandibular manipulation bilateral technique.[23,24] Both techniques are efficient and reproducible. The CR position is used as a diagnostic tool for differential diagnosis of true or pseudo-class III malocclusions.[25]

Pseudo-class III malocclusion is characterized by the forward shift of the mandible on closure, portraying a typical class III skeletal and dental pattern in maximum intercuspal position (MIP).[26] When the mandible is moved to the CR position, a class I skeletal pattern, normal facial profile, and a class I molar relation is present. With the mandible maintained in this position, the anterior teeth may be without contact, or in an edge-to-edge relation. A concurrent increase in the restored occlusal vertical dimension (OVD)[27] may be required, a clinically challenging rehabilitation. A clinical report of a patient presenting an apparent Angle's class III at the MIP position is described.

CLINICAL REPORT

A 55-year-old male patient (Fig 22.1) came to the Center of Continuing Education and Research in Implant Dentistry (Centro de Ensino e Pesquisa em Implantes Dentários [CEPID]) in the Department of Periodontology at the Federal University of Santa Catarina (Universidade Federal de Santa Catarina) for treatment. His chief complaint was the anterior position of the lower teeth and lack of posterior teeth, which compromised his esthetics and function.

After intra- and extraoral clinical exams, the patient was initially diagnosed with Angle's class III malocclusion. Periodontal examination was conducted, and the patient presented a highest probing depth of 3 mm. Clinical attachment loss ranged from 1 to 2 mm; bleeding on probing was absent. The periodontal diagnosis was chronic generalized slightly reduced periodontium. The patient had a history of tooth loss due to extensive carious lesions and to endodontically treated teeth that resulted in tooth fractures. Teeth #2, 3, 13, 14, 15, 18, 19, 20, 28, and 30 were absent at the initial appointment.

Despite the absence of most posterior teeth, the remaining occlusal contacts presented by the patient maintained the OVD in a position that allowed him to function with comfort. Next, the patient's jaw was manipulated in CR for differential diagnosis using the bilateral manipulation technique.[23] In

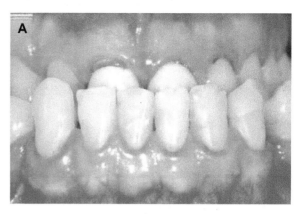

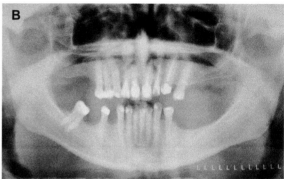

FIGURE 22.1   (A) Frontal view of patient in maximum habitual intercuspation. Note severe anterior and posterior crossbite. (B) Panoramic radiograph taken at initial appointment.

CR, there was contact between the right upper central incisor and the left central lower incisor, while the remaining anterior teeth were free from contact. Therefore, the OVD increased, indicating that the patient showed a pseudo-class III malocclusion. He was asked if his anterior crossbite was recent, and he stated that he always had the crossbite, which had always been a problem. The treatment plan was divided into two phases: preliminary and final. Alternative treatment options were presented to the patient at the initial consultation. The optimal treatment plan was dental implant rehabilitation for the missing teeth. Two additional treatment options were presented: (1) removable partial dentures (RPD) for the mandible and maxilla; or (2) combination of maxillary RPD with a mandibular fixed partial denture (FPD) from 27 to 31 and implant-supported prosthesis for 19 and 20. The patient rejected the last two options and chose the optimal treatment plan. He gave his informed consent to the treatment.

Preliminary Treatment

The master casts were mounted on a semi-adjustable articulator (Whip-Mix, 300 series; Whip Mix Corp., Louisville, KY) by means of a facebow. For the preliminary treatment

163

plan, an anterior stop CR record was fabricated. It is customary to use anterior deprogramming devices (permissive or restrictive splints), for example, Lucia Jig,[28] to deprogram the neuromuscular reflex. In this particular case, the anterior stop was made by the incisors, and therefore, the use of the Lucia Jig was not necessary. The dentist who prepared the record asked the patient to bite while conducting the bilateral mandibular manipulation technique. Next, the patient was asked to stay in that position to record the maxillomandibular relationship in CR with a thermoplastic bite wafer made from baseplate wax.

The preliminary treatment consisted of occlusal adjustment of premature contact using diamond tips (Intensiv; Grancia, Switzerland). During this process, other anterior teeth established contacts. Afterwards, occlusion was stabilized by means of light-cured composite resin (Filtek Z250; 3M/ESPE, São Paulo, Brazil) to add dental contacts in the anterior teeth and repair the incisal edges of the canine and premolar using adhesive technique for enamel[29] and dentine[30] (Fig 22.2). Invasion of the interocclusal space present after the occlusal adjustments and establishment of the occlusal contacts with composite resin were verified by asking the patient to say sibilant sounds without interferences. This space increased approximately 3 mm in the molar region. The patient did not use any provisional device to restore the absent posterior teeth. After adjusting the anterior guidance, canine disocclusion was established by occlusal adjustment, separating the posterior teeth during eccentric mandibular movements. The anterior horizontal overlap was 0.5 mm, and the vertical overlap was 1 mm. The patient received an anterior occlusal guard (AOG) in acrylic resin for routine use.[30] The use of occlusal splints to test the effect of change in occlusion on the temporomandibular joint (TMJ) and jaw muscle before extensive restorative treatment is recommended.[31] The AOG induces a therapeutic mandibular position that reduces stress in the disc/condyle complex.[32]

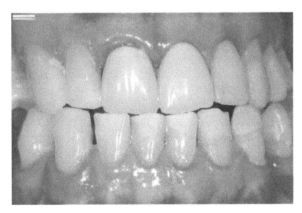

FIGURE 22.2 Frontal view of mandible in centric relation after occlusal adjustment and composite resin restoration of the incisal edges of the canine and premolar.

The AOG is typically placed in the maxillary arch with an anterior ramp. The ramp is designed to allow the disc/condyle complex to be altered temporarily while deprogramming muscle tone. The level of activation of the jaw elevator muscles decreases significantly during maximal clenching on an AOG with a bite ramp as compared to biting in MIP or clenching on a full-arch appliance.[33] Therefore, the authors indicate the use of an AOG customarily in extensive occlusal rehabilitations to protect the restored dentition. The patient was advised not to use the AOG constantly, but only when he was tense, to avoid the risk of over-eruption of the posterior teeth.

All of the aforementioned procedures were performed at the first dental visit. The patient was scheduled for the subsequent appointment 2 weeks thereafter.

In the second appointment, the patient showed a favorable response to the preliminary treatment outcome. He reported absence of TMJ discomfort or pain and expressed personal gratification. The outcome of the preliminary treatment was a stable occlusion and a more esthetic visual perception of the upper teeth.

Exams

Upper and lower casts were mounted on a semiadjustable articulator. A diagnostic wax-up and radiographic-surgical (RS) guides were fabricated. A cone beam computerized tomography scan was performed with the RS guides for analysis. Images showed the presence of sufficient bone for dental implant placement.

Definitive Treatment

External hex dental implants (Master Porous; Conexao Sistema de Protese; Sao Paulo, Brazil) were placed in the following sites:

- 3.75 × 11.5 mm: #2, 3, 14, 20, and 30;
- 3.75 × 13 mm: #28;
- 3.75 × 10 mm: #19.

In sites #13 and 14, the patient needed a sinus lift, which he refused. The treatment option of an angled implant for tooth #14 and an anterior cantilever for #13 was given, and the patient accepted. After the initial 3-month healing phase, a temporary implant-supported prosthesis and conventional prostheses were fabricated with thermo-cured composite resin according to the newly established vertical dimension reached after CR jaw manipulation and occlusal adjustment therapy.

Tooth #8 showed a questionable prognosis at the initial exam and resulted in root fracture at a follow-up appointment when it was extracted. The site was thoroughly debrided, decontaminated with tetracycline–HCl (at a 1:1 ratio with saline solution) for 3 minutes and thoroughly irrigated with saline solution. Next, a 5 × 13 mm implant (Master Porous) was immediately replaced. The implant-supported definitive prostheses were delivered 4 months after implants were activated with the interim prostheses. Meanwhile, the patient received a 4-unit temporary FPD. After the delivery of the first set of interim prostheses, an AOG was fabricated for use only at night.

The patient used the interim prostheses for a period of approximately 4 months. Castable plastic abutments with a metal collar (UCLA 056025; Conexão Sistema de Prótese) were used to fabricate crowns for sites presenting reduced interarch space. Additional occlusal adjustments were performed aiming to achieve more effective occlusal contacts. The patient's rehabilitation was adjusted and maintained to a canine guidance occlusal scheme. The patient was seen for monthly periodic adjustments and did not report any complaint for a period of 120 days. Impressions were made, and the casts were mounted in the articulator. Acrylic resin was placed in the incisal table, and customized with the guide pin to copy protrusive and lateral movements.

Porcelain-fused-to-metal conventional and implant-supported prostheses were then cemented, first on the maxilla and then the mandible (Fig 22.3). The horizontal overlap presented at the time of prosthetic delivery was approximately 1 mm. The patient's final profile remained the same as the profile registered at CR. The final OVD established after the delivery of the definitive prostheses was similar the initial OVD established after the initial occlusal adjustments were performed; however, 4 years after the definitive restorations were placed, a panoramic (Fig 22.4) radiograph shows stability of the peri-implant bone. The patient has not reported any pain or discomfort. Note that implant #30 could have been longer.

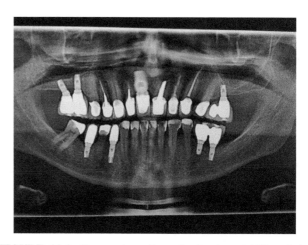

FIGURE 22.4 Panoramic radiograph showing stability of the peri-implant bone 4 years after final dental implant prosthetic delivery.

DISCUSSION

Pseudo-class III malocclusion occurs in less than 1% of the Caucasian population.[34] The treatment of this condition is approached early in life in order to correct the anterior displacement of the mandible by guiding the canines and premolars to erupt into class I with orthodontic therapy. In addition, early therapy provides a normal environment for maxillary growth and elimination of the anterior cross-bite.[35] This clinical report shows the management of an adult presenting pseudo-class III malocclusion. The patient did not report family history of pseudo-class III malocclusion. He did not receive early orthodontic therapy. The pseudo-class III malocclusion was diagnosed during the clinical exam while manipulating the patient's jaw to CR when the maxillary teeth were in tip-to-tip relation. This indicated that the pseudo-class III relationship was a positional malocclusion with an acquired neuro-muscular reflex.[6] The treatment option chosen by the patient was the least invasive; in addition, it showed more prompt results. After therapy, the patient functioned with more occlusal units anteriorly and posteriorly, eliminating the need for orthognatic surgery. This treatment option for patients who present the same diagnosis has been conducted for several patients at the CEPID with complete resolution and stabilization of the condition.

The postural rest position has a considerable range of adaptability to increases in the OVD; however, the range of comfort may vary considerably among individuals and even within a single individual under different conditions.[36] To evaluate if the temporized OVD was within the functional free space, interim prostheses were used to maintain the newly established OVD. They were fabricated with a slight overbite of approximately 1 mm, which established an anterior guidance to assist in posterior disocclusion. In addition,

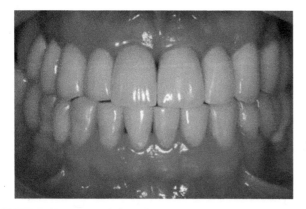

FIGURE 22.3 Frontal view of the porcelain-fused-to-metal definitive implant-supported and conventional prostheses.

an AOG was used to deprogram the muscle tone during the process of adaptation. In the present case, if the new OVD had caused pain or discomfort to the patient, the interim prosthesis would have been readjusted until a comfortable OVD was reached. The patient was followed up for 4 months prior to the delivery of the definitive prostheses to verify the muscular-articular behavior. The evaluation of the patient's response was favorable; therefore, the definitive prostheses followed the same parameters. The anterior guidance was then customized and transferred to the definitive prostheses.

There seems to be no apparent correlation between length of anterior cantilever and screw loosening; however, the ratio of posterior cantilever to the anteroposterior spread was significantly associated with screw loosening.[37] Therefore, an anterior cantilever was used in the FPD (teeth #13–14), to minimize or prevent screw loosening.

The association of malocclusions and occlusal interferences, as well as tooth contact patterns with clinical and subjective temporomandibular disorder (TMD) symptoms were studied.[38] The mechanical compression or tension of the TMJ is influenced by the magnitude of duration and adaptive capacities of the host.[39] Prolonged strains beyond the level of adaptation of the TMJ, the periodontium, and the dental occlusion, shifts in the fluids within the disc and retrodiscal tissues will result in an alteration of the architecture of the collagen and noncollagen proteins and ultimately a change in tissue morphology.[40] In the general population, TMJ disorders show a prevalence of 12% in clinical practice.[41]

Occlusal schemes have been discussed from different viewpoints; however, no scientific evidence encourages the use of one occlusal scheme over the other. Akoren and Karaagaçlioglu[42] compared the electromyographic activity of 30 individuals with canine guidance and group function. The patients were asked to chew gum during the electromyographic analysis. There was no statistical difference between patients presenting both occlusal schemes; however, canine guidance showed a narrower chewing model than group function, and reduced anterior temporal muscle activity during sliding. The authors suggested that in the presence of healthy canines, canine guidance occlusion would be preferable. In the presented report, canine guidance was selected as the occlusal scheme.

To our knowledge, this is the first report showing the management of adult pseudo-class III management with dental implant rehabilitation. Our rehabilitation strategy depended on the patient being able to be manipulated in CR; otherwise, the proposed treatment option would not have been available. The literature presents extensive management of class III malocclusion with an orthognathic surgery approach; however, we cannot determine if any of the reported cases could have been an undiagnosed pseudo-class III malocclusion.

CONCLUSION

It is known that there is only one "correct" diagnosis; however, there are several ways to treat a disease. For this patient, it is believed that the diagnosis was accurately reached, and that the treatment was properly performed. Other forms of treatment could have been proposed. For instance, orthognathic surgery, orthodontic treatment,[29] and the combination of these procedures in conjunction with prosthetic rehabilitations; however, such treatments would have been costly, traumatic, and certainly more time consuming. After the treatment was concluded, orthognathic and orthodontic treatments were no longer needed. Patient satisfaction in treatment outcome and comfort during therapy was our main goal.

REFERENCES

1. Xue F, Wong RW, Rabie AB: Genes, genetics, and Class III malocclusion. *Orthod Craniofac Res* 2010;13:69–74.
2. St-Jacques B, Hammerschmidt M, McMahon AP: Indian hedgehog signaling regulates proliferation and differentiation of chondrocytes and is essential for bone formation. *Genes Dev* 1999;13:2072–2086.
3. Delaire J: Maxillary development revisited: relevance to the orthopaedic treatment of Class III malocclusions. *Eur J Orthod* 1997;19:289–311.
4. da Silva Filho OG, Gomes Gloncalves RJ, et al: Sucking habits: clinical management in dentistry. *J Clin Pediatr Dent* 1991;15:137–156.
5. Ellis E, 3rd, McNamara JA, Jr: Components of adult Class III malocclusion. *J Oral Maxillofac Surg* 1984;42:295–305.
6. Moyers RE: *Handbook of Orthodontics*. London, Year Book Medical, 1988.
7. Rabie AB, Gu Y: Diagnostic criteria for pseudo-Class III malocclusion. *Am J Orthod Dentofacial Orthop* 2000;117:1–9.
8. Shanahan TE: Physiologic vertical dimension and centric relation. *J Prosthet Dent* 2004;91:206–209.
9. Kantor ME, Silverman SI, Garfinkel L: Centric-relation recording techniques: a comparative investigation. *J Prosthet Dent* 1972;28:593–600.
10. Lucia VO: *Modern Gnathological Concepts: Updated.* Chicago, Quintessence Publishing Co. Inc., 1983, p. 440.
11. Hobo S, Iwata T: Reproducibility of mandibular centricity in three dimensions. *J Prosthet Dent* 1985;53:649–654.
12. Wood GN: Centric relation and the treatment position in rehabilitating occlusions: a physiologic approach. Part II: The treatment position. *J Prosthet Dent* 1988;60:15–18.
13. Ash MM, Jr: Philosophy of occlusion: past and present. *Dent Clin North Am* 1995;39:233–255.
14. Tripodakis AP, Smulow JB, Mehta NR, et al: Clinical study of location and reproducibility of three mandibular positions in relation to body posture and muscle function. *J Prosthet Dent* 1995;73:190–198.

15. Rinchuse DJ: A three-dimensional comparison of condylar change between centric relation and centric occlusion using the mandibular position indicator. *Am J Orthod Dentofacial Orthop* 1995;107:319–328.

16. Utt TW, Meyers CE, Jr., Wierzba TF, et al: A three-dimensional comparison of condylar position changes between centric relation and centric occlusion using the mandibular position indicator. *Am J Orthod Dentofacial Orthop* 1995;107:298–308.

17. Baba K, Tsukiyama Y, Clark GT: Reliability, validity, and utility of various occlusal measurement methods and techniques. *J Prosthet Dent* 2000;83:83–89.

18. Keshvad A, Winstanley RB: An appraisal of the literature on centric relation. Part III. *J Oral Rehabil* 2001;28:55–63.

19. Keshvad A, Winstanley RB: Comparison of the replicability of routinely used centric relation registration techniques. *J Prosthodont* 2003;12:90–101.

20. Keough B: Occlusion-based treatment planning for complex dental restorations: part 1. *Int J Periodontics Restorative Dent* 2003;23:237–247.

21. Turp JC, Greene CS, Strub JR: Dental occlusion: a critical reflection on past, present and future concepts. *J Oral Rehabil* 2008;35:446–453.

22. Guichet NF: Biologic laws governing functions of muscles that move the mandible. Part I. Occlusal programming. *J Prosthet Dent* 1977;37:648–656.

23. Dawson PE: *Evaluation, Diagnosis and Treatment of Occlusal Problems*. St. Louis, Mosby, 1974, p. 633.

24. Cardoso AC: Oclusão Para Você e Para Mim. 1 ed. São Paulo, Editora Santos, 2003, p. 233.

25. Wood GN: Centric relation and the treatment position in rehabilitating occlusions: a physiologic approach. Part I: developing an optimum mandibular posture. *J Prosthet Dent* 1988;59:647–651.

26. Ngan P, Hu AM, Fields HW, Jr: Treatment of Class III problems begins with differential diagnosis of anterior crossbites. *Pediatr Dent* 1997;19:386–395.

27. Nakabayashi N, Kojima K, Masuhara E: The promotion of adhesion by the infiltration of monomers into tooth substrates. *J Biomed Mater Res* 1982;16:265–273.

28. Lucia VO: A technique for recording centric relation. *J Prosthet Dent* 1964;14:492–505.

29. Carlsson GE: Critical review of some dogmas in prosthodontics. *J Prosthodont Res* 2009;53:3–10.

30. Kochel J, Emmerich S, Meyer-Marcotty P, et al: New model for surgical and nonsurgical therapy in adults with Class III malocclusion. *Am J Orthod Dentofacial Orthop* 2011;139:e165–174.

31. Yadav S, Karani JT: The essentials of occlusal splint therapy. *Int J Prosthet Dent* 2011;2:12–21.

32. Maloney F, Howard JA: Anterior repositioning splint therapy. *Aus Dent J* 1986;31:30–39.

33. Fitins D, Sheikholeslam A: Effect of canine guidance of maxillary occlusal splint on level of activation of masticatory muscles. *Swed Dent J* 1993;17:235–241.

34. Nakasima A, Ichinose M, Nakata S: Genetic and environmental factors in the development of so-called pseudo- and true mesiocclusions. *Am J Orthod Dentofacial Orthop* 1986;90:106–116.

35. McNamara JA, Jr: Mixed dentition treatment. In Graber LW, Vanarsdall RL, Vig KWL (eds): *Orthodontics: Current Principles and Techniques*. St. Louis, Mosby, 1994, pp 507–541.

36. Rivera-Morales WC, Mohl ND: Relationship of occlusal vertical dimension to the health of the masticatory system. *J Prosthet Dent* 1991;65:547–553.

37. Brosky ME, Korioth TW, Hodges J: The anterior cantilever in the implant-supported screw-retained mandibular prosthesis. *J Prosthet Dent* 2003;89:244–249.

38. Mohlin B: Prevalence of mandibular dysfunction and relation between malocclusion and mandibular dysfunction in a group of women in Sweden. *Eur J Orthod* 1983;5:115–123.

39. Arnett GW, Milam SB, Gottesman L: Progressive mandibular retrusion-idiopathic condylar resorption. Part II. *Am J Orthod Dentofacial Orthop* 1996;110:117–127.

40. Harper RP: Clinical indications for altering vertical dimension of occlusion. Functional and biologic considerations for reconstruction of the dental occlusion. *Quintessence Int* 2000;31:275–280.

41. Carlsson GE: Epidemiology and treatment need for temporomandibular disorders. *J Orofac Pain* 1999;13:232–237.

42. Akoren AC, Karaaclioglu L: Comparison of the electromyographic activity of individuals with canine guidance and group function occlusion. *J Oral Rehabil* 1995;22:73–77.

PART V

MANAGEMENT OF PATIENTS WITH SURGICAL AND PROSTHODONTIC CHALLENGES

23

ALVEOLAR DISTRACTION OSTEOGENESIS OF THE SEVERELY ATROPHIC ANTERIOR MAXILLA: SURGICAL AND PROSTHETIC CHALLENGES

HANI BRAIDY, DMD[1] AND MARC APPELBAUM, DDS[2]

[1]Department of Oral Maxillofacial Surgery, University of Medicine and Dentistry of New Jersey, New Jersey Dental School, Newark, NJ
[2]Department of Prosthodontics, University of Medicine and Dentistry of New Jersey, New Jersey Dental School, Newark, NJ

Keywords

Distraction osteogenesis; anterior maxilla; atrophic alveolus.

Correspondence

Hani Braidy, Department of Oral Maxillofacial Surgery, University of Medicine and Dentistry of New Jersey, New Jersey Dental School, 110 Bergen St., Rm B-854, Newark, NJ 07101-1709. E-mail: braidyhf@umdnj.edu

Accepted April 9, 2010

Published in *Journal of Prosthodontics* February 2011; Vol. 20, Issue 2

doi: 10.1111/j.1532-849X.2010.00671.x

ABSTRACT

Significant maxillary anterior osseous defects are considered contraindications for fixed partial dentures. This clinical report discusses the surgical and restorative treatment protocol of a patient who sustained trauma to the premaxilla and was treated by distraction osteogenesis to provide an adequate restorative platform for an implant-retained fixed prosthesis.

HISTORY

Distraction osteogenesis (DO) is rooted in the 1940s and 1950s in Siberia with Dr. Ilizarov, a Russian orthopedic surgeon. Considered the father of DO, he treated World War II amputees with a revolutionary surgical technique that could "lengthen limbs." After performing a corticotomy in long bones, he would apply a four-ring distractor that could be activated several times a day after an initial healing interval of 5 to 7 days. The callus formed in the center of the corticotomy would then slowly be placed under the traction of the distractor, resulting in new bone formation (osteogenesis) over several weeks. In 1992, McCarthy et al[1] used this concept to treat hemifacial microsomia by distracting the mandible. In 1996, Block et al[2] subsequently described the first alveolar distraction in dogs, while Chin and Toth applied it to humans the same year.

Journal of Prosthodontics on Complex Restorations, First Edition. Edited by Nadim Z. Baba and David L. Guichet.
© 2016 American College of Prosthodontists. Published 2016 by John Wiley & Sons, Inc.

INDICATIONS FOR DO

The main indication for alveolar distraction is vertical augmentation of the ridge with or without soft-tissue deficiency. Compared to guided bone regeneration and onlay bone grafting, DO has proven to predictably gain more than 5 mm of alveolar height.[3,4,11] In addition to vertical bony growth, the mucosa also develops with a predictable increase of vestibular height. This technique may either be used to optimize esthetics in the anterior areas or to increase bony volume prior to implant placement in the posterior. Severe traumatic defects often result in complex multidimensional dentoalveolar and mucosal deficiencies best treated with a combination of DO and onlay bone grafting. In extremely atrophic areas, there may be minimal bone available to distract, requiring an onlay bone graft to be performed first. After 4 months of healing, the grafted area can then be vertically distracted. In cases where there is mild-to-moderate horizontal atrophy, the DO can be performed first, followed by an onlay bone graft.

CLINICAL REPORT

A 34-year-old male patient was first evaluated in the emergency department for maxillofacial injuries he sustained at work while operating heavy machinery. His medical history included an allergy to Penicillin and a history of tobacco use (one pack per day for the last 10 years). The upper anterior alveolus and teeth #7 through #12 were severely fractured and luxated, necessitating their extraction. After an initial healing period, he presented 12 weeks later for an evaluation, with the chief concern being replacement of the lost teeth. On examination, he had severe horizontal and vertical maxillary anterior alveolar deficiency (Fig 23.1), confirmed on a computed tomography (CT) scan reformatted with Simplant software (Materialise Dental, Leuven, Belgium) (Fig 23.2). The prosthetic options consisted of a fixed or removable

prosthesis. After carefully reviewing alternatives, complications, and benefits for each option, the patient opted for an implant-retained fixed prosthesis.

Based on our clinical exam, wax-up, and CT scan, it was determined that the patient's anterior maxilla needed to first be reconstructed with DO to gain vertical height, followed by onlay bone grafting to restore the deficient width. The patient underwent an anterior maxillary osteotomy with the placement of an alveolar distractor under general anesthesia. A Modus bidirectional distractor (Medartis, Basel City, Switzerland) with two independent central pins yielding vertical distraction of 0.25 mm per turn and a buccal tilt of 10° per turn was used. Through a vestibular incision, the distractor was first placed on the buccal alveolus and temporarily fixated before planning the osteotomies. Then, a horizontal and two divergent vertical osteotomies were carried out with sagittal and reciprocating saws under heavy normal saline irrigation with care to preserve the palatal pedicle prior to refixating the distractor (Fig 23.3).

After a latency period of 8 days, we began the distraction process at a rate of 0.5 mm/day. During a period of 36 days, the alveolus was vertically distracted a total of 10 mm; however, the activation was interrupted and decreased several times due to partial soft tissue dehiscence around the device (Fig 23.4). Ultimately, the dehiscence was primarily closed with nonresorbable sutures. In addition, the buccal segment was laterally tilted a total of 30°, split into three activations, spread 1 week apart.

During the activation period, it was also noted that the central pin, pulled lingually by the thick palatal tissue, impinged on the incisal surface of the lower anterior teeth. To remediate this situation, an acrylic occlusal splint was inserted on the maxillary arch accommodating the distractor to open the occlusal vertical dimension (OVD). Our patient was instructed to wear the splint continuously. Once the activation period was stopped, the pin was sectioned with a handpiece, and the occlusal splint removed.

Three months after removing the distractor, the patient was taken to the operating room for the placement of an onlay bone graft of the anterior maxilla using his anterior iliac crest as the donor site (Fig 23.5). Particulate cancellous bone chips were packed around the blocks and covered by a membrane. Then, a tension-free watertight closure was performed after releasing the flap and scoring the periosteum. A small bony dehiscence was noted 5 weeks later on the buccal aspect. It subsequently sequestered, and no treatment was needed.

After 5 months of graft maturation, a Simplant reformatted CT scan of the maxilla was repeated to plan placement of the implants. Despite marked graft resorption in some areas, it was determined that there was enough vertical and horizontal alveolar bone for fixture placement (Figs 23.6 and 23.7). Implants (Nobel Replace Select tapered, Nobel Biocare, Zurich, Switzerland) in the area of no. 7 (3.5 × 16 mm), no. 8 (3.5 × 13 mm), no. 9 (3.5 × 10 mm), no. 11 (3.5 × 16 mm),

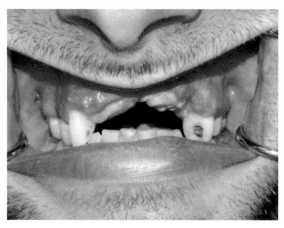

FIGURE 23.1 Vertical alveolar ridge defect.

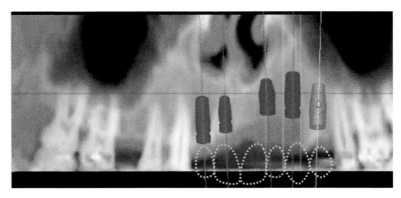

FIGURE 23.2   A panoramic reconstructed view of a CT scan. Note the apical position of the implants and the anticipated restorations. An unfavorable implant-to-crown ratio can be appreciated.

and no. 12 (3.5 × 13 mm) were placed (Fig 23.8). Although no implant threads were exposed, several buccal areas were noted to be very thin, prompting the need for localized guided tissue generation with Puros (RTI Biologics, Alachua, FL) covered with a Bio-Gide membrane (Osteohealth, Shirley, NY).

After a total of 6 months of integration, the implants were uncovered, and healing abutments placed. All implants were noted to be stable when manually torqued at 35 N cm before abutments were placed.

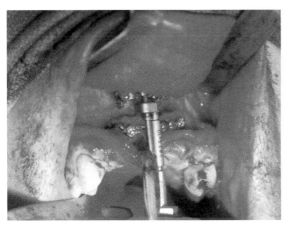

FIGURE 23.3   Osteotomies and the placement of the distractor.

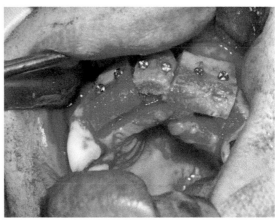

FIGURE 23.5   Anterior iliac crest bone graft to the maxilla. The blocks were subsequently rounded, and cancellous bone was added.

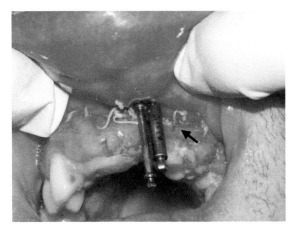

FIGURE 23.4   Intraoral photograph taken 13 days post-operatively, demonstrating a soft-tissue dehiscence around the device (black arrow).

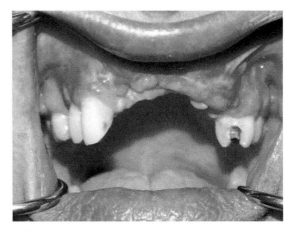

FIGURE 23.6   Morphology of the ridge 5 months after bone grafting. Note the improved vertical dimension of the alveolus (refer to Fig 23.1).

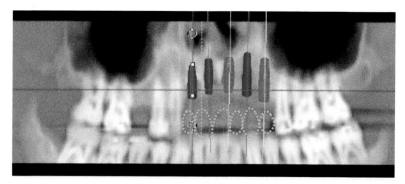

FIGURE 23.7   A panoramic reconstructed view of a CT scan taken 5 months after bone graft of the maxilla. Note the improved apico-coronal position of the implants and the anticipated restorations. An enhanced implant-to-crown ratio can be appreciated (refer to Fig 23.2).

The prosthodontic reconstructive phase of care consisted of a reevaluation of the implant fixture positions and axial inclinations, as well as the interarch distance and centric relation position of the mandible. The posterior maxillary teeth manifested neither mobility nor periodontal pocketing and were devoid of any significant restorative procedures. An Angle Class I molar relationship was present, and the centric relation and maximum intercuspation positions were coincident.

Closed tray impression copings were placed, radiographed, and stabilized with carbide burs luted to the copings with Triad Gel (Dentsply International, York, PA). The fixture level full-arch impression was made using polyvinyl siloxane (PVS) (Honigum, DMG, Hamburg, Germany). A facebow record facilitated the mounting of the maxillary cast to an arcon articulator (Teledyne Combi, Whip Mix, Louisville, KY). A wax interocclusal record was used to articulate the mandibular cast at the same vertical dimension. A diagnostic full-contour wax-up with labial flange incorporating temporary abutments was fabricated. The try-in allowed for evaluation and correction of lip support and incisal edge position in three planes. With the patient's approval of the esthetic arrangement of the teeth and flange-contour, the wax-up was transferred back to the master cast, and a labial

and lingual PVS lab putty (Sil-Tech Ivoclar, Buffalo, NY) index was made.

Although the anterior ridge height and width had been significantly enhanced, a labial flange on the fixed prosthesis was necessary to create a confluence from the natural dentition to the prosthetic replacement. Furthermore, to facilitate retrievability and removal during periodic prophylaxis, a screw-retained restoration was fabricated.

The framework was waxed in two segments, and at the try-in appointment, after radiographic verification of fit, the segments were luted with GC Pattern resin (GC America, Alsip, IL). The implant fixture in the area of the left central incisor (#9) was palatal to the arch (Fig 23.9). Porcelain was baked to the metal substructure in the area of the teeth. The labial and proximal soft tissue contours were reestablished with a resin flange (Figs 23.10 and 23.11). When reviewing tooth contours and shade, the patient brought photographs of himself prior to the accident but requested that the shade of the prosthetic teeth be lighter and more vibrant than his adjacent or opposing teeth.

The implant-retained fixed partial prosthesis was equilibrated in all excursions, ensuring an atraumatic mutually protected occlusal scheme. The prosthesis was repolished, and the setscrews were tightened to 20 N cm. The screw

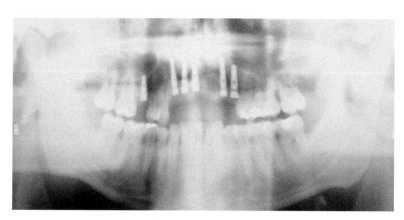

FIGURE 23.8   Panoramic radiograph depicting position of implants.

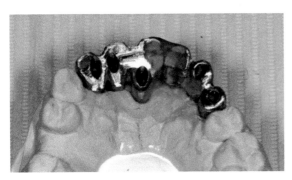

FIGURE 23.9 Cast metal substructure fabricated in two sections, luted with GC resin. Note the fixture in the #9 position is offset lingually.

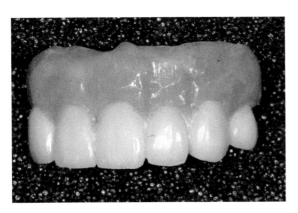

FIGURE 23.10 Porcelain baked to the tooth contours and soft tissue developed with a resin flange.

access holes were sealed with pellets of cotton and Tempit L/C (Centrix Corp., Shelton, CT). The patient has been followed for 6 months with no clinical complications (Fig 23.12). Radiographs of these implants will be taken every 18 months for the next 5 years to monitor bone resorption.

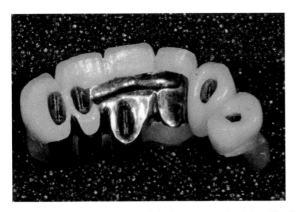

FIGURE 23.11 Lingual view of the implant-retained fixed bridge with metal incisal stops.

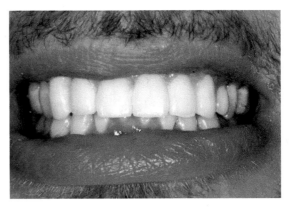

FIGURE 23.12 Frontal view of definitive prosthesis 6 months postinsertion.

DISCUSSION

As with any patient requiring dental implants to replace missing teeth, careful examination and treatment planning are critical. In extensive defects, a CT scan with a barium-coated radiographic guide may be used to evaluate ridge morphology, the vector of distraction, and the location of osteotomies in relation to neighboring roots, maxillary sinus, nasal cavity, inferior alveolar nerve, and inferior mandibular border. The segment being distracted should be at least 4 mm in height to prevent its resorption during the distraction phase. In the mandible, more than 9 mm of intact residual inferior border is necessary to prevent fractures.[5–9] To prevent damaging the adjacent teeth, the osteotomies are made 2 mm from the roots.

Careful assessment of occlusion is also critical to avoid interferences with the central pin protruding in the vestibule. When distracting the anterior maxilla, the pin may sometimes be camouflaged by a temporary prosthesis. Patient compliance is essential since the patient is responsible for activating the device two to three times per day by turning the pin clockwise. If this is not performed for a few days, there may be a risk for premature consolidation of the segments. Multiple follow-up appointments are recommended during the distraction phase to monitor the progress and treat occasional dehiscences of the devices or correct vector discrepancy.

In the case presented, we obtained approximately 5 mm of vertical augmentation and 3 mm of horizontal increase in the area of #7 through #12, as confirmed on the preimplant placement scans (Fig 23.7). The discrepancy between the initial amount of alveolus distracted (10 mm) and noted 5 months postgrafting (5 mm) is due to the prolonged treatment interval between the removal of the distractor and the placement of implants (9.5 months). In situations where no secondary grafting is needed, implants are usually placed at the time of distractor removal, thus minimizing the risks of resorption. Clinically, this bone loss translated into slight increase in crown-to-implant ratio.

Despite the great predictability of alveolar DO,[12-15] a high rate of surgical complications has been reported. In a comprehensive analysis of 37 patients with 45 ridge deficiencies, Enislidis et al[10] described a complication rate of 75.7%. The majority of these complications were categorized as "minor," and included soft-tissue dehiscences (37.8% of distracted sites), tilting of the segments, or occlusal interferences that did not impact adversely on implant survival (95.7%); however, "major" complications (21.6%) were reported as well, such as fracture of basal bone or the transport segment, breakage of the distractor, and severe mechanical problems, all resulting in treatment discontinuation.

In the clinical report presented, the patient experienced multiple minor complications during this multidisciplinary treatment plan. The soft-tissue dehiscence we experienced during the distraction period caused a total delay of more than 2 weeks and an additional surgical procedure to primarily close the site. Careful incision planning and good homecare can help prevent this complication. Unfortunately, the patient dehisced once again, 5 weeks postonlay bone grafting, resulting in partial loss of the graft and, ultimately, resulting in the palatal positioning of the fixtures.

Occlusal interferences by the central pin impinging on the lower incisors were also encountered in this case. To prevent excess trauma to the device, an acrylic occlusal splint was fabricated and inserted to slightly increase the OVD. Once the distraction phase was completed, the central pin was sectioned, relieving the occlusion. This minor complication is best avoided by careful preoperative planning, the use of articulated models, and precise placement of the device.[5] Orthodontic treatment and tilting of the segment can be achieved to relieve the occlusal interferences caused by a malposed distractor central pin.[10]

CONCLUSION

This case illustrates the multidimensional alveolar deficit frequently encountered after trauma and the different treatment modalities required to provide adequate site development for an implant-retained restoration. The vertical deficiency was first addressed with alveolar DO, followed by onlay bone grafting to correct the compromised width. Proper treatment planning, in conjunction with careful surgical technique and precise prosthetic rehabilitation are keys to minimizing complications and assuring long-term treatment success. DO is a viable treatment modality to expand the height of the residual ridge. This procedure does have several clinically limiting conditions and is not suitable for all patients. Careful consideration must be given to achieve proper lip support and lingual tooth morphology to ensure acceptable esthetics and anterior guidance.

REFERENCES

1. McCarthy JG, Schreiber J, Karp N, et al: Lengthening the human mandible by gradual distraction. *Plast Reconstr Surg* 1992;89:1-8; discussion 9-10.
2. Block MS, Chang A, Crawford C: Mandibular alveolar ridge augmentation in the dog using distraction osteogenesis. *J Oral Maxillofac Surg* 1996;54:309-314.
3. Chiapasco M, Romeo E, Casentini P, et al: Alveolar distraction osteogenesis vs. vertical guided bone regeneration for the correction of vertically deficient edentulous ridges: a 1-3-year prospective study on humans. *Clin Oral Implants Res* 2004;15:82-95.
4. Chiapasco M, Zaniboni M, Rimondini L: Autogenous onlay bone grafts vs. alveolar distraction osteogenesis for the correction of vertically deficient edentulous ridges: a 2-4-year prospective study on humans. *Clin Oral Implants Res* 2007;18:432-440.
5. Soares M: Alveolar distraction in the class V and VI edentulous mandible. In Jensen OT (ed): *Alveolar Distraction Osteogenesis.* Chicago, IL, Quintessence, 2002, pp. 77-88.
6. Lin Y, Wang X, Li J, et al: Clinical study of alveolar vertical distraction osteogenesis for implant. *Zhonghua Kou Qiang Yi Xue Za Zhi* 2002;37:253-256.
7. Garcia AG, Martin MS, Vila PG, et al: Minor complications arising in alveolar distraction osteogenesis. *J Oral Maxillofac Surg* 2002;60:496-501.
8. Fukuda M, Iino M, Ohnuki T, et al: Vertical alveolar distraction osteogenesis with complications in a reconstructed mandible. *J Oral Implantol* 2003;29:185-188.
9. Van Strijen PJ, Breuning KH, Becking AG, et al: Complications in bilateral mandibular distraction osteogenesis using internal devices. *Oral Surg Oral Med Oral Pathol Oral Radiol Endod* 2003;96:392-397.
10. Enislidis G, Fock N, Millesi-Schobel G, et al: Analysis of complications following alveolar distraction osteogenesis and implant placement in the partially edentulous mandible. *Oral Surg Oral Med Oral Pathol Oral Radiol Endod* 2005;100:25-30.
11. Saulacic N, Iizuka T, Martin MS, et al: Alveolar distraction osteogenesis: a systematic review. *Int J Oral Maxillofac Surg* 2008;37:1-7.
12. Rocchietta I, Fontana F, Simion M: Clinical outcomes of vertical bone augmentation to enable dental implant placement: a systematic review. *J Clin Periodontol* 2008;35:203-215.
13. Chiapasco M, Consolo U, Bianchi A, et al: Alveolar distraction osteogenesis for the correction of vertically deficient edentulous ridges: a multicenter prospective study on humans. *Int J Oral Maxillofac Implants* 2004;19:399-407.
14. Klug CN, Millesi-Schobel GA, Millesi W, et al: Preprosthetic vertical distraction osteogenesis of the mandible using an L-shaped osteotomy and titanium membranes for guided bone regeneration. *J Oral Maxillofac Surg* 2001;59:1302-1308.
15. Rachmiel A, Srouji S, Peled M: Alveolar ridge augmentation by distraction osteogenesis. *Int J Oral Maxillofac Surg* 2001;30:510-517.

24

REHABILITATION OF A COMPLETELY EDENTULOUS PATIENT WITH NONREDUCIBLE BILATERAL ANTERIOR DISLOCATION OF THE TEMPOROMANDIBULAR JOINT: A PROSTHODONTIC CHALLENGE—CLINICAL REPORT

MOATH MOMANI, BDS, MCLINDENT,[1,2,*] MOHAMED-NUR ABDALLAH, BDS, MSC,[2,1*]
DERAR AL-SEBAIE, BDS, MCLINDENT[1], AND FALEH TAMIMI, BDS, MSC, PHD[2]

[1]Royal Medical Services, Jordanian Armed Forces, Amman, Jordan
[2]Division of Restorative Dentistry, Faculty of Dentistry, McGill University, Montreal, Québec Canada

Keywords
Temporomandibular joint; bilateral anterior dislocation.

Correspondence
Faleh Tamimi, Room M/64, Faculty of Dentistry, McGill University, 3640 University St., Montreal, Québec H3A 0C7, Canada. E-mail: faleh.tamimimarino@mcgill.ca

* Both authors contributed equally.

Financial support from the Jordanian Armed Forces-Royal Medical Services, the Faculty of Dentistry of McGill University, and the Network for Oral and Bone Health Research (RSBO) (grant No. 5213).

The authors have no conflict of interest to declare.

Accepted February 2, 2015

Published in *Journal of Prosthodontics* July 2015

doi: 10.1111/jopr.12318

ABSTRACT

Nonreduced bilateral anterior dislocation of the temporomandibular joint (TMJ) is an extremely rare condition, and its prosthodontic rehabilitation is a clinical challenge, especially in patients who refuse to or cannot undergo surgery. There are no previous clinical reports of successful or standardized prosthetic rehabilitation approaches for patients with this condition. This clinical report describes the successful prosthodontic management of an edentulous patient with nonreduced bilateral anterior dislocation of the TMJ.

Typically, at rest, the condyle of the mandible is positioned in the most superior-posterior region of the glenoid fossa, and at maximum opening, the 12 o'clock position of the condyle is at the most inferior aspect of articular eminence on the zygomatic process of the temporal bone. Dislocation of the temporomandibular joint (TMJ) can be defined as the displacement of the head of the condyle from its normal position, and it can be partial (subluxation) or complete (luxation).[1] Subluxation is common and occurs mostly in patients with hypermobile joints. It may never cause any problems to the patients, and the joint always gets self-reduced back to its normal position by the patient upon closing the mouth. On the other hand, anterior dislocation occurs when the condyle is displaced anteriorly to the articular eminence and cannot be reduced by the patient.[2] Bilateral anterior dislocation of the TMJ is a rare condition most likely to occur in elderly, medically compromised, and edentulous patients,[3] with few clinical reports in the literature.[4-6]

The management approach of TMJ dislocations varies according to type of dislocation and its underlying cause. Various conservative and surgical methods have been described for managing TMJ dislocations.[1] The most conservative and first treatment option, especially in acute dislocations, is the manual reduction of the dislocated TMJ. Manual reduction can be done under local or general anesthesia, or analgesic control with or without sedation.[1] However, manual reduction frequently fails in patients with chronic dislocations who end up requiring alternative nonsurgical or surgical treatment modalities.[2,7]

Alternative nonsurgical techniques include intramuscular injection of botulinum toxin type A into the muscles of mastication to reduce muscular activity,[8,9] or intracapsular injection of a sclerosing agent (i.e., alcohol, rivanol, 5% sodium psylliate) or autologous blood[10,11] to induce fibrosis and limit jaw movement; however, these injections are not routinely used because the extent of their effect cannot be controlled and are contraindicated in patients with certain medical conditions.[1,8,12] In addition, the use of autologous blood is still debatable in young patients or those suffering from rheumatoid arthritis and articular degenerative diseases.[12-14] Other nonsurgical methods include using occlusal splints, physiotherapy (i.e., articular mobilization and home exercise programs) and intermaxillary fixation (IMF).[15,16]

Nonsurgical methods are not always successful in the treatment of chronic TMJ dislocations, and multiple surgical interventions have been tried, including osteotomy procedures (i.e., osteotomy of the articular eminence, mandibular ramus or coronoid process, and Dautrey's procedure) and grafting procedures to augment the articular eminence or restitute the capsular ligament.[1,12,17] These surgical procedures are invasive and not recommended for patients with significant comorbidities that render them unfit for surgery and/or general anesthesia. Moreover, these alternative nonsurgical and surgical interventions do not guarantee success, and the dislocation may relapse, leaving patients with the sole option of coping with the TMJ condition.[7]

In this clinical report, we describe the prosthodontic management of an edentulous patient with nonreducible bilateral anterior dislocation of the TMJ as a possible palliative treatment option. The prosthodontic management of these patients is a particularly challenging task and, to the best of the authors' knowledge, there are no previous clinical reports describing their prosthodontic management.

CLINICAL REPORT

Referral Details and History

An 83-year-old female patient was referred to the prosthodontic department of the hospital for complete denture fabrication, as she was fully edentulous without any previous maxillary or mandibular complete dentures. She had a history of cerebrovascular disease and chronic hypertension. Moreover, she had a previous history of pain in the TMJ area with recurrent dislocations. The patient was first referred by a dental clinic to the maxillofacial department of the nearest hospital because they were not able to reduce her TMJ into place. One week after the dislocation incident and during the first visit to the maxillofacial clinic, the patient complained of tenderness to palpitation in the periauricular region and difficulty opening her mouth and chewing food. She reported that before this incident she had previous episodes of dislocations in her TMJ and that she was always able to reduce the joint either by herself or by visiting a dental clinic; however, the dislocations were becoming more frequent and painful. After clinical and radiographic examination (panoramic radiograph and computed tomography [CT]), the patient was diagnosed with bilateral anterior dislocation of the TMJ. Three nonsurgical attempts for manual reduction of the dislocated joint were performed, but they all were unsuccessful. The first attempt was made after administering a muscle relaxant; 2 weeks later, a second attempt was performed under sedation, and the third and last attempt was performed under general anesthesia 1 week later. Although the patient suffered from severe pain in her TMJ during movement, she refused to undergo any further attempts to reduce her TMJ. After a month from the last reduction attempt, she suffered from severe malnutrition because she was not able to chew or eat properly and was hospitalized for IV solution intake for 3 weeks. To avoid a recurrence of malnourishment, she was instructed to eat a soft diet and increase her fluid intake. During the recall visit 3 months after of the last reduction attempt, she no longer reported severe pain in her TMJ during movement but still was complaining from her inability to chew food or eat properly. The patient refused to undergo any further reduction attempts and could not undergo any surgical intervention due to her age and compromised health status. Therefore, prosthodontic management was planned as a palliative treatment option to help her cope with the condition and to prevent further malnutrition episodes.

Patient Examination in the Prosthodontic Department

In the prosthodontic department, extraoral clinical examination revealed facial asymmetry with limited mouth opening (23 mm) and slight deviation to the right side on opening (Fig 24.1). The lips were competent at rest, and there was no impairment in speech. The patient had been completely edentulous for 2 years, and intraoral examination showed that her mandibular and maxillary ridges were well formed in a class III skeletal relationship. She did not wear any previous dentures, and she reported that her TMJ was dislocated during previous attempts at denture construction and was hesitant to undergo any further attempts. The diagnosis of bilateral TMJ dislocation was confirmed clinically and radiographically (Fig 24.1). Moreover, the radiographic examination showed erosion and flattening of the condylar head.

Prosthodontic Management

A review of the literature was conducted to search for any previous prosthodontic clinical reports involving the

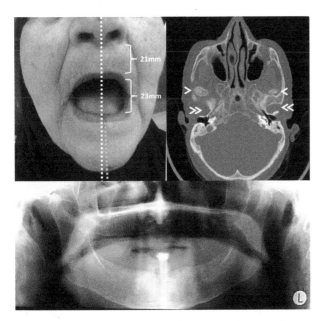

FIGURE 24.1 Clinical photograph showing the limited mouth opening (23 mm) and slight deviation of mandible to the right (gray dotted line) in relation to the midline (white dotted line) (top left), and a CT scan showing the anterior dislocation of the mandibular condyles (single arrow) in relation to the glenoid fossae (double arrows) (top right). Panoramic radiograph showing erosion and flattening of the condylar head (bottom).

treatment of edentulous patients with nonreducible bilateral anterior condylar dislocation. No previous reports were found; however, there are many successful reports of prosthetic rehabilitation of patients lacking condylar guidance, such as patients who went through mandibulectomy after radiotherapy.[18] In these cases, patients adapted to the new occlusal scheme by gradually applying modifications to the treatment dentures at specific time intervals. We hypothesized that the prosthetic rehabilitation of patients with nonreducible bilateral anterior TMJ dislocation could be successful using techniques used to treat patients lacking condylar guidance. These techniques depend on applying gradual modifications to treatment dentures at specific time intervals.[18]

Prosthodontic rehabilitation of edentulous patients suffering from TMJ dislocations usually commences after managing the dislocation, but in this clinical situation after the failed attempts to reduce the joint to its correct position, it was decided to start the prosthodontic rehabilitation as a palliative approach. The findings and management plan were discussed with the patient.

A clinical protocol was approved, and the patient's informed consent was obtained to proceed with the prosthodontic rehabilitation without reducing the TMJ. Preliminary and final impressions were made, and record bases with wax occlusal rims were fabricated. The maxillary wax rim was modified according to esthetics and phonetics,[19] and the Fox plane plate was used to adjust the denture occlusal plane by following the interpupillary and Camper's lines.[20] The mandibular wax rim was modified following the maxillary wax rim to obtain the compensating curves (curve of Spee and curve of Wilson), since the mandible is in an atypical position. Due to the atypical condylar position, the patient was repeatedly asked to swallow and relax, and the most consistent measurements were considered for vertical relations. The bite registration records were taken with the dislocated joints and were found to be repeatable. After bite registration, the record bases with the wax rims were mounted on a semiadjustable articulator to verify the occlusal relationship and the occlusal vertical dimension.

Treatment Denture Without Teeth

The next stage of treatment was the gradual adaptation of the neuromuscular system to the new occlusal scheme with atypical joint position. Accordingly, acrylic denture bases with acrylic occlusal rims (without teeth) were constructed (treatment denture) (Fig 24.2) and delivered to the patient. She was asked to wear the treatment dentures and to come back after 24 hours for occlusal adjustments; the occlusal rims were adjusted until a satisfactory balanced occlusion was achieved. This was achieved by the following steps: (1) performing a preocclusal/precentric record check, (2) remounting the treatment dentures on the semiadjustable

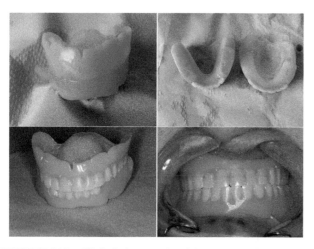

FIGURE 24.2   Clinical photographs of the treatment denture with acrylic occlusal rims for the maxilla and the mandible without teeth (top left), the maxillary and the mandibular acrylic occlusal rims with the added anterior teeth (top right), the maxillary denture with a complete set of teeth, and the mandibular denture with anterior teeth (bottom left), the maxillary and mandibular dentures with complete set of teeth in occlusion in the patient's mouth (bottom right).

articulator and removing any interferences during the simulation of the mandibular movements (centric, eccentric, and protrusive movements), and (3) reinsertion of the treatment dentures inside the patient's mouth and checking for any interferences during mandibular movements. After that, the patient was given appropriate postoperative instructions that included (1) wear the treatment dentures as much as possible; (2) take the dentures out at night and clean them; (3) insert food on both sides of the mandible and chew in hinge movements on both sides; (4) maintain a soft diet and avoid eating hard or sticky food; and (5) avoid voluntary extreme opening of the jaw and prevent involuntary openings (e.g., yawning) by pushing the chin upwards with the hand.

Gradual Addition of Teeth to the Treatment Dentures

The patient did not report any further complaints after 3 weeks of treatment denture delivery. Semianatomical artificial teeth were gradually added to the occlusal rims of the same treatment dentures based on neutral zone measurements, esthetics, and bite registration. The whole set of artificial teeth were added in four subsequent appointments 2 weeks apart (Fig 24.2). In the first appointment, the six maxillary anterior teeth were placed in the acrylic rim. In the second appointment, the mandibular anterior teeth were added. In the third appointment, the maxillary posterior teeth were added, so the patient had a maxillary complete set of teeth with the mandibular anterior teeth only. In the fourth appointment mandibular posterior teeth were added, so the patient finally had her complete dentures with the complete set of teeth (Fig 24.2).

Denture Delivery and Postinsertion Follow-up

The finalized complete denture was delivered, and the patient's progress was monitored for 1 year on regular monthly recall appointments. After 1 month of wearing the dentures, the extent of mouth opening increased and stabilized at 27 mm. This is probably due to the resolution of the TMJ inflammation that restricted its movement. After 1 year, the patient remained satisfied with her dentures and was able to wear them at all times and eat a wider range of foods efficiently without complaining of any pain or other complications.

DISCUSSION

To the best of the authors' knowledge, this is the first clinical report describing the prosthodontic management of an edentulous patient with a nonreducible bilateral anterior TMJ dislocation as a palliative treatment. Dislocation of the TMJ occurs due to a variety of predisposing and etiological factors, including tooth loss, trauma, dental treatments, medications, joint hyper-mobility, excessive mouth opening (i.e., excessive yawning), congenital joint weakness, and psychogenic and neurological disorders.[1,2,21] We were not able to pinpoint the factors that caused the bilateral anterior dislocation of the TMJ, but from the patient's history it is possible it might have occurred due to tooth loss and previous dental treatments.

Some of the potential long-term consequences of non-reducing the joint include bone remodeling of TMJ articular surfaces (erosion and flattening of the condylar head and posterior slope of the articular eminence) and degeneration of the articular disc.[22] In this case, manual attempts to reduce the TMJ were unsuccessful three times, and the patient was not medically fit to undergo any surgical procedures, leaving her with the sole option of coping with the condition. Despite the potential long-term consequences, the prosthodontic management was planned as palliative treatment and to prevent future episodes of severe malnutrition.

The prosthodontic management of an edentulous patient with mandibular dislocation is a particular challenge due to the loss of both anterior (teeth) and posterior guidance (condylar position). Accordingly, the occlusal pattern and tooth positioning of the dentures were based on esthetics and phonetics. Another challenge is the lack of specific standardized guidelines or previous clinical reports of prosthetic rehabilitation of such patients. Therefore, some steps of the prosthodontic management in this clinical report were based on a similarity with prosthetic rehabilitation of patients lacking condylar guidance such as patients who underwent mandibulectomy after radiotherapy,[4] which depends on applying gradual modifications to treatment dentures at specific time intervals.

After a 1-year follow-up, the patient adapted well to the dentures and was able to eat a wider range of foods without any complaints. Moreover, she showed improvement in tenderness in the TMJ region and maximal mouth opening despite the persistence of the dislocated joint. Therefore, this clinical report could emphasize the importance of muscular adaptation on the successful treatment of complete dentures, especially in patients suffering from dislocated TMJs. Moreover, this approach can be used as a palliative management of bilateral anterior dislocation of the TMJ in patients who are very old and/or not fit for surgical interventions.

CONCLUSIONS

Edentulous patients with nonreducible bilateral anterior mandibular dislocation can be managed with complete dentures as a palliative treatment. The prosthodontic management can be performed using esthetics and phonetics as guidance for tooth positioning and adjusting the occlusion gradually until the patient adapts to the new occlusal scheme.

REFERENCES

1. Akinbami BO: Evaluation of the mechanism and principles of management of temporomandibular joint dislocation. Systematic review of literature and a proposed new classification of temporomandibular joint dislocation. *Head Face Med* 2011;7:1–9.

2. Baur DA, Jannuzzi JR, Mercan U, et al: Treatment of long term anterior dislocation of the TMJ. *Int J Oral Maxillofac Surg* 2013;42:1030–1033.

3. Ugboko VI, Oginni FO, Ajike SO, et al: A survey of temporomandibular joint dislocation: aetiology, demographics, risk factors and management in 96 Nigerian cases. *Int J Oral Maxillofac Surg* 2005;34:499–502.

4. Goss AN: Bilateral anterior dislocation of the mandible. *N Z Dent J* 1968;64:29–30.

5. Cheng A, Al Hashmi A, Goss AN: Traumatic bilateral anterior dislocation of the mandible with impaction over the maxilla: a case report. *J Oral Maxillofac Surg* 2009;67:673–675.

6. Hynes SL, Jansen LA, Brown DR, et al: Bilateral temporomandibular joint dislocation with locked mandibular impaction. *J Oral Maxillofac Surg* 2012;70:E116–E118.

7. Ozcelik TB, Pektas ZO: Management of chronic unilateral temporomandibular joint dislocation with a mandibular guidance prosthesis: a clinical report. *J Prosthet Dent* 2008;99:95–100.

8. Ziegler CM, Haag C, Muhling J: Treatment of recurrent temporomandibular joint dislocation with intramuscular botulinum toxin injection. *Clin Oral Investig* 2003;7:52–55.

9. Fu KY, Chen HM, Sun ZP, et al: Long-term efficacy of botulinum toxin type A for the treatment of habitual dislocation of the temporomandibular joint. *Br J Oral Maxillofac Surg* 2010;48:281–284.

10. Daif ET: Autologous blood injection as a new treatment modality for chronic recurrent temporomandibular joint dislocation. *Oral Surg Oral Med Oral Pathol Oral Radiol Endod* 2010;109:31–36.

11. Machon V, Abramowicz S, Paska J, et al: Autologous blood injection for the treatment of chronic recurrent temporomandibular joint dislocation. *J Oral Maxillofac Surg* 2009;67:114–119.

12. Shakya S, Ongole R, Sumanth KN, et al: Chronic bilateral dislocation of temporomandibular joint. *Kathmandu Univ Med J* 2010;8:251–256.

13. Hasson O, Nahlieli O: Autologous blood injection for treatment of recurrent temporomandibular joint dislocation. *Oral Surg Oral Med Oral Pathol Oral Radiol Endod* 2001;92:390–393.

14. Kato T, Shimoyama T, Nasu D, et al: Autologous blood injection into the articular cavity for the treatment of recurrent temporomandibular joint dislocation: a case report. *J Oral Sci* 2007;49:237–239.

15. Stiesch-Scholz M, Fink M, Tschernitschek H, et al: Medical and physical therapy of temporomandibular joint disk displacement without reduction. *Cranio* 2002;20:85–90.

16. Januzzi E, Nasri-Heir C, Grossmann E, et al: Combined palliative and anti-inflammatory medications as treatment of temporomandibular joint disc displacement without reduction: a systematic review. *Cranio* 2013;31:211–225.

17. da Costa Ribeiro R, dos santos BJ Jr, Provenzano N, et al: Dautrey's procedure: an alternative for the treatment of recurrent mandibular dislocation in patients with pneumatization of the articular eminence. *Int J Oral Maxillofac Surg* 2014;43:465–469.

18. Jacob RF: Prosthodontic rehabilitation of the mandibulectomy patient. In Taylor TD (ed): *Clinical Maxillofacial Prosthetics*. Chicago, Quintessence, 2000.

19. Roumanas ED: The social solution-denture esthetics, phonetics, and function. *J Prosthodont* 2009;18:112–115.

20. Spratley MH: Simplified technique for determining the occlusal plane in full denture construction. *J Oral Rehabil* 1980;7:31–33.

21. Huang IY, Chen CM, Kao YH, et al: Management of longstanding mandibular dislocation. *Int J Oral Maxillofac Surg* 2011;40:810–814.

22. Kai S, Kai H, Tabata O, et al: Long-term outcomes of nonsurgical treatment in nonreducing anteriorly displaced disk of the temporomandibular joint. *Oral Surg Oral Med Oral Pathol Oral Radiol Endod* 1998;85:258–267.

25

PROSTHODONTIC REHABILITATION OF A SHOTGUN INJURY: A PATIENT REPORT

KIANOOSH TORABI, DMD, MSCD, AHMAD H. AHANGARI, DMD, MSCD, MAHROU VOJDANI, DMD, MSCD, AND FARNAZ FATTAHI, DMD, MSCD

Department of Prosthodontics, Faculty of Dentistry, Shiraz University of Medical Sciences, Shiraz, Islamic Republic of Iran

Keywords
Prosthodontic; rehabilitation; shotgun.

Correspondence
Farnaz Fattahi, Faculty of Dentistry, Shiraz University of Medical Sciences—Prosthodontics, Shiraz, Fars 71345, Iran.
E-mail: s.f.fattahi@gmail.com

Accepted November 18, 2009

Published in *Journal of Prosthodontics* December 2010;
Vol. 19, Issue 8

doi: 10.1111/j.1532-849X.2010.00645.x

ABSTRACT

This report describes the prosthodontic rehabilitation of a shotgun patient traumatized in the maxillary, mandibular, and nasal areas resulting in severe problems in her esthetics, phonetics, and mastication. The patient was treated with removable partial prostheses using tooth, soft tissue, and implant support.

Depending on the weight and velocity of the bullet, a shotgun may cause various tissue injuries. Shotgun injuries occur with a hunting rifle, while gunshot wounds occur with other gun types. A hunting rifle shot from a distance closer than 7 m would have the same effect as a gunshot and would be called a close-range shotgun injury.[1] Rehabilitation of these patients and those attempting suicide are still a challenge for prosthodontists.[1]

CLINICAL REPORT

A 23-year-old woman who had been shot by a hunting rifle in the submental area about 7 years ago presented for functional and esthetic rehabilitation to the Prosthodontic Graduate Department of Shiraz Dental School in southwest Iran. Her mandible, maxilla, and nose were severely traumatized (Fig 25.1). Her ACP Prosthodontic Diagnostic Index (PDI)

Journal of Prosthodontics on Complex Restorations, First Edition. Edited by Nadim Z. Baba and David L. Guichet.

for making impressions and photographs. Teeth #s 1, 6 to 12, 16 to 28, and 32 were missing. Teeth #s 4 and 5 were severely malpositioned, and due to resorption of the bone graft and lack of bone support, these two teeth and tooth #13 had 10- to 11-mm pocket depth and mobility grade II to III. Tooth #29 was supraerupted, interfering with the proper occlusal plane. Tooth #30 was severely damaged by caries, separating it into two roots.

The only occlusal vertical stop was on teeth #s2 and 31 (Fig 25.3). The patient was deeply concerned about her poor esthetics and impaired masticatory performance.

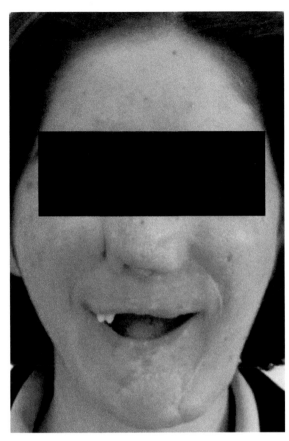

FIGURE 25.1   Frontal view of the patient.

was class IV. She had already undergone 13 reconstructive and plastic surgeries. Her mandible had been reconstructed using an iliac graft, and the maxilla had been repaired by a microvascular free flap from her forearm. Unfortunately, clinical and radiographic evaluations revealed extensive resorption of osseous tissue of the graft in the maxilla, leaving loose flabby tissue covered by skin, which was not a suitable bed for any kind of prosthetic rehabilitation.[2] In the radiographic and computerized tomography scan views of her mandible (Fig 25.2), presence of several screws and plates were noted.

Difficulty in speech was noted, and she wore a mask to hide her disfigured mouth. Due to widespread scars around the mouth, her mouth orifice was restricted, limiting access

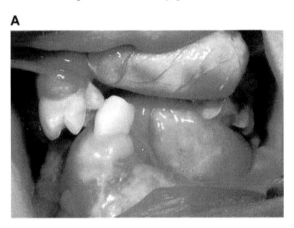

A

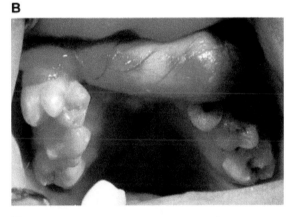

B

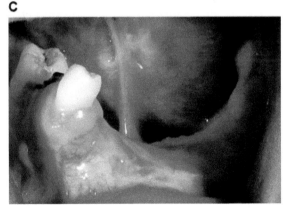

C

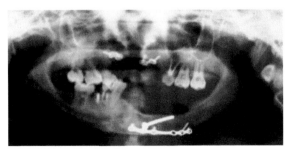

FIGURE 25.2   Preoperative panoramic X-ray.

FIGURE 25.3   Intraoral view. (A) Maximum intercuspation. (B) Maxillary arch. (C) Mandibular arch.

Maxillary and mandibular primary impressions were made using condensation silicone impression material (Speedex, Colten AG, Altstatten, Switzerland). Diagnostic casts were fabricated from type III dental stone (Dentstone, type III, Heraeus Kulzer, Armonk, NY) and mounted in a semi-adjustable articulator (Hanau H2, Teledyne Hanau, Buffalo, NY) using a facebow transfer and centric relation record bases for edentulous areas.

In the preprosthetic mouth preparation phase, teeth #s 4, 5, 13, and 30 were extracted. The mandibular right second premolar was treated endodontically, a crown-lengthening procedure was conducted, and the tooth was shortened to serve as an overdenture abutment. The flabby tissue in the premaxillary area was excised to provide a better prosthetic foundation.

All screws and plates were removed from the mandible to provide adequate space for implant placement and to prevent continuous corrosion.[2] Concomitantly, the skin graft from the maxilla was transferred to this area to provide needed keratinized tissue. Skin graft is an excellent base for a vestibuloplasty, particularly in combination with dental implants.[2] After vestibuloplasty of the lower anterior segment, interim prostheses were fabricated for both arches to temporarily restore lip support and esthetics.

Implant placement was initially considered for rehabilitation of the mandible. After 4 months of mandibular bone healing, the patient's interim prosthesis was duplicated into a surgical stent using a vacuum-formed shell (Temporary splint material, 0.02 thickness, Buffalo Dental Manufacturing Co., Syosset, NY) to insert three implants (5 mm diameter, 9 mm length, D3 Biohorizons, Birmingham, AL) in the anterior segment of the mandible in a tripod design.

Due to extensive bone deficiency for implant placement, a Kennedy class IV cobalt–chromium partial denture was planned for the maxilla. To provide the necessary retention in this edentulous configuration, the anterior-most and posterior-most teeth should be used.[2] Therefore, splinted and surveyed crowns were fabricated for teeth #s 2, 3, 14, and 15 as removable partial denture (RPD) abutments with parallel guiding planes. To provide better retention, extracoronal ball attachments at the mesial surfaces of 3 and 14 were planned.

On the distal sides and mesiobuccal surfaces of teeth #s 2 and 15, occlusal rests and proper retentive undercut areas, respectively, were planned (Fig 25.4A). For tooth #29, a gold coping was fabricated. For tooth #31, a surveyed metal ceramic restoration with a guiding plane, buccal retentive undercut, and lingual reciprocal ledge was fabricated (Fig 25.4B). To restore the partially edentulous area of the lower jaw, a Co–Cr RPD was considered.

Mandibular implants were uncovered after 4 months. After 1 week of soft tissue healing, a primary impression with indirect impression transfer coping and ball top screws

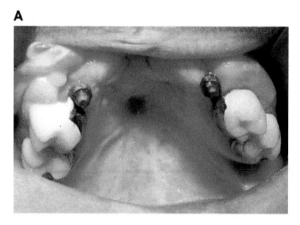

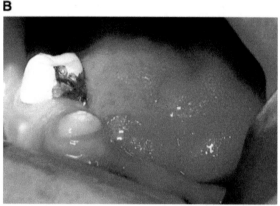

FIGURE 25.4   Intraoral view. (A) Maxillary arch. (B) Mandibular arch.

was made using condensation silicone impression material (Speedex) An open-top tray was fabricated with direct impression transfer coping and long screws, and a final impression was made with poly(vinyl siloxane) (PVS) impression material (Lastic Xtra, Kettenbach, Eschenburg, Germany).[3]

Implants were splinted by a bar with three ball attachments. The bar was checked for passivity by counterbalance method (Fig 25.5).[4] The impression for the RPD was made with PVS (Lastic Xtra) and an open-top tray for the mandible.

Crowns and the mandibular bar were picked up by the RPD impression. The RPD frameworks were fabricated (Fig 25.6) and checked in the mouth. Denture teeth were arranged to provide suitable lip support, esthetics, and phonetics. Maxillary and mandibular partial dentures are illustrated in Figures 25.7A to 25.7C.

Fixed and removable prostheses of the maxilla and mandible are shown in Figures 25.8A and 25.8B. Maximum intercuspation of the patient is presented in Figures 25.9A and 25.9B. An extraoral view of the final prostheses is shown in Figure 25.10. The postoperative panoramic X-ray is visible in Figure 25.11. The prostheses were delivered to the patient, and she was followed for 2 years.

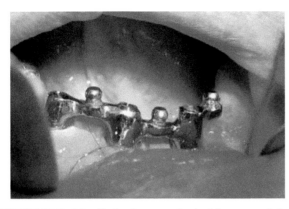

FIGURE 25.5 Mandibular bar was checked by counterbalance method.

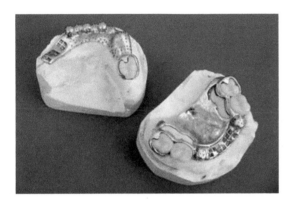

FIGURE 25.6 Maxillary and mandibular RPD frameworks.

DISCUSSION

Stevens et al[5] stated that the introduction of osseointegrated dental implants had significantly improved the overall reconstruction of patients with cranio-maxillofacial injuries. Siphai et al[6] restored a gunshot maxillofacial defect with dental implants and various attachments. They rehabilitated the patient by a fixed, full-arch, implant-supported prosthesis for the mandible and an obturator retained by bar/clip and ball attachments for the maxilla; however, in our patient, it was not possible to place any implants in the maxilla because there was inadequate bony tissue. Also because of extensive bone resorption of a previous microvascular free flap it was not a good recipient site for further bone grafting, so the patient rejected another bone grafting surgery. Therefore, there was no choice except to use the residual ridge and remaining teeth to support an RPD. In such a case with Kennedy class IV partial edentulism, the most-anterior and the most-posterior teeth should be used for prosthesis retention.[2] Therefore, retentive clasps were designed on the upper second molars, and extracoronal ball attachments were used on the upper first molars.

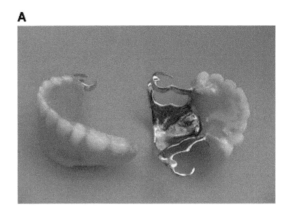

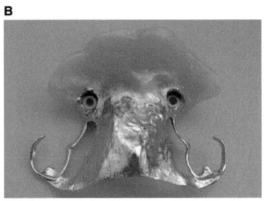

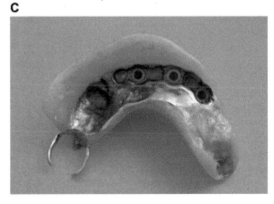

FIGURE 25.7 (A) Maxillary and mandibular RPDs. (B) Intaglio surface of maxillary RPD. (C) Intaglio surface of mandibular RPD.

The contact between teeth #s 2 and 31 provided an acceptable occlusal vertical dimension (OVD). During fabrication and adjustment of interim partial dentures, these teeth were in contact. Then during preparation of these two teeth and adjustment of their fixed prostheses, the interim partial dentures were in contact. Thus, OVD was maintained.

Mijiritsky and Karas[7] revealed that in situations where financial, systemic, or local conditions preclude the use of a fixed partial denture, a well-constructed RPD can be an excellent alternative. De Freitas et al[8] concluded that although the construction of an RPD may seem paradoxical

A

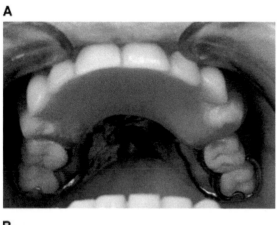

B

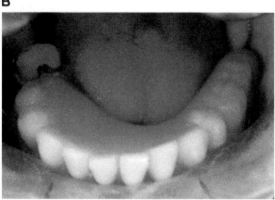

FIGURE 25.8 (A) Maxillary fixed and removable prosthesis in the mouth. (B) Mandibular fixed and removable prosthesis in the mouth.

A

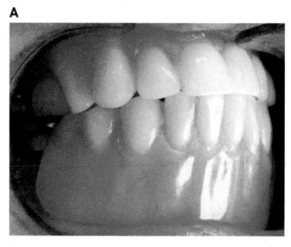

B

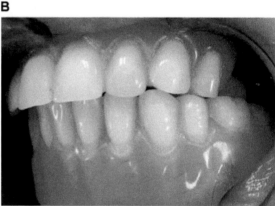

FIGURE 25.9 Intraoral view of maximum intercuspation. (A) Right lateral view. (B) Left lateral view.

when osseo-integrated implants are placed, in some cases, this option is best. In the mandibular reconstruction of our patient, there was no choice except an RPD with tooth, implant, and tissue support. Therefore, three implants were placed in a tripod configuration to stabilize the prosthesis and to minimize the bending moment. Implants were splinted with a bar with three ball attachments. The lower right second

premolar was used as an overdenture abutment to preserve the bony tissue, and the lower right second molar was used to provide support and retention for the prosthesis. A balance in the lip support and competency resulted in desirable esthetics, phonetics, and functional ability for the patient. This treatment plan provided a very acceptable rehabilitation for the patient.

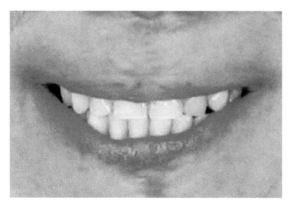

FIGURE 25.10 Extraoral view of maximum intercuspation of anterior teeth.

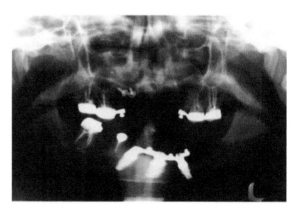

FIGURE 25.11 Postoperative panoramic X-ray.

REFERENCES

1. Brunicardi FC, Anderson DK, Billiar TR, et al: *Schwartz's Principles of Surgery (ed 8)*. New York, McGraw Hill, 2005.

2. Taylor TD: *Clinical Maxillofacial Prosthetics*. Chicago, Quintessence, 2000.

3. Misch CE: *Dental Implant Prosthetics (ed 1)*. St. Louis, Mosby, 2005.

4. Misch CE: *Dental Implant Prosthetics (ed 1)*. St. Louis, Mosby, 2005.

5. Stevens MR, Heit JM, Kline SN, et al: The use of osseointegrated implants in craniofacial trauma. *J Craniomaxillofac Trauma* 1998;4:27–34.

6. Siphai C, Ortakoglu K, Ozen J, et al: The prosthodontic restoration of a self-inflicted gunshot maxillofacial defect: a short-term follow-up case report. *Int J Prosthodont* 2007;20:85–88.

7. Mijiristsky E, Karas S: Removable partial denture design involving teeth and implants as an alternative to unsuccessful fixed implant therapy: a case report. *Implant Dent* 2004;13:218–222.

8. de Freitas R, Kaizer OB, Hamata MM, et al: Prosthetic rehabilitation of a bone defect with a teeth-implant supported, removable partial denture. *Implant Dent* 2006;15:241–247.

26

SURGICAL AND PROSTHODONTIC TREATMENT OF A PATIENT WITH SIGNIFICANT TRAUMA TO THE MIDDLE AND LOWER FACE SECONDARY TO A GUNSHOT WOUND: A CLINICAL REPORT

PAUL KELLY, DMD, MS[1,2] AND CARL J. DRAGO, DDS, MS[3–5]

[1]Arizona Maxillofacial Surgeons PC, Mesa, AZ

[2]Formerly, Chief Resident, Oral and Maxillofacial Surgery, Gundersen Lutheran Medical Center, LaCrosse, WI

[3]Director of Dental Research, Biomet 3i, Palm Beach Gardens, FL

[4]Adjunct Prosthodontic Faculty, Nova Southeastern University College of Dental Medicine, Ft. Lauderdale, FL

[5]Formerly, Prosthodontist, Gundersen Lutheran Medical Center, LaCrosse, WI

Keywords
Surgical treatment; facial gunshot wound; CAD/CAM bars; maxillary implant overdenture.

Correspondence
Carl J. Drago, 174 Via Veracruz, Jupiter, FL 33458. E-mail: cdrago@3implant.com

Accepted August 19, 2008

Published in *Journal of Prosthodontics* October 2009; Vol. 18, Issue 7

doi: 10.1111/j.1532-849X.2009.00483.x

ABSTRACT

Large defects of dentofacial structures may result from trauma, disease (including neoplasms), and congenital anomalies. The location and size of the defects are related to difficulties that patients report relative to speech, mastication, swallowing, facial esthetics, and self-image. This article reports on the evaluation and treatment of a patient who suffered significant trauma to the lower and mid-face secondary to a gunshot injury. It describes the initial presentation, life-saving procedures, and subsequent bone grafts, implant placement, and prosthetic treatments required to rehabilitate the patient to a condition that closely approximated his preoperative condition. This clinical report confirms that no matter the degree of complexity involved in treating the results of significant facial trauma, successful treatment is dependent on thorough physical and radiographic examinations, development of the appropriate diagnoses, and treatment based on sound prosthodontic and surgical principles.

Large defects of dentofacial structures may result from trauma, disease (including neoplasms), and congenital anomalies. The location and size of the defects are related to difficulties patients experience with speech, mastication, swallowing, facial esthetics, and self-image.[1–4] Patients who suffer from these facial defects often require multiple reconstructive surgeries over an extended period of time. Blood supply to the surgical sites may impact the postoperative results. Osseous and soft tissue contours may sometimes deviate significantly from normal. These patients may also demonstrate signs and symptoms consistent with anxiety, depression, or posttraumatic stress disorder.[5]

Treatments for major facial trauma are generally divided into three categories: life-saving procedures, surgical reconstruction, and definitive prosthodontic treatment. Numerous methods have been proposed for surgical reconstruction of pan-facial trauma.[6–11] The so-called bottom-up and inside-out, or more recently, top-down and outside-in, methods have been used for treatment and debated among surgeons.[7,8] Advances in facial-trauma management, including computerized tomography (CT), have enabled surgeons to visualize and successfully reconstruct complex panfacial injuries. Restoration of both preinjury facial esthetics and function is the goal of reconstructive surgery. An organized approach to these injuries begins at the maxillary and mandibular arches with progression to the vertical mandible. The nasoorbital-ethmoid complex should be stabilized to the cranium and bone grafted when indicated. The zygomatic complex is related medially, and orbital reconstruction is then performed. The facial architectural restoration is completed at the LeFort I level. this protocol enables surgeons to obtain reproducibly good results, even with the most extensive facial dislocations.[7]

Rigid fixation (ORIF) has also advanced in the field of oral and maxillofacial trauma reconstruction.[9] Despite excellent predicable results with various ORIF protocols, considerable debate still occurs in cases involving the traumatic avulsion of large volumes of hard and soft tissues. With severely comminuted jaw fractures, particularly of the mandible, stripping the periosteum from fractured, small pieces of remaining bone, for ORIF, may be counterproductive for achieving continuity of the mandible.[10,11]

The purpose of this article is to report on the evaluation and treatment of a patient who suffered significant trauma to the lower and mid-face secondary to a gunshot wound. This clinical report will briefly describe the patient's initial emergency room presentation, triage, and treatment for life-threatening injuries. The subsequent treatments with multiple surgeries, grafts, compromised nonoptimal endosseous implant placement, prosthodontic treatment, and plastic surgery procedures will also be illustrated.

CLINICAL REPORT

A 17-year-old malepatient presented to the Emergency Ward (EW) of the Gundersen Lutheran Medical Center, LaCrosse, WI, by helicopter, 45 minutes after extensive facial trauma from a self-inflicted gunshot wound (Fig 26.1). The patient's airway was stable, and he was not intubated at the time of EW admission. He had been hemodynamically stable during transportation. As per initial advanced trauma and life-support guidelines (ATLS), the patient was then intubated and studies were performed.[10,12] CT of the head and neck region was negative for intracranial penetration or other injury. The cervical spine had no radiographic or clinical signs of trauma. Fine cut (1 mm) axial and reconstructed coronal, sagittal, and 3D CT images were obtained for diagnostic and treatment-planning purposes. Radiographic studies showed extensive middle and lower face comminuted fractures with avulsion of multiple anterior teeth, hard palate, alveolar bone, nasal bone, nasal septum, and the maxillary and ethmoid sinuses. Zygomatic arches were intact bilaterally. The medial and lateral sides and floors of both orbits were violated.

The patient was taken to the operating room, where a tracheotomy and a percutaneous endoscopic gastronomy

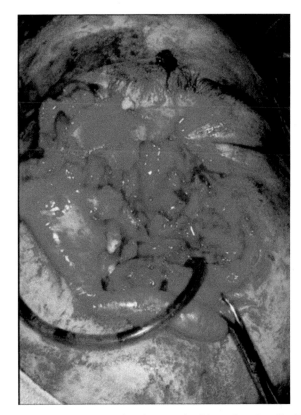

FIGURE 26.1 Preoperative photograph of the patient described in this report after being stabilized in the Emergency Ward. Note the extensive loss of hard and soft tissues in the middle and lower thirds of the face.

(PEG) were performed. Comprehensive evaluation of the hard and soft tissue injures to the face demonstrated significant avulsion of osseous and soft tissues. Given the extent of the comminuted fractures, a decision was made to not further disrupt the blood supply by stripping the periosteum from the segments with rigid fixation bone plates. A segmental arch bar and Ivy Loupes were placed to establish the occlusal vertical dimension (OVD). At this time, the patient's posterior teeth were in occlusion bilaterally. This was considered to be consistent with the patient's original OVD (Fig 26.2). The medial canthal ligaments were partially avulsed along with portions of the nasal and frontal bones. Twenty-five gauge transnasal wires were placed to reapproximate the medial canthal ligaments bilaterally. Intraoral and extraoral soft tissues were extensively explored, debrided, and closed. The patient's wounds were closed, and the remaining segments of the comminuted fractures in the maxilla and mandible were left with intact periosteum for consolidation. The patient was then taken to the intensive care unit (ICU) in a stable condition (Fig 26.3).

Reconstructive surgery with definitive prosthetic treatment planning began 15 months after the initial hospitalization. Due to the extensive loss of bone and soft tissue, including a major portion of the upper lip, and scarring with the loss of the anterior vestibules, the patient was unable to wear transitional removable partial dentures (RPDs). Reconstructive surgeries consisted of iliac bone grafts to the maxilla and mandible, followed by osseous healing[13–19] (Fig 26.4). Plastic surgical procedures were to be completed at the conclusion of prosthodontic treatment and included auricular cartilage grafting, paramedian forehead tube pedicle flap, and nasal tip revision.

Diagnostic prosthodontic procedures were accomplished after the bone grafts healed. Diagnostic casts and conventional record bases were made for the diagnostic articulator mounting, prior to the construction of diagnostic wax patterns (wax/acrylic resin denture bases and denture teeth) (Figs 26.5 and 26.6).

Trial dentures were fabricated to identify the optimal location of the missing teeth for construction of surgical

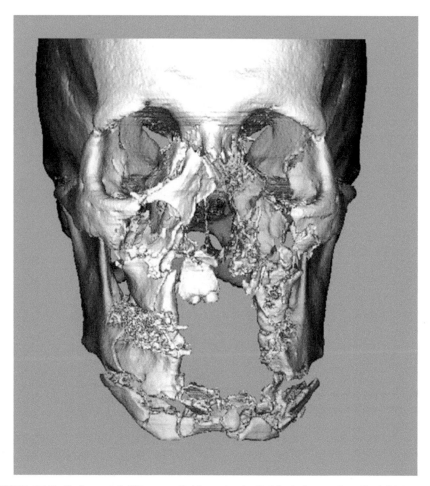

FIGURE 26.2 Reformatted CT scan of this patient's facial skeleton after the initial surgical procedures that included stabilization of the posterior segments. Note the significant loss of bone from the anterior maxilla and mandible, as well as the numerous comminuted mandibular segments.

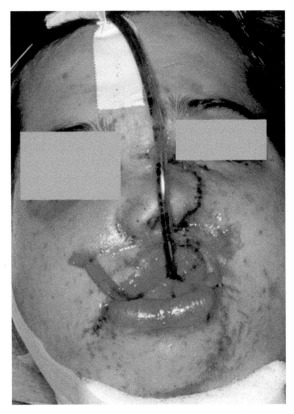

FIGURE 26.3 Postoperative photograph of the patient as he left the operating room 6 hours after admission.

guides prior to the placement of endossous implants. The OVD was maintained, consistent with the postoperative (surgical) condition. Esthetics, in terms of the amount of incisal display during speaking, smiling, and at rest, were not a significant consideration in maintaining the OVD, due to the large amount of soft tissue avulsion associated with the

original trauma. It was likely that more maxillary teeth would be visible at rest for this patient postoperatively (surgical and prosthetic) than would have been visible prior to the injury. The centric relation record was made with some difficulty as the mandibular left posterior segment had healed with a lingual inclination, and the mandibular left first molar had to be extracted approximately 5 months after the original presentation secondary to loss of attachment and mobility. The maxillary right first premolar was no longer in occlusion. In hindsight, this tooth should have been extracted and replaced with an endosseous implant. Even with multiple surgeries and perioral scarring, there was still a significant amount of interocclusal clearance between the jaws (Fig 26.7).

PROSTHODONTIC CLASSIFICATION

The American College of Prosthodontists has developed a classification system for partially edentulous patients based on diagnostic findings.[20] Four classes were identified with Class I representing uncomplicated clinical situations and Class IV representing complex clinical situations. Each class was differentiated by specific diagnostic criteria: location and extent of the edentulous areas, condition of abutment teeth, occlusion, and characteristics of the residual ridges.

Location and Extent of Edentulous Areas

Due to the significant amount of hard and soft tissue loss in the anterior maxilla and mandible and the quality of the soft tissues covering the edentulous ridges, this patient was identified as having severely compromised edentulous areas, because it was thought that implant placement into the

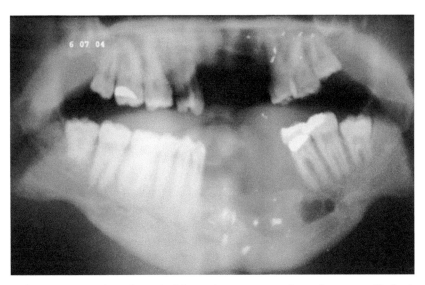

FIGURE 26.4 Panoramic radiograph 26 months posttrauma, just prior to mandibular implant placement.

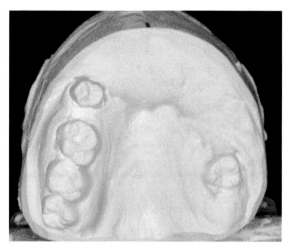

FIGURE 26.5 Maxillary diagnostic cast after osseous healing, before implant placement. Note the lack of vestibular depth in the anterior segment.

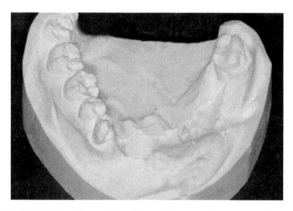

FIGURE 26.6 Mandibular diagnostic cast after osseous healing, before implant placement. Note the lack of a definitive residual ridge and vestibular extensions. The mandibular left first molar had been extracted several months prior to this photograph, secondary to the loss of attachment and mobility.

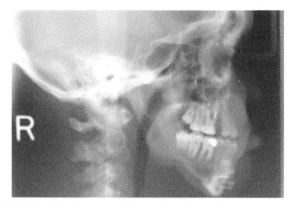

FIGURE 26.7 Lateral cephalometric radiograph taken 18 months posttrauma prior to the extraction of the maxillary right canine and right first premolar. Note the relative prominence of the lower lip and the amount of interocclusal distance between the anterior jaws.

preexisting edentulous areas would result in a nonoptimal implant placement and require a high level of patient compliance regarding oral hygiene and patient adaptation.

Condition of Abutments

As a result of the trauma, this patient's potential abutment teeth were assessed to have poor long-term prognoses due to their positions within the dental arches, the size/location of the edentulous ridges, and the dental/skeletal malocclusions. The teeth themselves were not deficient in terms of the remaining tooth structure; they were deemed compromised because of the amount of bone loss suffered as a direct result of the trauma and the location of the defects.

The mandibular left first molar was originally thought to be a viable tooth. It subsequently lost a large portion of its periodontal attachment, and developed acute irreversible pulpitis and mobility. It was extracted secondary to what was considered to be a hopeless prognosis. The maxillary right first premolar was asymptomatic and originally in a satisfactory position. During the healing process, it moved and was noted to be slightly above the occlusal plane relative to the opposing mandibular premolars. In hindsight, this tooth should have been extracted and replaced with an endosseous implant to more optimally restore the maxillary right posterior segment.

Occlusion

This patient was classified as having substantially compromised occlusal characteristics, because the occlusal scheme anterior to the mandibular right premolars had to be reestablished. The OVD was not altered from the immediate postoperative condition relative to the right posterior quadrants, because it was thought to be relatively stable. The anterior occlusion was missing.

Residual Ridge Characteristics

The edentulous ridges were characterized by the need for surgical revision of the supporting structures to permit adequate prosthodontic function.[21] There was adequate bone volume for implant placement in both jaws. The quality of the bone was unknown at this time. The quality of the soft tissues covering both edentulous areas was poor. The soft tissues were mucosa and nonkeratinized, and the depths of the vestibules were basically nonexistent. The vestibular tissues were coincidental with the maxillary palatal and mandibular lingual tissues, respectively. The potential for this patient to wear conventional removable prostheses was considered to be poor. There was not enough ridge height or width to resist lateral displacement for conventional RPDs. There were also psychosocial considerations that needed to be assessed relative to removable prostheses and the patient's self-image. The patient was adamant in his request that he not be treated with definitive RPDs.

Prosthodontic Classification

This patient was classified as Class IV because of the severely compromised location and extent of the edentulous areas. The remaining natural teeth were not considered to be adequate to serve as abutments for removable or fixed partial dentures. The occlusion required rehabilitation due to the absence of the anterior teeth, and the residual edentulous ridges were severely compromised.

COMPREHENSIVE SURGICAL AND PROSTHODONTIC TREATMENT PLAN

Due to the extensiveness of the patient's injuries, specifically the amount of horizontal and vertical bone loss in the maxillary anterior segment, the need for lip support, the lack of stable abutment teeth, and the lack of sufficient posterior occlusal contacts on the left side, implants would be required to support and retain a removable overdenture prosthesis in the maxilla. An overdenture was planned for the maxillary prosthesis, because the viable bone for implant placement was significantly palatal to the planned location of the maxillary teeth, and the patient required a significant amount of lip support. Due to the amount of upper lip lost, the patient could only achieve oral competence with slight straining. Lip competence is typically one of the significant factors in determining vertical dimension. In this case, lip competence was not thought to be obtainable with the patient at rest. While lip competence was desirable at the selected OVD, the lack of lip competence as a mitigating factor to success in this case was not considered to be significant in determining esthetics and OVD or rest positions. If lip competence was considered to be essential for success in this case, the OVD could have been reduced by adjusting and/or restoring the posterior teeth. A fixed implant-retained maxillary prosthesis was contraindicated secondary to the location of the supporting bone, the need for lip support, phonetics, and oral hygiene procedures.[22,23] For strength and additional retention and stability, a secondary casting that fitted precisely over the primary bar was planned for the removable maxillary overdenture prosthesis.[24]

A screw-retained, implant-supported fixed prosthesis was planned for the mandibular edentulous segment because the requisite bone for implant placement was much closer to normal, relative to the planned prosthetic arch form, and there was minimal need for lip support. Esthetics relative to space between the inferior borders of hybrid prostheses and mandibular edentulous ridges are generally not a concern. A screw-retained design was chosen for the mandibular prosthesis to permit easier access to the abutments for oral hygiene procedures as well as retrievability for prosthetic maintenance.[22]

The patient also suffered from a loss of tongue volume and function. It was estimated that approximately 10% of the anterior and anterior lateral tongue volumes were lost. The patient suffered some disability in terms of phonetics, especially prior to prosthetic replacement of the missing teeth, bone, and soft tissue. It also should be noted that he was not able to adapt to any type of transitional RPDs following the trauma and surgeries. Lewandowski reported on misarticulation following surgery for malignancies in the oral cavity.[25] Although the present clinical report illustrates the net result of a gunshot wound to the mid-face, the functional results were thought to be similar to patients who lost tongue function secondary to tumors.

Lewandowski reported that the underlying cause in his case series was dysfunction of the tongue due to partial or total resection, consequences of mandibular resection together with the oral cavity floor, or dysfunction of the lower lip. Anatomic alterations revealed themselves as shifts in the points of contact between structures of the articulation system noticeable on palatograms or linguograms.

In a study reported by Sun et al, the size of tongue tumors (T1, T2, T3) and the site of excision (anterior, middle, posterior) were responsible for significant differences between patients with T1- and T3-sized tumors ($p < 0.05$).[26] The speech intelligibilities of the patients with tumors in the anterior tongue were significantly lower than those with tumors in the middle or posterior tongue regions ($p < 0.05$). Patients with preservation of the tip of the tongue or floor of the mouth had higher intelligibilities ($p < 0.05$). They concluded that for patients after glossectomy within the range of 1/2 or less of the tongue, the tumor site or excision extent of the tongue followed by the tumor size may be key factors in determining the postoperative articulation intelligibility. In the present case, the design of the mandibular prosthesis and the arrangement of the mandibular artificial teeth were made consistent with the preexisting arch form and locations of the remaining mandibular teeth.

TREATMENT

Five maxillary and four mandibular implants were placed with two-stage surgical protocols. The mandibular implants were placed in the first surgical procedure; the maxillary implants were placed in a second, later procedure. All implants integrated without incident. The mandibular implants were placed consistent with the planned locations of the teeth in the trial denture setup and the surgical guides. The long-term prognoses of the endosseous implants in this case were thought to be less than prognoses that have been established for endosseous implants placed into healed edentulous sites.[27] At the time of this report (3 years after implant placement), all the implants have remained viable with less than 1 mm of bone loss noted on yearly radiographs.

The mandibular prosthesis was constructed first, since the anterior maxilla required additional healing time due to additional bone grafting at the time of implant placement. Abutments were placed (IOL Abutments, Biomet 3i, Palm Beach Gardens, FL), and abutment level impressions were required due to the significant amount of soft tissues covering/surrounding (4–6 mm) the mandibular implants. The mandibular anterior incisal plane was determined by identifying the level of the posterior occlusal plane (retromolar pads) and extending it anteriorly (Fig 26.8). Twenty-degree acrylic resin posterior teeth were used (Justi® Blend®, American Tooth Industries, Oxnard, CA).

The centric relation record, as defined by the *Glossary of Prosthodontic Terms*,[28] was difficult to obtain due to trauma, surgical procedures, and residual defects the patient experienced. The goal of the jaw relation records was to obtain a predictable jaw relationship at the predetermined OVD.

The mandibular wax denture and master cast were scanned for a CAD/CAM titanium alloy framework (CAM StructSURE Precision Milled Bar, Biomet 3i) (Fig 26.9). The mandibular prosthesis was finished in a conventional fashion and inserted.

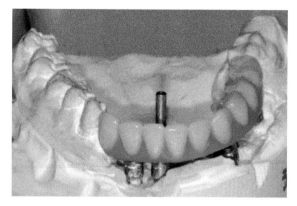

FIGURE 26.8 Laboratory facial occlusal view of mandibular waxed screw-retained prosthesis. The anterior incisal plane was at the same level (horizontal) as the posterior occlusal plane.

The maxillary implants were placed into the viable bone in the anterior maxilla; however, their locations were palatal to optimal implant positions as determined by the trial dentures and the surgical guide because the quality and quantity of bone in the anterior segment was deficient despite bone grafting. The implants were placed approximately 8 to 10 mm apart (Fig 26.10).

The peri-implant soft tissue depths of the maxillary implants were normal (2–3 mm) compared to the mandibular

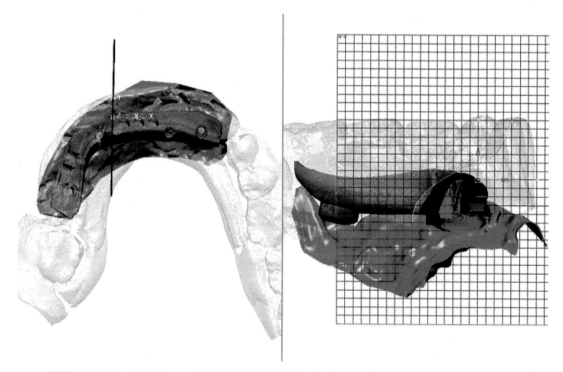

FIGURE 26.9 JPEG images of the CAD/CAM design for the mandibular framework. The location of the teeth in the wax denture can be visualized and verifies that the entire framework will be contained within the confines of the mandibular prosthesis. The screw access openings were lingual to the facial surfaces of the denture teeth in the prosthesis.

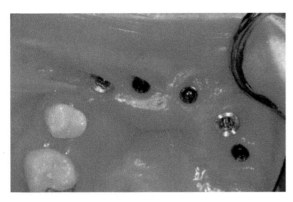

FIGURE 26.10 Maxillary intraoral occlusal image of five implants. Note the palatal positions of the implants relative to the arch form of the remaining natural teeth and the quality of the mobile mucosal tissues stretched with the lip retractors.

peri-implant tissues, and implant level impressions were made for fabrication of the master cast and verification index. A wax trial denture was fabricated and tried in for patient approval relative to the overall esthetic results, including lip support and incisal display at rest and smiling. At the selected OVD, lip competence was obtained with effort on the patient's part. The jaw relation record was verified. The casts and wax dentures were scanned, and a CAD/CAM framework was designed (CAM StructSURE Precision Milled Bar) (Fig 26.11). The maxillary primary bar was designed with a 2° taper and machined from a solid blank of titanium alloy (Fig 26.12).

The bar was designed to be used with two anterior Bredent 2.2 VKS-OC Stud-head screws (XPdent Corporation, Miami, FL) that screwed directly into the tapped sites prepared after the bar was milled. These attachments are designed for use in multiple clinical situations and the female, plastic portions of the attachments are replaceable chairside.

The posterior attachment was a 6-mm SwissLoc attachment (Attachments International, Burlingame, CA). This SwissLoc NG Next Generation attachment consisted of an extracoronal locking pin/plunger designed to prevent lift-off, a common problem reported with bar overdentures. The design incorporated positive in-and-out positions, which prevented the attachment from disengaging unintentionally during function. It was screwed directly into the preexisting tapped site in the primary bar.

The secondary casting was fabricated with type IV gold alloy (North Shore Dental Laboratories, Lynn, MA). Frameworks were tried in and noted to fit well. The maxillary prosthesis was entirely implant supported and did not feature any palatal coverage or tooth support. The palatal portion of

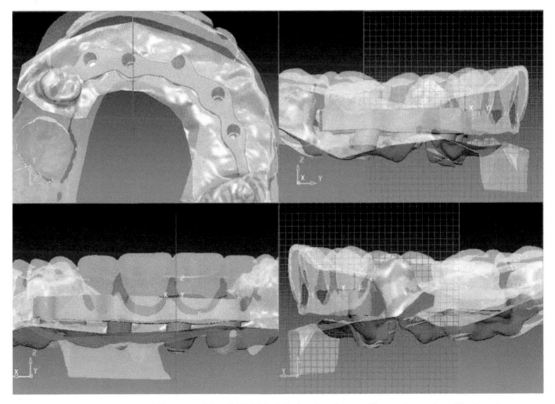

FIGURE 26.11 JPEG images of the CAD/CAM design for the maxillary primary bar. The location of the teeth in the wax denture can be visualized and verifies that the entire primary bar will be contained within the confines of the maxillary overdenture.

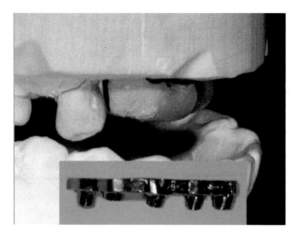

FIGURE 26.12 Laboratory image of the articulated casts. The maxillary cast has both the primary bar and secondary casting in place. The milled bar is offset in the bottom of the image.

the maxillary prosthesis was contoured to be consistent with the contours of the patient's posterior palate. These contours were arbitrary, and the patient was advised that adjustments could be required to optimize his phonetics with the prosthesis in place. The maxillary overdenture prosthesis was completed in a conventional fashion (Figs 26.13–26.20). When the patient returned for the 2-week postinsertion clinical appointment, he reported minimal difficulties in adapting to the prostheses while speaking and chewing. He reported that he was extremely pleased with the esthetic and functional results.

This patient has been followed for 3 years and is comfortable with the prosthetic and surgical rehabilitation. He has experienced no long-term significant problems regarding mastication, oral hygiene, or phonetics. There has been minimal bone loss visualized around the implants in both jaws (Fig 26.21). His long-term prognosis relative to the osseointegrated implants and prosthetics is thought to be favorable.

DISCUSSION

Surgical correction of facial defects may be hampered from the lack of adequate quality and quantities of hard and soft tissues.[6,11] Trauma to the mid-face (hard palate, maxillary sinus, nasal cavity, zygomatic processes, infraorbital rims) may result in varying degrees of maxillary defects,

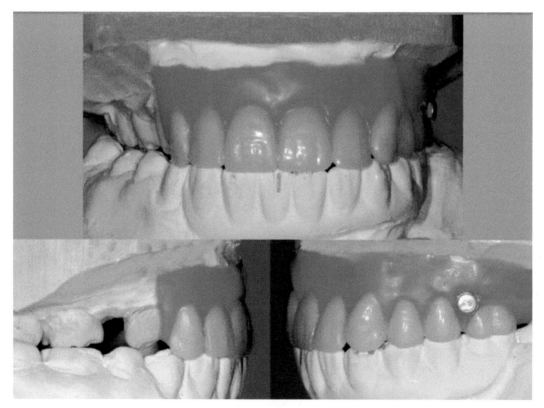

FIGURE 26.13 Laboratory images of the maxillary wax implant prosthesis prior to processing. The mandibular prosthesis (mandibular cast) was completed first to accommodate the increased healing time required for the second maxillary bone grafting procedures. The posterior attachment is in the locked, or "in," position (center: anterior; lower left: right posterior segment; lower right: left posterior segment).

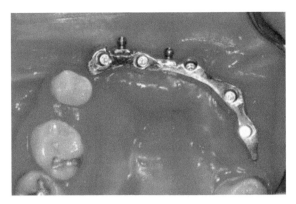

FIGURE 26.14 Maxillary intraoral occlusal image with the primary bar in place. The two anterior attachments are visible on the labial surface of the anterior segment.

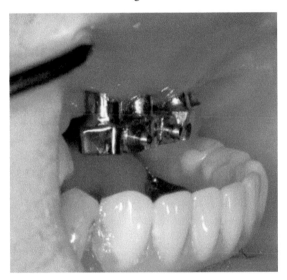

FIGURE 26.15 Lateral clinical image with the maxillary primary bar in place. Note the amount of horizontal distance between the bar and the labial surfaces of the mandibular screw-retained, implant-supported fixed prosthesis.

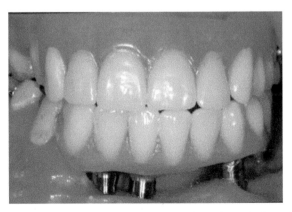

FIGURE 26.16 Anterior clinical view of centric occlusion with both prostheses in place. The large horizontal discrepancy between the location of the maxillary implants and the optimal location of the artificial teeth has been compensated for with the maxillary overdenture.

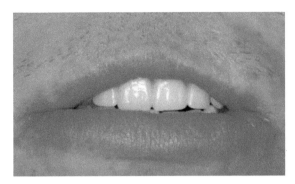

FIGURE 26.17 Clinical image with both prostheses in place. The patient did not have lip competence at rest.

depending on the velocity and etiology of the injury. Due to the anatomic complexity of the mid-facial region and the almost endless potential for defect size, shape, and location, there are an unlimited number of potential disconfigurations, and there is no universally accepted definition of panfacial fractures in the literature. Aramany has published a classification of these defects.[14] Markowitz and Manson have also described panfacial trauma.[15] Applying no one definition or classification, the patient presented in this article had no frontal bone defect, yet otherwise had severely comminuted facial fractures bordered superiorly by the naso-orbito-etmoid

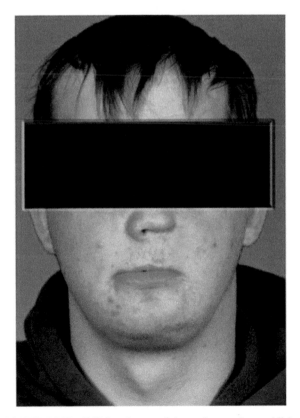

FIGURE 26.18 Full-face image of the patient at the established OVD with a forced effort to establish lip competency.

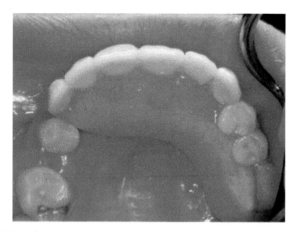

FIGURE 26.19   Clinical image of the partially edentulous maxilla with the overdenture prosthesis in place. Note the atypical contours of the palatal soft tissues.

complex and continuing throughout the mid-face to the inferior extent of the mandible.

Trauma to the mandible can be just as challenging to clinicians as maxillary defects, depending on the volume and location of the defect(s). The muscles of mastication and facial expression attach to the mandible in an extremely complex fashion and also give form to the lower third of the face. Discontinuity defects have the potential to impact negatively on any one of a number of critical functions associated with these structures. This case was particularly challenging because of the loss of significant amounts of

bone and soft tissue, along with loss of vestibular depth in both jaws. This raised the level of difficulty in providing the patient with adequate amounts of bone and soft tissue prior to definitive prosthodontic treatment. Another challenge was that the quality of the intraoral tissues was not ideal in that the tissues surrounding the implant abutments were quite mobile and nonkeratinized.

Debate also exists over where and when to begin treatment in panfacial trauma.[7–10] In this case, the surgical protocol consisted of debridement and primary closure, healing, multiple bone grafts, and additional healing prior to the placement of endosseous implants.

Authors have also differed on the methods of fixation of severe, comminuted mandibular fractures.[16–19] With extensive avulsion-type injuries, rigid fixation of severely comminuted fractures has been problematic. In this case, decisions were made to minimize the risk of infection and decrease the operating time by obtaining closure without rigid fixation.

This case demonstrated the importance of a team approach in comprehensive treatment planning. Initially, the foremost concern was that the patient be stabilized. This was prior to deciding on the definitive surgical and prosthetic treatment plans required to complete the rehabilitative treatment. This patient is now approximately 5 years posttrauma and approximately 3 years postprosthodontic reconstruction. None of the attachments have had to be replaced. The implants and prosthetic treatments have remained stable, and the long-term prognosis for continued success is good.

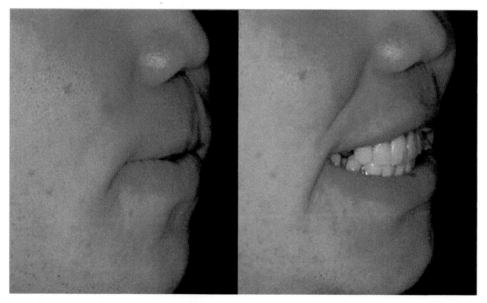

FIGURE 26.20   Profile views of the patient with the prostheses in place 2 weeks postprosthesis insertion. The patient still had to strain slightly to obtain lip competence at rest (rest vertical dimension, left; smiling, right). The anterior/posterior deficiency of the mid-face has been compensated for with the labial flange and tooth positions of the maxillary overdenture prosthesis. The esthetic result in the right posterior maxillary quadrant was slightly compromised due to the retention of the maxillary first premolar.

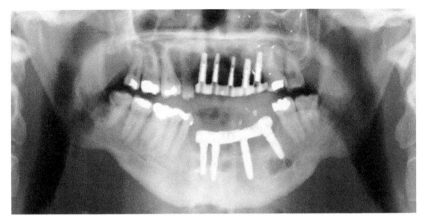

FIGURE 26.21   Panoramic radiograph 3 years postocclusal function. All implants have stable bone levels, without radiolucencies.

REVIEW

This clinical report illustrated the devastating injuries secondary to a self-inflicted gunshot wound to the face. The patient survived the life-threatening injuries while receiving excellent trauma and surgical care immediately posttrauma. Numerous surgeries were required to provide satisfactory bases for long-term prosthodontic success. Endosseous implants were placed into the available, viable maxillary and mandibular bone and became osseointegrated. The patient was restored with a primary maxillary bar, retained by screws in the endosseous implants, and a maxillary overdenture prosthesis. The mandibular defect was restored with a screw-retained, implant-supported fixed prosthesis. Both prostheses have been viable for over 3 years. Despite the clinical success of the treatment noted above, there were several compromises that had to be taken into consideration: the mid-face was deficient horizontally, including lack of soft tissue volume (lips); complete lip competence was not achieved without straining by the patient; an end-to-end anterior tooth arrangement was used to decrease the upper lip volume; the maxillary primary implant-retained bar was not in the position of the maxillary anterior teeth, but was within the anterior articulation zone of the anterior hard palate; and there was a loss of tongue volume and tongue mobility secondary to the original injury. Fortunately in this case, the patient proved to be quite adept at adapting to the compromises noted above, and continues to function without phonetic deficits. The long-term prognosis for this patient is acceptable, both in terms of continued survival of the endosseous implants and the prostheses.

ACKNOWLEDGMENTS

The authors wish to acknowledge the surgical expertise of Dr. Larry Kent, former attending surgeon of Oral and Maxillofacial Surgery, Gundersen Lutheran Medical Center, LaCrosse, WI, and the laboratory assistance of Andrew Gingrasso, Department of Prosthodontics, Gundersen Lutheran Medical Center and Thomas Peterson, CDT, MDT, President, NorthShore Dental Laboratories, Lynn, MA.

REFERENCES

1. Desjardins R: Early rehabilitative management of the maxillectomy patient. *J Prosthet Dent* 1977;38:311–318.
2. Kornblith A, Zlotolow I, Gooen J, et al: Quality of life of maxillectomy patients using an obturator prosthesis. *Head Neck* 1996;18:323–334.
3. Rogers S, Lowe D, McNally D, et al: Health-related quality of life after maxillectomy: a comparison between prosthetic obturation and free flap. *J Oral Maxillofac Surg* 2003;61:174–181.
4. Devlin H, Barker G: Prosthetic rehabilitation of the edentulous patient requiring a partial maxillectomy. *J Prosthet Dent* 1992;67:223–227.
5. Taylor TD (ed): *Clinical Maxillofacial Prosthetics*. Chicago, IL, Quintessence, 2000, p. 6.
6. Vinzenz K, Schaudy C, Wuringer E: The iliac prefabricated composite graft for dentoalveolar reconstruction: a clinical procedure. *Int J Oral Maxillofac Implants* 2006;21:117–123.
7. Markowitz BL, Manson PN: Panfacial fractures: organization of treatment. *Clin Plast Surg* 1989;16:105–114.
8. Mason PN, Clark N, Robertson B, et al: Sub-unit principles in midface fractures: the importance of sagittal buttresses, soft tissue reductions and sequencing treatment of segmental fractures. *Plast Reconstr Surg* 1999;103:1287–1306.
9. Mercuri LG, Steinberg MJ: Sequencing of care for multiple maxillofacial injuries. In Peterson LJ (ed): *Principles of Oral and Maxillofacial Surgery*. Philadelphia, PA, Lippincott, 1992, pp. 615–622.
10. Kelly J: *War Injuries to the Jaws and Related Structures*. Washington, DC, US Government Printing Office, 1978.

11. Gruss JS, Phillips JH: Complex facial trauma: the evolving role of rigid fixation and immediate bone graft reconstruction. *Clin Plast Surg* 1989;16:93–104.

12. *American College of Surgeons: Advanced Trauma and Life Support for Doctors (ed 7)*. Chicago, Il., American College of Surgeons, 2004.

13. Shockley W, Weissler M: Reconstructive alternatives following segmental mandibulectomy. *Am J Otolaryngol* 1992;13:156–165.

14. Aramany M: Basic principles of obturator design for partially edentulous patients. Part I: classification. *J Prosthet Dent* 1978;40:554–561.

15. Markowitz BL, Manson PN: Panfacial fractures: organization of treatment. *Clin Plast Surg* 1989;16:105–114.

16. Benson PD, Marshall MK, Engelstad ME, et al: The use of immediate bone graft in reconstruction of clinically infected mandibular fractures: bone grafts in the presence of pus. *J Oral Maxillofac Surg* 2006;64:122–126.

17. Finn RA: Treatment of comminuted mandible fractures by closed reduction. *J Oral Maxillofac Surg* 1996;54:320–327.

18. Ellis E. III, Muniz O, Anand K: Treatment considerations for comminuted mandibular fractures. *J Oral Maxillofac Surg* 2003;61:861–870.

19. Kazanjian VH: An outline of the treatment of extensive comminuted fractures of the mandible. *Am J Orthod Oral Surg* 1942;28:265.

20. McGarry TJ, Nimmo A, Skiba JF, et al: Classification system for partial edentulism. *J Prosthodont* 2002;11:181–193.

21. McGarry TJ, Nimmo A, Skiba JF, et al: Classification system for complete edentulism. *J Prosthodont* 1999;8:27–39.

22. Goodacre CJ, Kan JY, Rungcharassaeng K: Clinical complications of osseointegrated implants. *J Prosthet Dent* 1999;81:537–552.

23. Brägger U, Aeschlimann S, Bürgin W, et al: Biological and technical complications and failures with fixed partial dentures (FPD) on implants and teeth after four to five years of function. *Clin Oral Implants Res* 2001;12:26–34.

24. Kiener P, Oetterli M, Mericske E, et al: Effectiveness of maxillary overdentures supported by implants: maintenance and prosthetic complications. *Int J Prosthodont* 2001;14:133–140.

25. Lewandowski L: Palatograms and linguograms for studying misarticulation following surgery for tumors of the tongue and oral cavity floor. *Ann Acad Med Stetin* 2006;52(Suppl 3): 13–16.

26. Sun J, Weng Y, Li J, et al: Analysis of determinants on speech function after glossectomy. *J Oral Maxillofac Surg* 2007;65:1944–1950.

27. Krennmair G, Krainhöfner M, Piehslinger E: Implant-supported maxillary overdentures retained with milled bars: maxillary anterior versus maxillary posterior concept—a retrospective study. *Int J Oral Maxillofac Implants* 2008;23:343–352.

28. The glossary of prosthodontic terms. *J Prosthet Dent* 2005;94:10–92.

27

TREATMENT OF HEMI-MANDIBULECTOMY DEFECT WITH IMPLANT-SUPPORTED TELESCOPIC REMOVABLE PROSTHESIS: A CLINICAL REPORT

Athanasios Ntounis, dds, ms,[1] Michael Patras, dds, ms,[2] Stavros Pelekanos, dds, dr. med. dent,[3] and Gregory Polyzois, dds, mscd, dr. dent[4]

[1]Prosthodontist, Resident in Graduate Periodontology Clinic, University of Alabama, Birmingham, AL

[2]Prosthodontist, Clinical Assistant, Department of Prosthodontics, Dental School, University of Athens, Greece

[3]Assistant Professor, Department of Prosthodontics, Dental School, University of Athens, Greece

[4]Associate Professor and Chief of Maxillofacial Prosthetics Unit, Dental School University of Athens, Greece

Keywords

Fibula free flap; telescopic; removable dental prosthesis; implants.

Correspondence

Athanasios Ntounis, 1530 3rd Avenue South; SDB 412, Birmingham, AL 35294. E-mail: thanosnt@uab.edu

The authors deny any conflicts of interest.

Accepted October 8, 2012

Published in *Journal of Prosthodontics* August 2013; Vol. 22, Issue 6

doi: 10.1111/jopr.12012

ABSTRACT

Excision of head and neck tumors (benign or malignant) often leads to large segmental resections of the mandible. The following clinical report describes the oral rehabilitation of a 60-year-old Caucasian man after partial mandibulectomy due to primary oral leiomyosarcoma. Treatment consisted of a free fibula flap and an implant-supported telescopic removable prosthesis.

Oral cancer is an important public health concern and has presented an alarming global increase during the last few decades. Statistics show oral cancer to be one of the most common forms of the disease.[1,2] Primary oral leiomysarcoma is an extremely rare malignant mesenchymal carcinoma with only 70 cases reported worldwide.[3] Farman and Kay estimated an incidence of 0.064% for primary smooth muscle tumors with oral appearance.[4] The tumor presents aggressive behavior with local or distal metastasis and high recurrence.[5] Traditional treatment modalities primarily include surgical interventions by means of oncologic tumor resection.

Contemporary advances in surgical techniques and grafting procedures have enabled surgeons to correct tumor postablative defects with predictable and effective means. Large volumes of autogenous combined soft- and hard-tissue grafts can be transferred from various donor sites and used for the reconstruction of deficiencies.[6,7] Among the numerous available options, the osteocutaneous free fibula flap (FFF) represents a widely used treatment modality for the reconstruction of mandibular defects and allows for repair of the mandibular continuity.[8–11]

After reconstructive surgery, drastic changes in oral anatomy as well as the establishment of new anatomical relationships make dental rehabilitation with a conventional prosthesis challenging.[11–14] Although removable prostheses can adequately support the facial soft tissues, the new denture-bearing surfaces occasionally fail to provide ideal retention and stability.[11,12,15] During the last few decades, osseointegrated implants have become a very important adjunct treatment option for tumor patients. Their placement significantly adds to the retention and support of the prostheses, thus improving chewing efficiency and comfort.[12,15] Numerous studies report favorable survival rates for implants inserted in FFFs and indicate long-term success of the corresponding restorations.[14,16,17] Implant-supported prostheses can help restore facial contours and function.[15,18,19]

Implant-supported telescopic restorations (also referred to as "double crown" or "conical crown" retained removable prostheses) may fulfill the requirements for a successful treatment concept.[14,20,21] The objective of this clinical report is to describe the oral rehabilitation of a patient who underwent a mandibular resection due to a leiomyosarcoma. The prosthetic rehabilitation included the use of implants in conjunction with conical crowns to support a removable dental prosthesis (RDP).

CLINICAL REPORT

A 60-year-old Caucasian man presented to the Maxillofacial Prosthetics Unit, University of Athens, Greece, to restore his missing dentition. His chief complaint was, "I want to get teeth on the bottom right side." The patient reported a history of leiomyosarcoma on the lower right side a year previous. He had been treated with a segmental mandibulectomy, followed by chemotherapy. The defect was reconstructed at the time of surgery with an FFF, and 1 year later three Bicon (Bicon, Boston, MA) implants were placed.

Initial intraoral examination revealed partial edentulism, a Siebert class III defect[22] on the lower right side, and the presence of three nonparallel Bicon implants. Interestingly, plastic impression copings were present over the implants at initial presentation (Fig 27.1). In addition, lack of keratinized periimplant mucosa was noted. Radiographic evaluation revealed good integration of the implants in the free fibula graft with no signs of radiographic bone loss.

Following data collection and preliminary impressions using alginate (Jeltrate, Denstply, York, PA), a facebow transfer (Denar Mark II Earbow, Whip Mix Corp., Louisville, KY) and jaw registration with a lower occlusal rim facilitated mounting of the study casts in a semiadjustable articulator (Denar Mark II Plus articulator, Whip Mix Corp.). A design cast was fabricated using type III dental stone (Microstone, Whip Mix Corp.) and surveyed (Ney Surveryor, Dentsply). Treatment options, including a proposed soft-tissue grafting procedure to increase the width of keratinized mucosa around the implants, were discussed with the patient, who declined to have any further surgical interventions. The restorative treatment plan included the fabrication of double conical crowns on the malaligned implants and an RDP to restore both function and esthetics. The prosthesis was designed to achieve combined tooth and implant support and retention.

A #6 round bur (Brasseler USA, Savannah, GA) was used to prepare occlusal rest seats. The occlusal rest seats were prepared on the distal lingual aspect on the occlusal surface of the second molar as well as the embrasure space between the premolars, extending on the adjacent interproximal marginal ridges and occlusal surfaces. A natural guide plane was present on the mesial surface of the left mandibular canine, and preparation was not necessary. Prior to final impression of the lower arch, an interocclusal record was made using

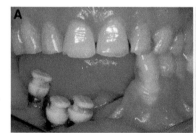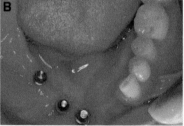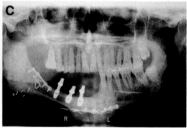

FIGURE 27.1   (A) At initial clinical presentation, a severe Siebert class III defect[26] can be appreciated. Note the plastic impression copings on the abutments, and lack of implant parallelism. (B) Occlusal view of the implant abutments after removal of the impression copings. (C) Orthopantomograph revealed the restored continuity of the mandible with the FFF and good bone integration of three Bicon implants.

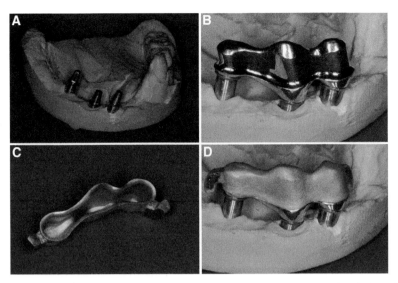

FIGURE 27.2   (A) Working cast. Bicon uses one-piece implant replicas. (B) After the insertion path of the RPD was determined, the primary component of the telescopic prosthesis was fabricated. The milled primary coping corrected the unfavorable inclination of the implant abutments, thus establishing an agreement with the insertion path of the RPD. (C) Intaglio surface of the secondary copings. Two extensions were fabricated to connect the telescopic superstructure and the RDP framework. (D) Secondary coping in place on the working cast. The external surface was sandblasted to enhance mechanical retention of the acrylic resin.

vinylpolysiloxane (Regisil, Dentsply) over the plastic impression copings. An acrylic custom tray was fabricated using Triad Blue Tray material (Dentsply), and conventional border molding was performed using green stick modeling compound (Impression Compound; Kerr Corp, Orange, CA). An impression was made using polyether impression material (Impregum; 3M ESPE, Monrovia, CA). The impression captured the implant positions and ensured maximum extension of the acrylic base. The working cast was fabricated using type IV dental stone (Silky-Rock, Whip Mix Corp.). The working cast incorporated one-piece implant analogs of the specific implant system (Bicon) (Fig 27.2A). The cast was surveyed (Ney Surveyor) to accurately determine the most favorable path of insertion and aid in the final framework design.

Unfavorable implant positioning required the fabrication of three primary copings (conical crowns). The primary copings were splinted in a one-piece superstructure using a type III gold alloy (Degulor C, Degussa, Hanau, Germany). The superstructure corrected the inclination of the implant abutment and was milled to match the insertion path of the RDP (Fig 27.2B). The axial walls of the primary superstructure were fabricated with a 4° convergence, to achieve at least 10 N retention force.[23] Finally, a secondary superstructure was fabricated of the same alloy (Figs 27.2C and 27.2D). Retention was tested with the use of a special instrument (Koni-Meter, Krupp, Essen, Germany). Partial denture design consisted of a lingual bar major connector,

occlusal rests in the premolar region, and a circumferential clasp on the lower left second molar. A guide plane mesial to the lower left canine was added to provide additional stability of the final prosthesis. The final Co–Cr alloy cast (Vitallium 2000 Plus, Austenal, Dentsply) was then connected to the secondary coping by laser welding (LaserStar 8000 Series, Crafford-LaserStar Technologies, Orlando, FL) (Fig 27.3).

Framework try-in took place, and passive fit was verified using Occlude disclosing medium (Pascal Company, Bellevue, WA) (Fig 27.4). Custom shades were selected for the

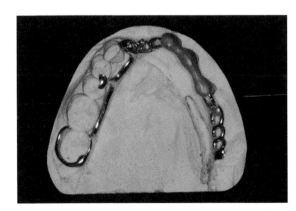

FIGURE 27.3   Complete framework on master cast. The telescopic component was laser welded to the major and minor connectors of the RPD framework.

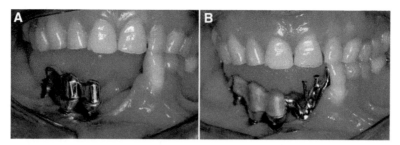

FIGURE 27.4   (A) Try-in of primary coping. (B) Clinical view of secondary coping and RDP framework seated. Note the proximal guide plate mesial to the lower left canine, as well as the incisal projections of the framework to compensate for the vertical defect and to provide additional acrylic support.

teeth (Vita 3D-Master Shade Guide) and mucosa (Naturcryl, GC America Inc, Alsip, IL). Digital photos were taken and sent to the laboratory. Multilayered teeth (Visio.Lign veneering system, Bredent GmbH & Co. KG, Senden, Germany) were used for ideal color matching and long-lasting esthetics. During the setup appointment, esthetic factors and phonetics were evaluated, and patient approval was obtained (Fig 27.5). Conventional processing of the superstructure followed.

At the time of delivery of the implant-supported partial overdenture, the primary crowns were luted on the abutments with resin cement (C&B Cement, Bisco, Schaumburg, IL) and the RDP immediately seated, thereby ensuring accurate fit of all parts of the restoration (Fig 27.6). The patient was seen for follow-up appointments for minor occlusal adjustments. The patient was provided with prosthesis care and oral hygiene instructions. Subsequent recall visits were scheduled. The patient adapted to the removable prosthesis easily and did not require any further revision. Remarkable stability of the prosthesis, enhanced facial support, and improved overall appearance were reported by the patient.

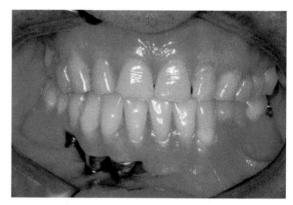

FIGURE 27.6   Final prosthesis in place. Note the enhanced esthetics provided by multilayered teeth and optimal color matching of the pink acrylic.

DISCUSSION

In recent years there have been significant advances in treatment options for oral rehabilitation of the cancer patient through a multidisciplinary team approach.[13] With contemporary surgical interventions, excellent results can be accomplished with the resection of malignant lesions and simultaneous reconstruction by means of osteocutaneous free flap tissue transplants.[4,6,7] This method has become an established treatment modality that predictably restores the continuity of resected mandible.[6,7] Sufficient length, good vascularization, and good bone quality are some of the significant advantages provided by FFF.[6,7] However, the resulting height of the hard tissue in sites restored with the FFF is usually deficient. This is critical in cases of partial mandibular resection where the contralateral side is unaffected and the occlusal plane is found further cranially,[11] and an unfavorable "crown-to-implant ratio" is introduced to the implant-supported restoration. To overcome this disadvantage, several techniques have been proposed, such as

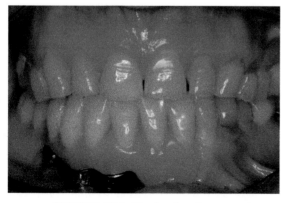

FIGURE 27.5   Try-in of teeth setup.

the "double barrel" fibula transfer[24] or the use of vertical distraction osteogenesis[25] to improve bone height.

For the present patient, a large discrepancy between the fibula transplant and the unaffected area was present. Important considerations included the nonideal implant positioning as well as the need for tissue support to restore normal facial contours.[26] In addition, the designed prosthesis should be able to facilitate optimal hygiene around the implants. A removable instead of a fixed prosthesis was selected, since it can provide better support of the buccal mucosa and underlying musculature, thus restoring facial appearance. Removable prostheses can also accommodate comfortable hygiene practices that ensure long-term periimplant tissue health.[26] This is critical since the patient refused to undergo gingival augmentation to increase the width of periimplant keratinized tissue. In the vast majority of similar cases, a loss or absence of keratinized mucosa is observed.[17] Although clinical evidence on the role of keratinized mucosa on implant survival is still a point of discussion,[27–29] it has been shown that an adequate zone of keratinized mucosa is associated with less gingival inflammation.[27,28] However, another study concluded that acceptable periimplant tissue health can be maintained even in the absence of keratinized mucosa when optimal oral hygiene is performed.[29]

Dental implants provide considerable solutions as supporting elements, where lack of adequate support and retention from the remaining teeth and compromised edentulous areas exist.[11,12,15] Implants placed in FFFs have been shown to achieve adequate osseointegration and comparable long-term success to implants placed in native bone.[8,14,15–17] However, the literature supports the notion that the estimated lower implant survival rates in cancer patients may be attributed to grafting, unfavorable anatomic relationships, compromised surgical field, or contributory medical history.[8,12,17,30]

The use of implant-supported removable prostheses makes treatment more feasible for rehabilitation of orofacial defects.[12] Various clinical studies and case reports have demonstrated the use of different clip and bar designs, stud attachments, or magnets[11,30] for such cases. The use of a double crown system (conical crowns) on implants, in combination with an overdenture, has been shown to be very successful.[31] The aforementioned conical connection provides increased stability, retention, and reciprocation due to the friction between the primary and the secondary copings.[32] This type of connection also provides axial implant loading and can potentially eliminate the increased maintenance needs of stud attachments and bar/clip connections, while providing comparable stability and retention of the prosthesis.[33] It is also a flexible design that can be combined with other retentive elements once an insertion path is established. In this case, the use of friction-fit copings was successfully combined with a conventional RDP design.

The design selected provided cross-arch stabilization, thus eliminating potential lateral forces on the implants, as well as equally distributing the functional loads between teeth and implants.[26] The disadvantages of this prosthesis design are the increased cost due to the gold alloy used for the coping fabrication, as well as the technically sensitive laboratory procedures that require a highly trained and experienced dental technician.[34,35]

CONCLUSION

The primary objective of prosthetic treatment following an ablative oncologic surgery is to create a functional and esthetic dentition. In addition to restoring function and esthetics, oral rehabilitation addresses social disability parameters and plays a key role in providing an acceptable quality of life.[6] In this case, prosthetic rehabilitation included the use of implants in conjunction with conical crowns to support an RDP.

ACKNOWLEDGMENTS

The authors would like to thank George Pasias, CDT, for the laboratory stages of the presented case and Dr. Lillie Pitman, DMD, for constructive criticism during editing this article.

REFERENCES

1. Parkin DM, Bray F, Ferlay J, et al: Global cancer statistics, 2002. *CA Cancer J Clin* 2005;55:74–108.
2. de Camargo Cancela M, Voti L, Guerra-Yi M, et al: Oral cavity cancer in developed and in developing countries: population-based incidence. *Head Neck* 2010;32:357–367.
3. Izumi K, Maeda T, Cheng J, et al: Primary leiomyosarcoma of the maxilla with regional lymph node metastasis. Report of a case and review of the literature. *Oral Surg Oral Med Oral Pathol Oral Radiol Endod* 1995;80:310–319.
4. Farman AG, Kay S: Oral leiomyosarcoma. Report of a case and review of the literature pertaining to smooth-muscle tumors of the oral cavity. *Oral Surg Oral Med Oral Pathol* 1977;43:402–409.
5. Nikitakis NG, Lopes MA, Bailey JS, et al: Oral leiomyosarcoma: review of the literature and report of two cases with assessment of the prognostic and diagnostic significance of immunohistochemical and molecular markers. *Oral Oncol* 2002;38:201–208.
6. Moscoso JF, Keller J, Genden E, et al: Vascularized bone flaps in oromandibular reconstruction. A comparative anatomic study of bone stock from various donor sites to assess suitability for enosseous dental implants. *Arch Otolaryngol Head Neck Surg* 1994;120:36–43.

7. Iizuka T, Häfliger J, Seto I, et al: Oral rehabilitation after mandibular reconstruction using an osteocutaneous fibula free flap with endosseous implants. Factors affecting the functional outcome in patients with oral cancer. *Clin Oral Implants Res* 2005;16:69–79.

8. Smolka K, Kraehenbuehl M, Eggensperger N, et al: Fibula free flap reconstruction of the mandible in cancer patients: evaluation of a combined surgical and prosthodontic treatment concept. *Oral Oncol* 2008;44:571–581.

9. Reychler H, Iriarte Ortabe J: Mandibular reconstruction with the free fibula osteocutaneous flap. *Int J Oral Maxillofac Surg* 1994;23:209–213.

10. Cordeiro PG, Disa JJ, Hidalgo DA, et al: Reconstruction of the mandible with osseous free flaps: a 10-year experience with 150 consecutive patients. *Plast Reconstr Surg* 1999;104:1314–1320.

11. Dalkiz M, Beydemir B, Günaydin Y: Treatment of a microvascular reconstructed mandible using an implant-supported fixed partial denture: case report. *Implant Dent* 2001;10:121–125.

12. Schoen PJ, Reintsema H, Raghoebar GM, et al: The use of implant retained mandibular prostheses in the oral rehabilitation of head and neck cancer patients. A review and rationale for treatment planning. *Oral Oncol* 2004;40:862–871.

13. Moroi HH, Okimoto K, Terada Y: The effect of an oral prosthesis on the quality of life for head and neck cancer patients. *J Oral Rehabil* 1999;26:265–273.

14. Weischer T, Mohr C: Implant-supported mandibular telescopic prostheses in oral cancer patients: an up to 9-year retrospective study. *Int J Prosthodont* 2001;14:329–334.

15. Kramer FJ, Dempf R, Bremer B: Efficacy of dental implants placed into fibula-free flaps for orofacial reconstruction. *Clin Oral Implants Res* 2005;16:80–88.

16. Foster RD, Anthony JP, Sharma A, et al: Vascularized bone flaps versus nonvascularized bone grafts for mandibular reconstruction: an outcome analysis of primary bony union and endosseous implant success. *Head Neck* 1999;21:66–71.

17. Cheung LK, Leung AC: Dental implants in reconstructed jaws: implant longevity and peri-implant tissue outcomes. *J Oral Maxillofac Surg* 2003;61:1263–1274.

18. Weischer T, Mohr C: Ten-year experience in oral implant rehabilitation of cancer patients: treatment concept and proposed criteria for success. *Int J Oral Maxillofac Implants* 1999;14:521–528.

19. Balshi TJ: Implant rehabilitation of a patient after partial mandibulectomy: a case report. *Quintessence Int* 1995;26:459–463.

20. Bergman B, Ericson A, Molin M: Long-term clinical results after treatment with conical crown- retained dentures. *Int J Prosthodont* 1996;9:533–538.

21. Behr M, Hofman E, Rosentritt M, et al: Technical failure rates of double crown-retained removable partial dentures. *Clin Oral Invest* 2000;4:87–90.

22. Seibert JS: Reconstruction of deformed, partially edentulous ridges, using full thickness onlay grafts. Part I: technique and wound healing. *Compend Contin Educ Dent* 1983; 4:437–453.

23. Bayer S, Kraus D, Keilig L, et al: Changes in retention force with electroplated copings on conical crowns: a comparison of gold and zirconia primary crowns. *Int J Oral Maxillofac Implants* 2012;27:577–585.

24. Bähr W, Stoll P, Wächter R: Use of the "double barrel" free vascularized fibula in mandibular reconstruction. *J Oral Maxillofac Surg* 1998;56:38–44.

25. Chiapasco, M, Brusati, R, Galioto S: Distraction osteogenesis of a fibular revascularized flap for improvement of oral implant positioning in a tumour patient: a case report. *J Oral Maxillofac Surg* 2000;58:1434–1440.

26. Jacob RF, King GE: Partial denture framework design for bone-grafted mandibles restored with osseointegrated implants. *J Prosthodont* 1995;4:6–10.

27. Schrott AR, Jimenez M, Hwang JW, et al: Five-year evaluation of the influence of keratinized mucosa on peri-implant soft-tissue health and stability around implants supporting full-arch mandibular fixed prostheses. *Clin Oral Implants Res* 2009;20:1170–1177.

28. Adibrad M, Shahabuei M, Sahabi M: Significance of the width of keratinized mucosa on the health status of the supporting tissue around implants supporting overdentures. *J Oral Implantol* 2009;35:232–237.

29. Esper LA, Ferreira SB Jr, de Oliveira Fortes Kaizer R, et al: The role of keratinized mucosa in peri-implant health. *Cleft Palate Craniofac* 2012;49:167–170.

30. Shaw RJ, Sutton AF, Cawood JI, et al: Oral rehabilitation after treatment for head and neck malignancy. *Head Neck* 2005;27:459–470.

31. Romanos GE, May S, May D: Treatment concept of the edentulous mandible with prefabricated telescopic abutments and immediate functional loading. *Int J Oral Maxillofac Implants* 2011;26:593–597.

32. Hoffmann O, Beaumont C, Tatakis DN, et al: Telescopic crowns as attachments for implant supported restorations: a case series. *J Oral Implantol* 2006;32:291–299.

33. Eitner S, Schlegel A, Emeka N, et al: Comparing bar and double-crown attachments in implant-retained prosthetic reconstruction: a follow-up investigation. *Clin Oral Implants Res* 2008;19:530–537.

34. Halterman SM, Rivers JA, Keith JD, et al: Implant support for removable partial overdentures: a case report. *Implant Dent* 1999;8:74–78.

35. Kaufmann R, Friedli M, Hug S, et al: Removable dentures with implant support in strategic positions followed for up to 8 years. *Int J Prosthodont* 2009;22:233–241.

PART VI

MANAGEMENT OF COMPLETELY EDENTULOUS PATIENTS USING NEW CERAMIC MATERIAL

28

THE USE OF CUSTOM-MILLED ZIRCONIA TEETH TO ADDRESS TOOTH ABRASION IN COMPLETE DENTURES: A CLINICAL REPORT

JOANNE M. LIVADITIS[1] AND GUS J. LIVADITIS, DDS[2]

[1]Student, University of Maryland, College Park, MD
[2]Private Practice, Baltimore, MD

Keywords
Zirconia; dentures; removable prosthodontics.

Correspondence
Gus J. Livaditis, Ste. 100, 1206 York Rd., Baltimore, MD 21093. E-mail: LivaditisDDS@aol.com

The authors deny any conflicts of interest.

Accepted August 11, 2012

Published in *Journal of Prosthodontics* April 2013; Vol. 22, Issue 3

doi: 10.1111/j.1532-849X.2012.00943.x

ABSTRACT

A patient exhibited severe abrasion of resin posterior denture teeth including perforation of the denture base. New dentures were provided to explore the application of zirconia teeth for complete dentures. [Correction added to online publication 07 November 2012: "Zirconium" corrected to "Zirconia."] Traditional denture procedures were combined with fixed prosthodontic CAD/CAM procedures to fabricate custom-designed four-tooth posterior segments in hollow crown form to reduce weight and with a retentive form for interlocking to the denture base. The new dentures were successful in reducing wear of the denture teeth over the short-term follow-up period.

Zirconia is currently used in numerous applications, including crowns, fixed dental prostheses (FDPs), dowels, cores, implants, implant abutments, and orthodontic brackets.[1-3] Of these applications, fixed prosthodontic restorations are the most relevant for complete dentures. Due to its compression resistance of approximately 2000 MPa,[1] zirconia has been shown to be effective for posterior teeth of fixed prostheses supported by and/or opposing natural teeth or implant-supported restorations. Given that soft-tissue-supported prostheses experience less masticatory force, the application of zirconia to dentures can be reasonably extrapolated from the use of zirconia in current practice.

Zirconia stabilized with 3% Y_2O_3 (3Y-TZP) is the form most commonly used for dental restorations.[1] In the following clinical report, the Y-TZP zirconia system included an alloy of 5% Y_2O_3 with 3% HfO_2 and less than 1% Al_2O_3

(crystal diamond high translucency YZ zirconia, DLMS-crystal zirconia). As reported by the manufacturer, this type of zirconia has a flexural strength of 950 MPa. The posterior tooth segments for this denture application were formed entirely in zirconia as there was no specific functional or esthetic advantage for layering porcelain.

Zirconia has numerous characteristics that make it attractive for use in dental restorations, including the proposed denture application. Zirconia is neither cytotoxic nor mutagenic, and it has been shown to induce a smaller inflammatory response in tissues and less bacterial colonization than other restorative materials.[3,4] Zirconia is tooth-colored and opaque, providing a desirable alternative to fabricating less-esthetic porcelain-fused-to-metal frameworks. Unlike most brittle, moderately strong ceramic materials that are subject to failure, zirconia ceramic has been shown to inhibit crack growth.[5] It also has been shown to wear less than other ceramic materials when opposed by zirconia during testing[6] and to cause less wear on antagonists than other ceramics do.[7]

CLINICAL REPORT

A 50-year-old patient with 13.5-month-old complete maxillary and mandibular dentures was referred for evaluation and treatment. The dentures exhibited normal contact of the anterior teeth but extreme wear in the posterior areas, with a higher degree of wear on the left side than on the right. The patient's occlusal vertical dimension (OVD) was maintained by the anterior teeth, which exhibited no abrasion. The degree of abrasion on the posterior teeth resulted in a 5 to 7 mm interocclusal space in the most severe areas. Abrasion occurred to the extent that the maxillary denture was perforated through the denture base with an opening of approximately 7 × 20 mm (Fig 28.1). The referring dentist reported that the patient's previous dentures also exhibited a similar degree of abrasion over a period of 27 months. Both sets of dentures consisted entirely of resin-based denture teeth.

During the initial consultation, the patient reported having numerous teeth extracted immediately before the first dentures.

He described wearing the dentures at night and using denture adhesive throughout the 40-month denture-wearing period. No unusual habits such as holding or biting objects with the teeth were identified. Upon reviewing his diet, the patient reported no unusual patterns except for frequent snacking on sourdough pretzels. He also reported being told that he had a bruxing habit.

The oral examination revealed prominent ridge form on both arches. The patient's current dentures were evaluated and found to be well adapted and stable on the ridges. Retention could not be adequately assessed in light of the large perforation. The absence of posterior occlusion was

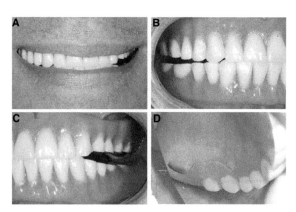

FIGURE 28.1   (A) Anterior teeth displayed no wear and maintained the OVD. (B) Tooth abrasion resulted in lack of occlusion of posterior teeth. (C) Greater wear occurred on patient's preferred chewing side. (D) Wear pattern extended beyond tooth surfaces resulting in perforation of the denture base.

considered to be a significant reason for the reliance on denture adhesive, as functioning only on anterior teeth would dislodge the dentures. The soft tissues appeared normal, and there were no indications of tissue irritation, tissue indentations, or pressure spots as might be seen with clenching or bruxing. Except for the extreme wear of the dentures, the patient was evaluated as a class I patient based on the Prosthodontic Diagnostic Index.[8]

The wear pattern on the dentures was consistent with localized abrasion, which could not be attributed to attrition, as there was no potential for frictional contact of the posterior teeth after the initial wear (Figs 28.1B and 28.1C). Since significant abrasion only occurred on the posterior teeth, the cause of abrasion was likely due to a material or object large enough to account for the 5 to 7 mm spaces in the posterior areas. The patient reported consuming three 16-oz bags of sourdough pretzels (Utz Quality Foods, Inc., Hanover, PA) per week during the 40-month period. Sourdough pretzels are characterized by thick loops of dough, a hard inner consistency, and a rigid crust with exposed large salt granules. The width of the pretzel loops (approximately 13–15 mm) was sufficient to have caused the posterior tooth wear. The projecting salt granules could have served as an abrasive material, and the large granule size (approximately 1–2 mm in diameter) may have increased abrasion due to a prolonged period needed to dissolve the salt.

Once the abrasion was attributed to the pretzels, the recommendation was made to the patient to reduce his consumption. When planning new dentures, the use of resin-based, including composite-based, posterior denture teeth was ruled out. Implant-supported prostheses were not acceptable to the patient. Other alternatives considered to prevent similar abrasion included the use of porcelain denture teeth or metal onlay denture teeth; however, potential chipping or fracturing of porcelain teeth was a concern, and metal onlay teeth were regarded as esthetically unacceptable. The patient was informed that zirconia is used for restorations on natural teeth and on dental implants and may be an abrasion-resistant option for complete dentures. The patient was receptive to the possibility of obtaining more durable dentures and retained the option for conventional dentures in the event the effort was unsuccessful. This patient provided an opportunity to explore the application of zirconia teeth in complete denture procedures.

Various macromechanical forms are possible to provide retention of the teeth in the denture base. For this patient, retention was accomplished by drilling several holes in the subgingival areas of the zirconia teeth during the presintered stage (Fig 28.2). This method was used instead of bonding the denture base to the zirconia, because zirconia is typically not amenable to bonding without additional preparation of the zirconia surface. Bonding may be beneficial, however, to prevent potential leakage and staining at the interface of the denture base and teeth. Several procedures have been investigated to create a retentive and active surface on zirconia for bonding. These include (1) fusing a slurry of zirconia powder and "pore former" to the surface of the pre- or postsintered

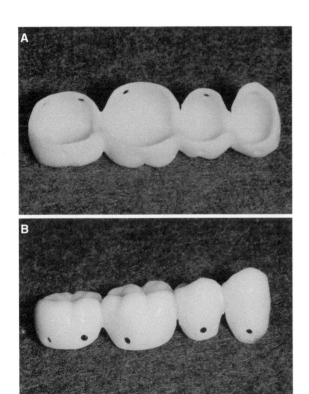

FIGURE 28.2 (A) Zirconia teeth were milled in four-tooth segments. The teeth were milled in a hollow form to reduce the weight of the zirconia teeth. (B) Holes were created in subgingival areas of the segments in the presintered stage to provide retention to the denture base.

zirconia and later burning off the "pore former" to create a micromechanical surface for bonding,[9,10] and (2) using selective infiltration etching whereby a glass-containing compound is heated to molten stage for diffusion along grain boundaries. Upon cooling, the glass would be dissolved in an acid bath, exposing a retentive surface.[11,12] A third procedure involves fusing etchable porcelain to the zirconia, followed by etching the porcelain with hydrofluoric acid to create micromechanical retention to resin.[13–16] Additionally, two systems are commercially available for embedding silica on the surface of zirconia using air abrasion with aluminum trioxide particles modified with silica. A laboratory version uses 110 μm silica-coated alumina particles (Rocatec, 3M ESPE, St. Paul, MN), while a chairside system uses 30 μm particles (CoJet, 3M ESPE).[17–21] Both systems embed silica onto the zirconia surface, making the surfaces chemically reactive to resin with silane coupling agents. In this denture procedure, there was no compelling need to incorporate micromechanical retention in the denture teeth unless staining at the interface had been observed to occur. The custom milling process and the hollow form of the teeth provided a reliable and efficient means for retention of the teeth to the denture base. Micromechanical retention and/or chemical adhesion features are more valuable for fixed prosthodontic restorations.

Hollow denture teeth, similar in form to conventional crowns or FDPs (Fig 28.2), were considered to be preferable to solid teeth to reduce the weight of the denture teeth without sacrificing strength. Zirconia is substantially heavier than traditional porcelain or resin; even in a hollow form, the zirconia teeth were approximately three times the weight of porcelain teeth and five times the weight of resin-based teeth. A potential complication of the hollow design could have been discoloration, if the moderately translucent zirconia teeth were filled and processed with a pink denture base resin; however, this problem was avoided by filling the zirconia teeth with tooth-colored resin immediately prior to processing the denture bases (Fig 28.3).

Denture teeth were not available in zirconia molds or shades, and no computer software program designed to fabricate denture teeth in zirconia was known to the authors at the time of this procedure. Such a computer program likely would have provided not only the mechanism for designing and milling the zirconia teeth, but also a method for accurately positioning the zirconia teeth on the denture base throughout the process. A software program and milling equipment designed for fixed prosthodontic procedures were used to the extent possible, and laboratory procedures were adapted as needed.

Clinical and Laboratory Procedures

The clinical phase for the zirconia dentures followed traditional complete denture procedures for the preliminary and

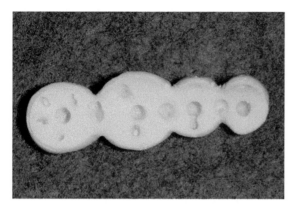

FIGURE 28.3 The zirconia segments were filled with tooth-colored composite to prevent discoloration by the pink denture base resin. Additional retention was created in the composite filler.

master impressions, as well as for refinement of the occlusal rims and for interocclusal records. The new zirconia dentures were designed to include resin-based anterior teeth since no wear occurred in the anterior areas of the previous dentures. Denture teeth were set to create a customized arrangement, which was checked intraorally for optimal esthetics and occlusion (Fig 28.4). Laboratory procedures also paralleled traditional complete denture procedures, except for the fabrication and processing of the zirconia teeth.

The zirconia teeth were processed in four-tooth posterior segments. A customized arrangement of the teeth for trial dentures was completed prior to scanning; therefore, no benefit would have been derived by milling 16 individual teeth. A CAD/CAM system for fixed prosthodontic zirconia restorations was used to design and fabricate the zirconia denture tooth segments (DLMS-Crystal Zirconia, Scottsdale, AZ). First, a scan was made of the posterior segments of the trial tooth arrangement to generate the full contours

and occlusal anatomy of the zirconia teeth. Next, an impression was made of the posterior segments of the trial tooth arrangement, the impression was poured in stone, and a vacuum-formed shell was created for each segment. The posterior teeth were removed from the trial denture bases, and indexing areas were formed in the trial bases for eventual repositioning of the segments. Using the vacuum-formed shells, the posterior segments were replicated in a semirigid polyether impression material (Ramitec, 3M ESPE) on the denture bases while registering the indexing areas. The posterior segments, formed with a material (Ramitec) with properties that facilitated carving (Fig 28.5), were removed and carved to simulate tooth preparation form for crowns. The carved segments were repositioned on the denture bases using the indexing areas. Then, the carved segments were scanned to serve as prepared dies for the design of crown segments by the computer program. The computer program integrated the initial scan of fully contoured teeth onto the tooth preparation scan to enable the designing, processing, and milling of each four-tooth fixed-prosthodontic-type restoration.

All segments were milled to provide zirconia thickness of approximately 1.5 mm except for the margin areas (Fig 28.2). The segments were formed using zirconia (DLMS) and milled (CBMS, Cercon, Dentsply Intl, York, PA). After milling and prior to sintering the segments, perforations were made in the subgingival areas of the teeth for retention of the segments within the denture base. The segments were then stained, sintered, further stained, and glazed.

The zirconia segments were repositioned in the trial denture bases and were evaluated intraorally to confirm

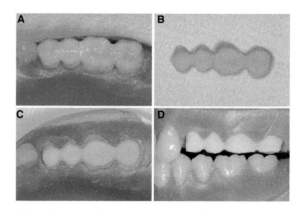

FIGURE 28.5 (A) Impressions were made of the posterior segments of the trial denture. The segments were replicated in a material for trimming. The segments were indexed to the denture base for accurate repositioning. (B) The segments were trimmed to fixed prosthodontic abutment form. (C) The prepared abutment segments were repositioned in the denture base for scanning. (D) The prepared abutment segments were scanned and the abutment scans were merged with the full-contour scans to generate the zirconia tooth segments.

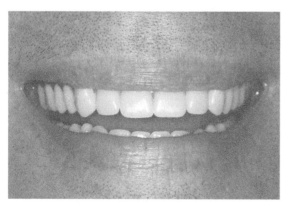

FIGURE 28.4 Trial insertion with resin denture teeth set in a customized arrangement. Posterior teeth were scanned to generate the full-contour pattern for milling the zirconia teeth.

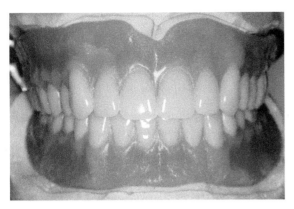

FIGURE 28.6 The milled, sintered, and glazed segments were repositioned in the denture base with the anterior teeth. Occlusion and patient acceptance of the esthetic arrangement were verified during a trial insertion.

proper occlusal relationship (Fig 28.6). The soft tissue areas of the dentures were refined in the trial dentures and prepared for processing. After flasking the dentures and eliminating the denture base wax, the zirconia segments were filled with tooth-colored resin (Vita Zeta, Vita Zahnfabrik, Bad Säckingen, Germany). Additional retention was created in

the resin that filled the segments (Fig 28.3). The dentures were processed, removed from the flasks, cleaned, and polished. They were provided to the patient with routine checks and adjustments. Occlusal adjustments were made using conventional diamond burs and polished with rubber wheels (Dedeco Classic #4950 and #4960, Dedeco Intl., Long Eddy, NY) (Fig 28.7).

The patient was followed for 8 months prior to this publication. At the 8-month visit, the patient reported having ended consumption of the sourdough pretzels. Within the 8-month period, the zirconia dentures had been exposed to the sourdough pretzels for 4.5 months. The dentures exhibited loss of luster and slight wear of the denture base in the areas adjacent to the teeth; however, the zirconia teeth exhibited no abrasion or loss of the glazed surface (Fig 28.8). The patient reported being very satisfied with the dentures. When informed about possible "clicking" of the teeth, as is sometimes encountered with porcelain teeth, the patient indicated no such awareness. The patient has continued to use denture adhesive as he has from the time of extractions, and to wear the dentures at night. The patient continues to be monitored for changes in the zirconia teeth and abrasion of the adjacent denture base.

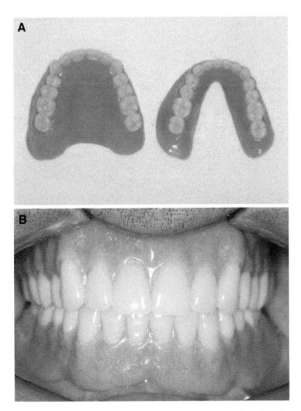

FIGURE 28.7 (A) The dentures were processed, refined, and polished. (B) The dentures were provided to the patient after routine adjustments.

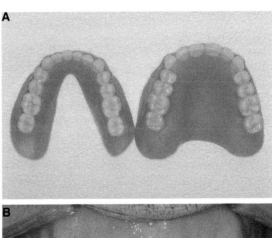

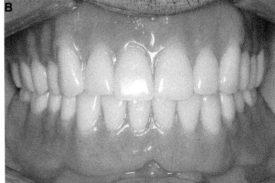

FIGURE 28.8 (A) At 8 months, dentures show loss of luster on the denture base areas. Teeth exhibit no wear. (B) The patient at 8 months depicting dentures with intact posterior occlusion.

DISCUSSION

During this treatment period, two methods for using zirconia teeth in future complete denture procedures were envisioned: (1) premanufactured denture teeth, and (2) CAD/CAM fabricated teeth custom-designed for each patient. With the first option, zirconia teeth could be manufactured and made accessible in a variety of molds similar to currently available denture teeth. Through a manufacturing process that would produce high volume in a factory setting, the mass production of zirconia teeth could integrate features, such as hollow form, optimal thickness to balance strength and weight considerations, tooth-colored resin internally, and retention for interlocking with denture base resin.

With the second option, laboratory computer programs for designing and milling could provide a wide range of tooth molds or patterns, avoiding an extensive inventory of manufactured teeth. Ideally, a CAD/CAM program would automate the process of creating denture tooth segments while simultaneously including retentive features in the zirconia teeth; however, a combination of new clinical procedures and modifications to existing computer technology would be needed. A combined clinical and laboratory program would enable several features: (1) virtual customized tooth arrangements milled in resin material for trial insertion, and (2) evaluation of tooth arrangement by the clinician and patient with an option for virtual alteration before or after trial insertion. Since the fabrication of zirconia teeth consumed a substantial portion of the laboratory effort for the patient described in this report, the development of a software program designed specifically for complete denture applications would significantly reduce the effort required to fabricate customized denture tooth arrangements.

Shortly after treatment of this patient, two computer-generated denture systems (Dentca CAD/CAM Denture, Dentca, Inc, Los Angeles, CA; and Avadent Digital Dentures, Global Dental Science LLC, Scottsdale, AZ) were introduced commercially. Both systems incorporate commercially available premanufactured resin-based teeth, and both systems mill denture bases by scanning traditional impressions provided by the dentist. Teeth are selected from a library of tooth molds; then, computer programs arrange the teeth in occlusion and relation to each denture base from clinical data provided by the dentist. Additional anatomical data are obtained from the scanned impressions and from the occlusal devices, which relate the arches in centric relation at the selected OVD. Denture teeth may be trimmed to accommodate limited interocclusal space, to refine the occlusion, and to provide esthetic modifications. Neither system currently offers the capability for custom-milled denture teeth regardless of the tooth material; however, these systems incorporate advances in denture fabrication that have been available in fixed conventional and implant prosthodontics for several years. The application of custom-milled denture teeth in removable complete dentures is only a matter of time and demand.

SUMMARY

The patient described in this report presented with a severe degree of denture tooth abrasion. Tooth abrasion in complete dentures remains a significant concern, particularly with commonly used resin-based denture teeth. Porcelain denture teeth are resistant to abrasion but susceptible to fracture. Zirconia is anticipated to improve resistance to abrasion, result in fewer tooth fractures, and provide a longer useful life than other materials used for teeth in complete dentures. In conclusion, zirconia denture teeth may serve as a valuable alternative to existing denture teeth, provided that procedures for designing, fabricating, orienting, and processing the teeth are comparable to or improvements on traditional procedures.

ACKNOWLEDGMENT

The authors would like to acknowledge the assistance of George Diacoloukas, CDT of Friendship Dental Laboratory, Baltimore, MD, for the design and fabrication of the zirconia teeth.

REFERENCES

1. Zarone F, Russo S, Sorrentino R: From porcelain-fused-to-metal to zirconia: clinical and experimental considerations. *Dent Mater* 2011;27:83–96.
2. Koutayas SO, Vagkopoulou T, Pelekanos S, et al: Zirconia in dentistry: part 2. Evidence-based clinical breakthrough. *Eur J Esthet Dent* 2009;4:348–380.
3. Vagkopoulou T, Koutayas SO, Koidis P, et al: Zirconia in dentistry: part 1. Discovering the nature of an upcoming bioceramic. *Eur J Esthet Dent* 2009;4:130–151.
4. Manicone PF, Iommetti PR, Raffaelli L: An overview of zirconia ceramics: basic properties and clinical applications. *J Dent* 2007;35:819–826.
5. Giordano R, Sabrosa CE: Zirconia: material background and clinical application. *Compend Contin Educ Dent* 2010;31: 710–715.
6. Albashaireh ZS, Ghazal M, Kern M: Two-body wear of different ceramic materials opposed to zirconia ceramic. *J Prosthet Dent* 2010;104:105–113.
7. Ghazal M, Yang B, Ludwig K, et al: Two-body wear of resin and ceramic denture teeth in comparison to human enamel. *Dent Mater* 2008;24:502–507.
8. McGarry TJ, Nimmo A, Skiba JF, et al: Classification system for complete dentures. *J Prosthodont* 1999;8:27–39.
9. Phark JH, Duarte S Jr, Blatz M, et al: An in vitro evaluation of the long-term resin bond to a new densely sintered high-purity

zirconium-oxide ceramic surface. *J Prosthet Dent* 2009; 101:29–38.

10. Duarte S Jr, Phark JH, Tada T, et al: Resin-bonded fixed partial dentures with a new modified zirconia surface: a clinical report. *J Prosthet Dent* 2009;102:68–73.

11. Aboushelib MN, Kleverlaan CJ, Feilzer AJ: Selective infiltration-etching technique for a strong and durable bond of resin cements to zirconia-based materials. *J Prosthet Dent* 2007; 98:379–388.

12. Aboushelib MN, Feilzer AJ, Kleverlaan CJ: Bonding to zirconia using a new surface treatment. *J Prosthodont* 2010;19: 340–346.

13. Everson P, Addison O, Palin WM, et al: Improved bonding of zirconia substructures to resin using a "glaze-on" technique. *J Dent* 2012;40:347–351.

14. Ntala P, Chen X, Niggli J, et al: Development and testing of multi-phase glazes for adhesive bonding to zirconia substrates. *J Dent* 2010;38:773–781.

15. Valentino T, Borges G, Borges L, et al: Influence of glazed zirconia on dual-cure luting agent bond strength. *Oper Dent* 2012;37:181–187.

16. Fushiki R, Komine F, Blatz MB, et al: Shear bond strength between an indirect composite layering material and feldspathic porcelain-coated zirconia ceramics. *Clin Oral Investig* 2011;16:1401–1411.

17. Atsu SS, Kilicarslan MA, Kucukesmen HC, et al: Effect of zirconium-oxide ceramic surface treatments on the bond strength to adhesive resin. *J Prosthet Dent* 2006;95:430–436.

18. Attia A, Lehmann F, Kern M: Influence of surface conditioning and cleaning methods on resin bonding to zirconia ceramic. *Dent Mater* 2011;27:207–213.

19. Blatz MB, Chiche G, Holst S, et al: Influence of surface treatment and simulated aging on bond strengths of luting agents to zirconia. *Quintessence Int* 2007;38:745–753.

20. Smith RL, Villanueva C, Rothrock JK, et al: Long-term microtensile bond strength of surface modified zirconia. *Dent Mater* 2011;27:779–785.

21. Tsukakoshi M, Shinya A, Gomi H, et al: Effects of dental adhesive cement and surface treatment on bond strength and leakage of zirconium oxide ceramics. *Dent Mater J* 2008;27: 159–171.

29

RETRIEVABLE METAL CERAMIC IMPLANT-SUPPORTED FIXED PROSTHESES WITH MILLED TITANIUM FRAMEWORKS AND ALL-CERAMIC CROWNS: RETROSPECTIVE CLINICAL STUDY WITH UP TO 10 YEARS OF FOLLOW-UP

Paulo Malo, dds,[1] Miguel de Araujo Nobre, rdh,[2] Joao Borges, dds,[3] and Ricardo Almeida, dds[3]

[1]Department of Oral Surgery, Malo Clinic, Lisbon, Portugal
[2]Department of R&D, Malo Clinic, Lisbon, Portugal
[3]Department of Prosthodontics, Malo Clinic, Lisbon, Portugal

Keywords
Implant-supported prosthesis; metal framework; Procera copings; zirconia; retrievable.

Correspondence
Miguel de Araújo Nobre, Malo Clinic–R&D, Avenida dos Combatentes, 43, 8 Edificiio Green Park, Lisboa 1600-043, Portugal. E-mail: mnobre@maloclinics.com

Accepted August 13, 2011

Published in *Journal of Prosthodontics* June 2012; Vol. 21, Issue 4

doi: 10.1111/j.1532-849X.2011.00824.x

ABSTRACT

Purpose: The purpose of this study was to report on the outcome of metal ceramic implant-supported fixed prostheses with milled titanium frameworks and all-ceramic crowns.

Materials and Methods: The clinical study included 108 patients (67 women, 41 men), mean age of 58.6 years (range: 34–82), and followed between 9 months and 10 years (postocclusal loading). The mean follow-up time for all patients in the study was 5 years. A total of 125 prostheses were fabricated. The data were divided into two groups. Development group (DG): 52 patients with 66 prostheses (28 maxillary, 38 mandibular) fabricated with individual Procera crowns (Alumina copings, Nobel Biocare AB) and Allceram ceramics (Ducera Dental GmbH) cemented onto a CAD/CAM fabricated Ti framework (Nobel Biocare AB) with pink ceramic (Duceram, Ducera Dental GmbH) that replicated the missing gingival tissues. Routine group (RG): 56 patients with 59 prostheses (49 maxillary, 10 mandibular) fabricated with individual Procera crowns (Zirconia copings and Nobel Rondo Zirconia Ceramic; Nobel Biocare AB) cemented onto a CAD/CAM-fabricated Ti framework (Nobel Biocare AB) with pink acrylic resin (PallaXpress Ultra, Heraeus Kulzer GmbH) that replicated the missing gingival tissues. Primary outcome measures were prosthetic survival and mechanical complications. Secondary outcome measures were biological complications testing the retrievability characteristic of the prosthesis. Survival estimates were calculated on the patient level with the Kaplan–Meier product limit estimator (95% confidence intervals [CI]). Data were analyzed with descriptive and inferential analyses.

Results: The cumulative survival rates for the implant-supported fixed prostheses were 92.4% for the DG at 10 years and 100% for the RG at 5 years (overall 96%) (Kaplan–Meier). Mechanical complications occurred in 44 patients (DG: 29 patients, 36 prostheses; RG: 15 patients, 16 prostheses); the large majority were crown fractures, occurring in 48 patients (DG: 33 patients, 36 prostheses; RG: 15 patients, 16 prostheses). In the DG, univariate analysis of logistic regression disclosed the presence of a metal ceramic implant-supported fixed prosthesis opposing dentition as a risk factor for crown fracture (OR = 1.97). Biological complications occurred in 33 patients (DG: 18 patients; RG: 15 patients), the majority being peri-implant pathologies in 19 patients (DG: 9 patients, RG: 10 patients). All situations were resolved except one in the DG that led to fixture and prosthesis loss.

Conclusions: The results of this study indicated that, within the limitations of this study, the CAD/CAM protocol is acceptable for definitive prosthetic rehabilitation. This protocol provided these patients with a good prognosis on a middle-to-long-term basis (5 years).

Implant-supported fixed prostheses have increasingly been the first-choice treatment for the rehabilitation of edentulous areas.[1–3] Replacement of complete dentures with fixed implant-retained prostheses has achieved predictable high cumulative survival rates.[4] It is the authors' opinion that additional research should focus on types of frameworks, fabrication techniques, and their predictability. This should coincide with the development of new prosthetic solutions for treating edentulous patients with improved quality of materials, esthetics, biomechanics, facilitation of hygienic maintenance, retrievability, and long-term prognoses for patients and prostheses.

Economically, it has also proved to be important for new technologies to be cost effective, as well as accurate and predictable. Goals related to developing and using new technologies should include using state of the art dental technology, reliable materials, and solutions to problems previously encountered with preexisting technology. Implant frameworks should be biocompatible, have excellent physical properties in terms of strength, fit accurately to implants and abutments,[5] and be compatible with esthetic veneering materials such as ceramic and acrylic resins. A passive fit of implant-supported prostheses is considered a prerequisite for the prevention of mechanical complications,[6] and therefore prosthetic success. Two main reasons emerge for complications in the prosthesis framework or veneer: lack of passive fit between the restoration and the abutment and destructive occlusal contacts.[7]

Because implants lack the stress release associated with a periodontal ligament, impact loading to restorative materials and the crestal bone remains potentially more damaging with implant-supported restorations.[8] It is therefore believed that dental implants may be more prone to occlusal overloading, which is often regarded as one of the potential causes of peri-implant bone loss and failure of the implant/implant prosthesis.[9] Overloading factors that may negatively influence implant longevity include large cantilevers, parafunctions, improper occlusal designs, and premature contacts.[9] In this field and among other factors, porcelain fractures[10] and marginal bone resorption[11] seem to be significantly associated with opposing implant-supported metal ceramic restorations.

Two basic methods are currently used in the fabrication of implant frameworks: the conventional lost wax/casting technique[12] and CAD/CAM milling procedures where frameworks are milled from solid blanks of titanium, titanium alloy, or ceramic materials such as zirconia.[13] The benefits of the lost wax/casting technique include the ability to create optimal esthetics due to the proven technology associated with porcelain fused to metal,[14] high biocompatibility with gold alloys,[15,16] and the ability of most commercial dental laboratories to fabricate implant frameworks with this proven technology. The limitations of the lost wax/casting technique include the precision of fit, described by numerous researchers.[17–19] It is not uncommon to have to section cast metal frameworks to obtain precise, passive fits between frameworks and implants. The sections must then be connected via welding or soldering.[20–22]

The rigid connectors are known to be the weakest parts of these castings.

Several advantages are associated with CAD/CAM systems (Ti alloy with ceramic applied to it):[13,23,24] biocompatibility,[25] highly precise fit,[13] the possibility of extended cantilever lengths (due to characteristics of Ti/zirconia, which can be shaped only by CAD/CAM systems),[26] the lack of rigid connectors such as solder or welded joints within the CAD/CAM framework, and that it is machine manufactured,[25] thus less susceptible to human error. A potential limitation associated with CAD/CAM technologies is that ceramics do not bond well to Ti or Ti alloy.[27] However, both technologies have limitations. A potential disadvantage might be the physical properties associated with the metal castings including limited cantilever lengths and increased expense due to the recent increases in prices for noble metals. Both technologies are limited when deficiencies are noted regarding insufficient metal to support the prosthesis.

For both technologies the management of ceramics is also a concern. This may be due to technique sensitivity.[28]

Dealing with ceramic fractures is another disadvantage present in both technologies. Fractures may be repaired by adding additional ceramic and refiring the prosthesis; however, this may increase the probability of damaging the non-rigid connectors (in the lost wax/casting technique) and potentially damaging the ceramics due to too many baking cycles (in both technologies).[29] Difficulty in masking screw access openings is another disadvantage present in both technologies.

Evidence supports the use of full ceramics on implant prostheses.[30,31] The constant evolution of ceramics includes several advantages including excellent esthetics,[31] high fracture resistance, maintenance of vertical dimension, increased longevity,[32] better hygiene,[33] better stain resistance,[34] and greater ability to customize.[35]

The theoretical rationale for developing implant-supported fixed prostheses with CAD/CAM-fabricated frameworks (Procera) and individualized crowns incorporates the advantages of both technologies while minimizing the disadvantages. By using a framework produced by one specific CAD/CAM system (Procera), the authors sought to use the following advantages: high precision of fit,[36] longer cantilever lengths, use of fewer implants to support the prostheses,[1] biocompatibility, elimination of rigid connectors, frameworks less susceptible to human error, and standardized fabrication procedures.

The authors designed the prostheses with individual Procera-crowns to use the following advantages: high esthetics,[37–39] high capacity of repair (by individually cementing the crowns it is possible to repair without removing the whole structure). This allows the benefits of repairability (repairing without removing the whole structure) and cushion effect. Additionally, if any misjudgment is made in the vertical dimension or position of the teeth, it is easily solved by the double scan characteristic of the Procera system,[40] which offers a good prognosis in the medium and long term.[30,41]

Several reports, including a review focused on the prosthodontic survival outcome of these types of rehabilitation, report survival rates ranging between 87 and 92.1% with a follow-up between 5 and 15 years.[42–47] This methodology was designed for patients in need of a rehabilitation solution for a full metal ceramic implant-supported fixed prosthesis using the advantages of different concepts and materials to ensure consistently high-quality prostheses. The purpose of this clinical study was to document the clinical and laboratory procedures to fabricate implant-supported standardized fixed metal ceramic prostheses. The null hypothesis was that there would be no differences in the survival and complication outcomes of the implant-supported treatments using the current protocol or other CAD/CAM technologies.

MATERIALS AND METHODS

This clinical study was performed in a private center (Malo Clinic), in Lisbon, Portugal, and included 108 completely edentulous patients (67 women, 41 men), with an average age of 58.6 years (range: 34–82), rehabilitated through implants in immediate function. Inclusion criterion was patients in need of definitive implant-supported fixed rehabilitations having successfully overcome the osseointegration period. Exclusion criteria were patients who did not overcome the osseointegration period and the presence of compromised implants that could affect the survival outcome at the time of the definitive prosthesis manufacture. Regarding systemic conditions, 17 patients had cardiovascular problems, 4 patients had thyroid problems, 1 patient had diabetes, and 1 patient was immunocompromised. Eighty-five patients were healthy. A total of 634 implants (Branemark system, Nobel Speedy; Nobel Biocare AB, Göteborg, Sweden) were placed. Multi-unit straight and 30° angulated abutments (Nobel Biocare) were used in the rehabilitations. Six months after the surgical procedure, the patients were rehabilitated with 125 definitive dental prostheses (77 maxillary, 48 mandibular). The same team performed the surgical and prosthodontic treatments. The first prosthesis was placed in January 2000; the last prosthesis was placed in February 2007. The patients were followed between 9 months and 10 years, with a mean follow-up of 5 years.

Patients were treated at one rehabilitation center (Malo Clinic); all patients were in need of definitive full-arch dental prostheses. The study was approved by an independent ethical committee, and written informed consent to participate in this study was obtained for all patients. The cohort was divided into two groups, with a development group and a routine group. The development group consisted of 52 patients (23 women, 29 men), with an age range of 38 to 81 years (mean: 59.5 years). Sixty-six prostheses (28 maxillary, 38 mandibular) were fabricated for the development group using the CAD/CAM protocol (Table 29.1), with a mean follow-up of 78 months (range: 9–127 months).

The routine group included 56 patients (35 women, 21 men), with an age range of 34 to 82 years (mean: 57.6 years). Fifty-nine prostheses (49 maxillary, 10 mandibular) were fabricated, with a mean follow-up of 46 months (range: 12–67 months; Table 29.1).

Regarding the laboratory protocol, prostheses in the development group had the following characteristics:

TABLE 29.1   **Population and Methods (development and routine groups)**

Population and methods	Development group	Routine group
Number of patients	52	56
Gender distribution	23 women, 29 men	35 women, 21 men
Mean age (range)	59.5 years (38–81)	57.6 years (34–82)
Number of prostheses (distribution per arch)	66 (28 maxillary, 38 mandibular)	59 (49 maxillary, 10 mandibular)
Type of titanium framework	Procera Titanium framework (Nobel Biocare AB)	
Technology		CAD/CAM
Type of copings	Alumina copings (Nobel Biocare AB)	Zirconia copings (Nobel Biocare AB)
Type of ceramic used to fabricate the crowns	Allceram (Ducera Dental)	Nobel Rondo Zirconia Ceramic (Nobel Biocare AB)
Type of material replicating gingival tissues	Duceram (Ducera Dental)	PalaXpress Ultra (Heraeus Kulzer GmbH)

12–14 individual Procera crowns (Alumina copings, Nobel Biocare AB) with Allceram ceramics (Ducera Dental GmbH, Rosbach, Germany) cemented onto a Procera Titanium framework (Nobel Biocare AB) with pink ceramic (Duceram, Ducera Dental GmbH) replicating the missing gingival tissues. The criteria for doing 12 or 14 crowns, anterior–posterior spread, and number of implants per arch were based on the degree of jaw atrophy. A minimum of 12 crowns and a maximum of 14 crowns were placed. If the emergence position of the most posterior implant was on the second premolar, two cantilevers were included in the prosthesis. If the emergence position of the implant was located on the first molar, one cantilever was included, and if the emergence position of the implant was the second molar, no cantilevers were included. The mean number of implants per arch was five (range: 4–11 implants), with the following distribution: 81 prostheses supported by four implants; 5 prostheses supported by 5 implants; 16 prostheses supported by 6 implants; 6 prostheses supported by 7 implants; 14 prostheses supported by 8 implants; 2 prostheses supported by 10 implants; and 1 prosthesis supported by 11 implants.

Interocclusal space and vertical dimension were maintained if the patient presented with teeth prior to the rehabilitation process. If the patient presented with removable dentures, the vertical dimension was maintained, and the interocclusal space was maintained when possible.

In the routine group, the changes implemented were related to the materials used [alumina copings were replaced by zirconia copings with Nobel Rondo Zirconia Ceramic (Nobel Biocare AB), and pink acrylic resin (PalaXpress Ultra, Heraeus Kulzer GmbH, Hanau, Germany) was used instead of pink ceramic]. Regarding the protocol, no differences existed between the clinical procedures used on the patients in both groups. The authors designed the intaglio surfaces of the prostheses to improve the ease of oral hygiene procedures by the patients.

To avoid esthetic and/or functional compromises, screw access openings were positioned as palatal as possible on the occlusal surfaces of posterior teeth or on the false palatal interdental papilla of the anterior teeth, preventing a visible vestibular screw access opening that could compromise esthetics. In some situations, the angulation of some implants dictated the use of angulated abutments (17° or 30° multi-unit angulated abutments, Nobel Biocare AB) to achieve a non-visible screw access opening.

All definitive impressions were achieved in two steps. The first step was to splint together multi-unit impression copings (Nobel Biocare AB) or fixture-level impression copings (Nobel Biocare AB) with stainless-steel bars and a low contraction autopolymerizing acrylic resin (GC Pattern Resin, GC Co, Alsip, IL). Definitive impressions were made with custom, open trays and addition reaction silicone impression material (Light Body and Putty Soft, fast setting; Zhermack Co, Rovigo, Italy).

The dental laboratory used the tooth arrangement on the interim implant-supported fixed prostheses as a starting point to manufacture the definitive prostheses. First, an acrylic resin screw-retained pattern of the interim implant-supported fixed prosthesis was made on the master cast to plan the future Ti framework. This acrylic resin pattern was fabricated with individual crown preparations (12–14) to accommodate the corresponding individual ceramic crowns (Nobel Biocare AB; Fig 29.1). After the pattern was completed, the pattern was ready to be scanned and read by the Procera software

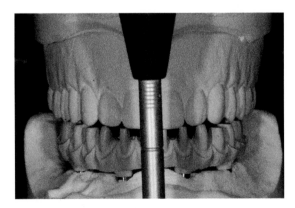

FIGURE 29.1   Production of the titanium framework. Acrylic duplicate prepared to be scanned.

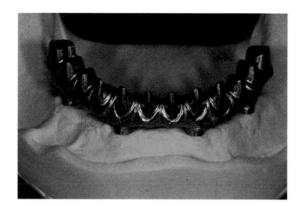

FIGURE 29.2   Titanium framework finished and polished.

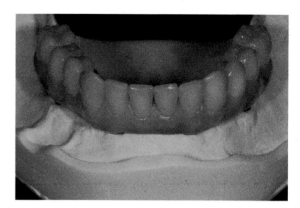

FIGURE 29.4   The crowns were cemented to the framework extraorally.

(Nobel Biocare AB). The data were transferred digitally to a milling machine for fabrication of the Ti framework (Fig 29.2).

Once the Ti frameworks were milled, the ceramic copings were fabricated. Silicone impressions were made of the preparations within the frameworks. The copings were then milled.

The ceramic was applied individually to each coping (Allceram for the development group; Nobel Rondo Zirconia Ceramic for the routine group). Finally, after all the crowns were glazed, the implant-supported fixed prostheses were completed. The crowns were cemented to the preparations using a definitive cement (Fig 29.3), the screw access openings were opened, and the customized acrylic gingiva (Unifast TRAD, GC Co, Tokyo, Japan) was applied and polymerized around the crowns and in the inferior portion of the prosthesis (Fig 29.4).

For the routine group, all implant-supported fixed prostheses were placed without trial placements or any other type of extra visits apart from the final connection of the prosthesis (Fig 29.5). All prosthetic screws were given a final torque of 15 N/cm. The prosthetic screw access holes were sealed using cotton pellets and composite material (Fig 29.5),

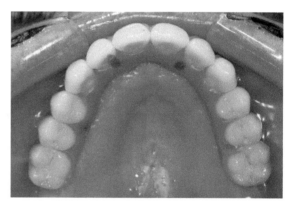

FIGURE 29.5   Occlusal view of the prosthesis.

and the occlusion was evaluated respecting the following occlusion scheme: in the excursive movement, disclosure in anterior teeth; lateral movement of the mandible was a canine function with absolutely no prematurities; the excursion of canines and lower incisors was in a slope of less than 10° when possible. Due to the tendency of these patients to slightly modify the occlusion pattern, occlusion was checked according to these guidelines, especially in the first 6 months.

Canine guidance was based on lateral eccentric movements, incisive guidance on protrusive movements and balanced contacts in maximal intercuspation (Fig 29.6). The follow-up examinations were scheduled at the connection of the prosthesis and after 2 and 6 months, 1 year, and thereafter each year.

Complication parameters were assessed. *Mechanical complications*: fracture or loosening of mechanical and prosthetic components (using magnifying glasses and a probe to check for small chips or cracks), lack of passive fit (by placing the fixed partial denture [FPD] over the implants making sure there was no pressure on the soft tissue and using only one prosthetic screw attached to the implants. The verification was done with magnifying glasses at the FPD/abutment interface and using a probe or radiologically if

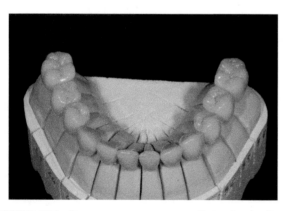

FIGURE 29.3   Procera crowns were manufactured according to the interim prosthesis and the prosthodontist's specifications.

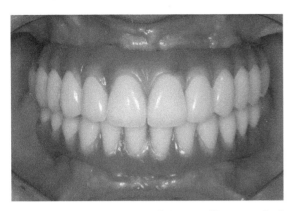

FIGURE 29.6 Intraoral view of the maxillary prosthesis in occlusion.

the interface between prosthesis and abutment was not visible). *Biological complications*: soft tissue inflammation, fistula formation, pain or peri-implant pathology; *Esthetic complications*: esthetic complaints of the patient or dentist; *Functional complications*: phonetic complaints, masticatory complaints, and comfort complaints; *Oral hygiene complications*: low levels of oral hygiene. Descriptive statistics were used to analyze the outcome of complications in both groups.

The survival criteria implemented in this study were based on the functionality of the prosthesis. A prosthesis was considered a success if it remained in function and did not need to be substituted. The survival estimate was calculated on patient level through the Kaplan–Meyer product limit estimator with 95% confidence intervals (CI).

The association between the variables "presence or absence of metal ceramic implant-supported prosthesis as opposing dentition" and "crown perforation" (crowns with screw access openings versus crowns without screw access openings) and the outcome variable "incidence of fractured crowns" was evaluated by unconditional logistic regression to estimate odds ratios (ORs) and corresponding 95% CIs. The effect of each variable was assessed both in univariate (crude) analysis and after adjustment for the other variables of interest. The level of significance considered was 5%. The statistical analysis was performed using the Statistical Package for Social Sciences (SPSS) version 19.0 (2009; SPSS Inc., Chicago, IL).

RESULTS

Twelve patients were lost to follow-up during the completion of this study, representing 11% of the sample size. The overall survival rate of the implant-supported fixed prostheses was 96% at 10 years of follow-up (Kaplan–Meier). The overall survival estimate for the implant-supported fixed prostheses was 120.9 months 95% CI: 115.5 to 126.3 months (maximum follow-up registered was 127 months).

The development group rendered a 92.4% survival rate at 10 years of follow-up (Kaplan–Meier). Five prostheses in this group were replaced by acrylic resin prostheses due to recurrent crown fractures. Mechanical complications occurred in 29 patients and 36 prostheses, ranging from crown fracture (between 1 and 91 months of follow-up; anterior crowns—12 prostheses; posterior crowns—15 prostheses; anterior and posterior crowns—6 prostheses; in a total of 33 prostheses with crown fractures: 29 with complete fractures and 4 with chipped ceramics), abutment loosening (2 in 29 prostheses), and chipping of the ceramic gingiva (3 in 36 prostheses). In 2 patients, more than one incidence of mechanical complications occurred. From the 33 prostheses with crown fractures, 24 prostheses' opposing dentition was a metal ceramic implant-supported fixed prosthesis. Presence of a metal ceramic implant-supported fixed prosthesis as opposing dentition was found to be a risk factor for the incidence of mechanical complications in the development group in the logistic regression model both in univariate analysis (OR = 2.04) and after adjusting for "crown perforation" (OR = 1.97; Table 29.2). No further mechanical complications were registered in the development group.

The routine group rendered a 100% survival rate at 5 years of follow-up (Kaplan–Meier; Tables 29.3 and 29.4; Fig 29.7). Mechanical complications occurred in 15 patients and 16 prostheses, consisting of crown fractures (between 4 and 54 months of follow-up; anterior crowns—6 prostheses; posterior crowns—4 prostheses; anterior and posterior crowns—4 patients; in a total of 14 prostheses with fractured crowns: 13 with complete fractures and 1 with chipped ceramics), abutment loosening (1 patient), and abutment substitution (1 patient).

No significant effects were revealed in the logistic regression analysis for the outcome "incidence of mechanical complications." No further mechanical complications occurred in the routine group.

For both groups, the ceramic fractures that implicated removing the crown were repaired immediately in the mouth by the dentist with a provisional crown, and later a ceramic crown was manufactured and cemented. The Procera software saves the files of previously scanned dies, making it possible to produce a new coping with the exact same characteristics. The implant-supported fixed prostheses were never removed from the mouth nor baked again during this process. The repairing process ended with the manufacture of a night-guard. The abutment loosening was solved by adjusting the patients' occlusion and manufacturing an occlusal night-guard.

The chipping of the ceramic gingiva in the development group (that created a gap on the affected prosthesis) was repaired by the clinician using a special pink-colored resin composite (Gradia Gum, GC Company, Tokyo, Japan). No further mechanical complications were registered during the follow-up of this study.

TABLE 29.2 **Odds Ratio (OR) with 95% Confidence Intervals (CI) for Opposing Dentition and Crown Status**

Factor	OR	Sig.	95% CI	OR[a]	Sig.	95% CI
				Development group		
Opposing dentition						
Non-ceramic	1.0					
Ceramic	2.04	0.01	1.18–3.54	1.97	0.016	1.14–3.43
Crown status						
Not perforated	1.0					
Screw access opening	1.53	0.100	0.92–2.54	1.45	0.156	0.87–2.41
				Routine group		
Opposing dentition						
Non-ceramic	1.0					
Ceramic	0.36	0.163	0.08–1.52	0.36	0.165	0.08–1.53
Crown status						
Not perforated	1.0					
Screw access opening	1.65	0.204	0.76–3.59	1.65	0.207	0.76–3.59

[a]OR from logistic regression analysis with opposing dentition and crown status included as explanatory variables.

In the development group, the univariate and adjusted analyses disclosed a significant effect for opposing dentition as a risk factor for the incidence of mechanical complications, which remained significant after adjusting for crown status effect.

In the routine group, no relevant effects were found in the univariate or adjusted analysis, meaning that variable (opposing dentition or crown status) had a relevant effect on the model.

The incidence of biological complications registered in the development group occurred in 18 patients, including peri-implant pathology (9 patients), soft tissue inflammation (7 patients), and implant loss (2 patients). The peri-implant pockets were solved through nonsurgical therapy (removal of the prosthesis, mechanical debridement, and pocket irrigation with a chlorhexidine gel in six patients) and surgical therapy (open flap debridement and soft tissue

TABLE 29.3 **Estimated Fractions for Survival Using the Kaplan–Meier Product Limit Estimator for the Prostheses in the Development Group**

Time (months)	Status (0 = non failure; 1 = failure)	Cumulative proportion surviving at the time		N of cumulative events	N of prostheses at risk
		Estimate	Std. Error		
0	0	–	–	0	66
12	0	–	–	0	64
13	1	0.984	0.016.	1	63
24	0	–	–	1	63
30	1	0.968	0.022	2	61
36	0	–	–	2	60
48	0	–	–	2	57
53	1	0.952	0.027	3	56
60	0	–	–	3	52
72	0	–	–	1	45
73	1	0.930	0.034	4	44
84	0	–	–	4	22
89	1	0.883	0.056	5	19
96	0	–	–	5	11
108	0	–	–	5	3
120	0	–	–	5	2
122	0	–	–	5	1
127	0	–	–	5	0

TABLE 29.4   Estimated Fractions for Survival Using the Kaplan–Meier Product Limit Estimator for the Prostheses in the Routine Group

Time (months)	Status (0 = non failure; 1 = failure)	Cumulative proportion surviving at the time		N of cumulative events	N of prostheses at risk
		Estimate	Std. Error		
0	0		–	0	59
12	0		–	0	59
24	0		–	0	56
36	0		–	0	52
48	0		–	0	25
60	0		–	0	4
61	0		–	0	2
62	0		–	0	1
67	0		–	0	0

repositioning in two patients). In one patient the situation led to the loss of the implants and the prosthesis (unaccounted for the survival estimate), with a new prosthesis manufactured to connect to both the remaining implants and the new implants inserted. In another patient who lost implants, the prosthesis was attached to the remaining implants without further insertion of implants.

The incidence of biological complications registered in the routine group occurred in 15 patients, ranging from peri-implant pathology (10 patients) to soft-tissue inflammation (5 patients). The peri-implant pockets were solved through non-surgical therapy (10 patients) using the same method as described in the development group. No implants were lost after the connection of the prosthesis in the routine group.

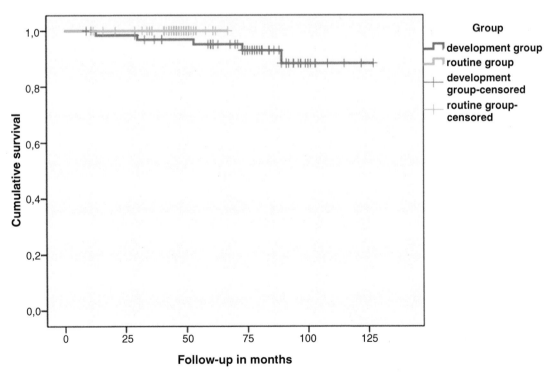

Survival functions

FIGURE 29.7   Prosthesis survival using Kaplan–Meier product limit estimator.

Aside from the cases of peri-implant pathology and soft-tissue inflammation, poor oral hygiene was diagnosed in another six patients of the development group and five patients in the routine group. These patients received mechanical debridement and chemical therapy (chlorhexidine) together with reinforcement of the oral hygiene recommendations.

Common to all therapies for solving the biological complications was the possibility to remove and reconnect the prosthesis (retrievability of the prosthesis), which was possible due to the existing screw access openings in the definitive crowns. No functional, esthetic, or comfort complications were registered during the follow-up of this study in the development or the routine group.

DISCUSSION

The survival of the prosthesis in both the development and routine groups is comparable to other rehabilitations of completely edentulous arches,[42–47] and therefore allow us not to reject the null hypothesis. These findings continue to build on the issue of long-term outcomes of implant-supported metal ceramic prostheses manufactured using CAD/CAM technology.

The lower survival rate achieved in the development group is related to the incidence of mechanical complications (most of them crown fractures). This finding influenced the treatment planning in the routine group, where with the introduction of zirconia crowns and controlling for the possible effect of the opposing dentition (excluding metal ceramic implant-supported fixed prostheses), led to a low number of fractures. It was possible to identify the absence of a negative effect of perforating the crowns (screw access openings) on the outcome of the rehabilitations. The survival of the crowns can be compared with other reports that analyzed all-ceramic crown survival in the medium and long term.[30,41] The concept's independence from technique sensitivity (allowing a standardized production) accounts for a higher probability of success and increased predictability in the clinical setting.[28]

The accurate precision of fit in these rehabilitations was related to the welded Ti framework used in this concept, which is described in the literature as achieving superior results when compared to the frameworks made with cast gold alloy.[36] All-ceramic crowns with Procera laminates resulted in a high esthetic result, judged by the absence of esthetic complaints registered in our study. Previous reports acknowledged a superior esthetic level with this concept when compared to the metal ceramic crowns.[38,39] The ceramic fractures were easily repaired due to the concept's flexibility. Those fractures implicating removal of the crown were repaired immediately in the mouth by the dentist with a provisional acrylic crown, and later a ceramic crown was made and cemented. The Procera software saves the files of previously scanned dies, making it easy to manufacture a new coping. The prostheses were never removed from the mouth due to ceramic fractures and most important, not baked again, which would have brought negative consequences for the ceramic. Also, this capacity of repair demonstrated by the structure was an important factor for the patient, as the protocol applied assured a rapid and comfortable repairing.

The reasons for crown fractures (ceramic failures) may be related to technical failure in the manufacturing process, occlusion failure in controlling the occlusion following the guidelines previously presented,[9,10] or parafunctional movements by the patient.[9,10] All these possible causes could act independently or in association; however, there was a twofold increase in the probability of crown fracture when the opposing dentition was an implant-supported metal ceramic FPD, a situation acknowledged in previous reports,[10] which could imply a lack of proprioception by the patient and/or the lack of shock-absorbing capacity by the prosthesis. It is important to control implant occlusion within physiologic limits and thus provide optimal implant load to ensure long-term implant success, but currently there is no evidence-based implant-specific concept of occlusion.[9] The precision of fit is another important factor to prevent mechanical complications,[6] and our results (taking into consideration the absence of misfit incidences registered in our study) are supported by other studies stating that using CAD/CAM technologies should allow a more uniform passive fit to the prosthesis.[5,48] The method for repairing the chipping of the ceramic gingiva (that created a gap on the affected prosthesis) using a special pink-colored resin composite (Gradia Gum) is not satisfactory in terms of longevity, and future research should focus on better methods to resolve this complication.

The biological complications registered in our study were most likely related to low levels of oral hygiene. Apart from the necessary high levels of oral hygiene self-care from the patient that influence the outcome,[49] the necessity of removing the prostheses in these situations further expresses the need for easy retrievability of these structures, facilitating access to the implants for accurate diagnosis or therapeutic interventions.

The limitations of the study are related to the retrospective design, only one clinical center involved, the shorter follow-up time of the routine group, and the lack of randomization. The methodology implemented with a development and a routine group, was integrated in a concept of rehabilitation with several phases of conception, experiment, evaluation (development group), reconception, and reexperiment (routine group), to resolve the weak points identified in the development group.

The 12 patients lost to follow-up (11% of the sample) account for the good methodological quality of the study, representing less than 20% of the sample size,[50] thus reducing the probability of bias. Future research should focus on the documentation of fixed implant-supported rehabilitations using CAD/CAM technology with long-term outcomes (more than 10 years of follow-up).

CONCLUSIONS

Within the limitations of this study, the outcome of a metal ceramic implant-supported fixed prosthesis with a Ti framework and all-ceramic crowns is valid, with a survival estimate of 96.4% overall, 92.4% for the development group at 10 years, and 100% for the routine group at 5 years. The absence of esthetic complaints or misfit, the independence from technique sensitivity (allowing a standardized production), retrievability, and capacity of repairing characteristics prove the viability of this fixed prosthetic solution. When planning the rehabilitation, the existing opposing dentition should be considered, as the presence of a metal ceramic implant-supported fixed prosthesis resulted in a twofold-increased probability of crown fractures. This type of fixed rehabilitation should be further investigated to evaluate its survival with 10 years of follow-up using the current protocol.

ACKNOWLEDGMENTS

The authors would like to thank Mr. Sandro Catarino for all the help with data collection.

REFERENCES

1. Malo P, Rangert B, Nobre M: All-on-4 immediate-function concept with Brånemark System implants for completely edentulous mandibles: a retrospective clinical study. *Clin Implant Dent Relat Res* 2003;5:S2–S9.

2. Malo P, Rangert B, Nobre M: All-on-4 immediate-function concept with Brånemark System implants for complete edentulous maxillae: a 1-year retrospective clinical study. *Clin Implant Dent Relat Res* 2005;7:S88–S94.

3. Friberg B, Raghoebar GM, Grunert I, et al: A 5-year prospective multicenter study on 1-stage smooth-surface Brånemark System implants with early loading in edentulous mandibles. *Int J Oral Maxillofac Implants* 2008;23:481–486.

4. Malo P, De Araújo Nobre M, Lopes A, et al: A longitudinal study of the survival of all-on-4 implants in the mandible with up to 10 years of follow-up. *J Am Dent Assoc* 2011;142:310–320.

5. Mericske-Stern R: Prosthetic considerations. *Aust Dent J* 2008;53:S49–S59.

6. Greven B, Luepke M, von Dorche SH: Telescoping implant prostheses with intraoral luted galvano mesostructures to improve passive fit. *J Prosthet Dent* 2007;98:239–244.

7. Kohavi D: Complications in the issue of integrated prostheses components: clinical and mechanical evaluation. *J Oral Rehabil* 1993;20:413–422.

8. Curtis DA, Sharma A, Finzen FC, et al: Occlusal considerations for implant restorations in the partially edentulous patient. *J Calif Dent Assoc* 2000;28:771–779.

9. Kim Y, Oh TJ, Misch CE, et al: Occlusal considerations in implant therapy: clinical guidelines with biomechanical rationale. *Clin Oral Implants Res* 2005;16:26–35.

10. Kinsel RP, Lin D: Retrospective analysis of porcelain failures of metal ceramic crowns and fixed partial dentures supported by 729 implants in 152 patients: patient-specific and implant-specific predictors of ceramic failure. *J Prosthet Dent* 2009;101:388–394.

11. Naert I, Quirynen M, van Steenberghe D, et al: A study of 589 consecutive implants supporting complete fixed prostheses. Part II: prosthetic aspects. *J Prosthet Dent* 1992;68:949–956.

12. Puri S: Techniques used to fabricate all-ceramic restorations in the dental practice. *Compend Contin Educ Dent* 2005;26:519–525.

13. Jemt T, Petersson A: Precision of CNC-milled titanium frameworks for implant treatment in the edentulous jaw. *Int J Prosthodont* 1999;12:209–215.

14. Segal BS: Prospective assessment of 546 all-ceramic anterior and posterior crowns in general practice. *J Prosthet Dent* 2001;85:544–550.

15. Craig RG, Hanks CT: Cytotoxicity of experimental casting alloys evaluated by cell culture tests. *J Dent Res* 1990;69:1539–1542.

16. Kansu G, Aydin AK: Evaluation of the biocompatibility of various dental alloys: part I–toxic potentials. *Eur J Prosthodont Restor Dent* 1996;4:129–136.

17. Carr AB, Stewart RB: Full-arch implant framework casting accuracy: preliminary *in vitro* observation for *in vivo* testing. *J Prosthodont* 1993;2:2–8.

18. Tan KB, Rubenstein JB, Nicholls JL, et al: Three-dimensional analysis of the casting accuracy of one-piece, osseointegrated implant-retained prostheses. *Int J Prosthodont* 1993;6:346–363.

19. Jemt T, Lie A: Accuracy of implant-supported prostheses in the edentulous jaw: analysis of precision of fit between cast gold-alloy frameworks and master casts by means of a three-dimensional photogrammetric technique. *Clin Oral Implants Res* 1995;6:172–180.

20. Hobo S, Ichida E, Garcia LT: *Osseointegration and Occlusal Rehabilitation*. Chicago, Quintessence, 1989, p. 176.

21. Klineberg IJ, Murray GM: Design of superstructures for osseointegrated fixtures. *Swed Dent J* 1985;28:S63–S69.

22. Parel S: Modified casting technique for osseointegrated fixed prosthesis fabrication: a preliminary report. *Int J Oral Maxillofac Implants* 1989;4:33–40.

23. Ortorp A, Jemt T: Clinical experiences of CNC-milled titanium frameworks supported by implants in the edentulous jaw: 1-year prospective study. *Clin Implant Dent Relat Res* 2000;2:2–9.

24. Ortorp A, Jemt T: Clinical experience of CNC-milled titanium frameworks supported by implants in the edentulous jaw: a 3-year interim report. *Clin Implant Dent Relat Res* 2002;4:104–109.

25. Drago CJ, del Castillo RA: Treatment of edentulous and partially edentulous patients with CAD-CAM frameworks: a pilot case study. *Pract Proced Aesthet Dent* 2006;18: *665-671; quiz 672*

26. Strub JR, Rekow ED, Witkowski S: Computer-aided design and fabrication of dental restorations. Current systems and future possibilities. *J Am Dent Assoc* 2006;137:1289–1296.

27. Suansuwan N, Swain MV: New approach for evaluating metal-porcelain interfacial bonding. *Int J Prosthodont* 1999;12: 547–552.

28. Cho CG, Donovan TE: Rational use of contemporary all-ceramic crown systems. *J Cal Dent Assoc* 1998;2:1–11.

29. Yanikoglu N: The repair methods for fractured metal-porcelain restorations: a review of the literature. *Eur J Prosthodont Restor Dent* 2004;12:161–165.

30. Fradeani M, D'Amelio M, Redemagni M, et al: Five-year follow-up with Procera all-ceramic crowns. *Quintessence Int* 2005;36:105–113.

31. Lang BR, Malo P, Guedes CM, et al: Procera All Ceram Bridge. *Appl Osseointegration Res* 2004;4:13–21.

32. Ödman P, Andersson B: Procera AllCeram crowns followed for 5 to 10.5 years: a prospective clinical study. *Int J Prosthodont* 2001;14:504–509.

33. Sundh B, Köhler B: An *in vivo* study of the impact of different emergence profiles of procera titanium crowns on quantity and quality of plaque. *Int J Prosthodont* 2002;15:457–460.

34. Koksal T, Dikbas I: Color stability of different denture teeth materials against various staining agents. *Dent Mater J* 2008;27:139–144.

35. Graha L: The essence of restorative care: long-term tooth preservation. *Compend Contin Educ Dent* 2005;26:S28–S33.

36. Takahashi T, Gunne J: Fit of implant frameworks: an *in vitro* comparison between two fabrication techniques. *J Prosthet Dent* 2003;89:256–260.

37. Hegenbarth E: *Quintessence Dental Technology.* Chicago, Quintessence, 1996, pp. 23–34.

38. Hager B, Oden A, Andersson B, et al: Procera AllCeram laminates: a clinical report. *J Prosthet Dent* 2001;85:231–232.

39. Chu FC, Andersson B, Deng FL, et al: Making porcelain veneers with the Procera AllCeram system: case studies. *Dent Update* 2003;30:454–460.

40. Andersson M, Razzoog ME, Oden A, et al: Procera: a new way to achieve an all-ceramic crown. *Quintessence Int* 1998;29: 285–296.

41. Zarone F, Sorrentino R, Vaccaro F, et al: Retrospective clinical evaluation of 86 Procera AllCeram™ anterior crowns on natural and implant-supported abutments. *Clin Implant Dent Relat Res* 2005;7:S95–S103.

42. Parel SM: The single-piece milled titanium implant bridge. *Dent Today* 2003;22:96–99.

43. Jemt T, Bergendal B, Arvidson K, et al: Implant-supported welded titanium frameworks in the edentulous maxilla: a 5-year prospective multicenter study. *Int J Prosthodont* 2002;15: 544–548.

44. Jemt T, Johansson J: Implant treatment in the edentulous maxillae: a 15-year follow-up study on 76 consecutive patients provided with fixed prostheses. *Clin Implant Dent Relat Res* 2006;8:61–69.

45. Ortorp A, Jemt T: Early laser-welded titanium frameworks supported by implants in the edentulous mandible: a 15-year comparative follow-up study. *Clin Implant Dent Relat Res* 2009;11:311–322.

46. Gualini F, Gualini G, Cominelli R, et al: Outcome of Branemark Novum implant treatment in edentulous mandibles: a retrospective 5-year follow-up study. *Clin Implant Dent Relat Res* 2009;11:330–337.

47. Lambert FE, Weber HP, Susarla SM, et al: Descriptive analysis of implant and prosthodontic survival rates with fixed implant-supported rehabilitations in the edentulous maxilla. *J Periodontol* 2009;80:1220–1230.

48. Eliasson A: On the role of number of fixtures, surgical technique and timing of loading. *Swed Dent J Suppl* 2008;197:3–95.

49. Quirynen M, De Soete M, van Steenberghe D: Infectious risks for oral implants: a review of the literature. *Clin Oral Implants Res* 2002;13:1–19.

50. NCBI Bookshelf: U.S. Preventive Services Task Force Evidence Syntheses, formerly Systematic Evidence Reviews: SCREENING for Human Immunodeficiency Virus, Appendix 1. Quality Rating Criteria. Available at http://www.ncbi.nlm.nih.gov/bookshelf/br.fcgi?book=es46&part=A34812 (accessed on November 2, 2010).

30

IMPLANT-SUPPORTED FIXED DENTAL PROSTHESES WITH CAD/CAM-FABRICATED PORCELAIN CROWN AND ZIRCONIA-BASED FRAMEWORK

MASAYUKI TAKABA, SHINPEI TANAKA, YUICHI ISHIURA, AND KAZUYOSHI BABA, DDS, PHD
Department of Prosthodontics, Showa University School of Dentistry, Tokyo, Japan

Keywords
Dental implants; fixed dental prostheses; CAD/CAM; zirconia framework; porcelain crown.

Correspondence
Masayuki Takaba, Showa University, Prosthodontics, 2-1-1 Kitasenzoku Ohta-ku, Tokyo 145-8515, Japan. E-mail: mtakaba@dent.showa-u.ac.jp

The authors deny any conflict of interest.

Accepted October 20, 2012

Published in *Journal of Prosthodontics* July 2013; Vol. 22, Issue 5

doi: 10.1111/jopr.12001

ABSTRACT

Recently, fixed dental prostheses (FDPs) with a hybrid structure of CAD/CAM porcelain crowns adhered to a CAD/CAM zirconia framework (PAZ) have been developed. The aim of this report was to describe the clinical application of a newly developed implant-supported FDP fabrication system, which uses PAZ, and to evaluate the outcome after a maximum application period of 36 months. Implants were placed in three patients with edentulous areas in either the maxilla or mandible. After the implant fixtures had successfully integrated with bone, gold–platinum alloy or zirconia custom abutments were first fabricated. Zirconia framework wax-up was performed on the custom abutments, and the CAD/CAM zirconia framework was prepared using the CAD/CAM system. Next, wax-up was performed on working models for porcelain crown fabrication, and CAD/CAM porcelain crowns were fabricated. The CAD/CAM zirconia frameworks and CAD/CAM porcelain crowns were bonded using adhesive resin cement, and the PAZ was cemented. Cementation of the implant superstructure improved the esthetics and masticatory efficiency in all patients. No undesirable outcomes, such as superstructure chipping, stomatognathic dysfunction, or periimplant bone resorption, were observed in any of the patients. PAZ may be a potential solution for ceramic-related clinical problems such as chipping and fracture and associated complicated repair procedures in implant-supported FDPs.

Dental implants are now widely recognized as a viable treatment option for prosthetic replacement of missing teeth. After implant fixtures are successfully placed and abutments are connected, implant-supported fixed dental prostheses (FDPs) are fabricated on the abutments. Porcelain is the material of choice for most FDPs, and metal ceramic restorations are widely used for FDPs because of their clinically acceptable biological stability, esthetics, and mechanical properties. Previous reports suggest that porcelain-fused-to-metal (PFM) crowns[1,2] and FDPs[3,4] exhibit excellent long-term prognosis, and metal ceramics have thus also been applied to implant-supported FDPs. On the other hand, metal ceramic FDPs are opaque, and the gingival marginal area is often discolored due to the metallic framework. In addition, they may induce metallic allergy,[5] although the number of such patients is not very high. The increasing demand for metal-free prostheses with better translucency that mimic the natural dentition has led to the recent development of several esthetically pleasing and biocompatible ceramics.[6,7] Feldspathic ceramics meet patient esthetic demands but do not provide adequate structural integrity, especially for implant-supported posterior FDPs.

In recent years, FDPs using a zirconia framework produced by a new fabrication system combined with computer-assisted fabrication (CAD/CAM) systems have attracted much attention and emerged as a popular treatment modality.[8,9] While zirconia ceramic FDPs exhibited a survival rate similar to metal ceramic FDPs after 3 years of function,[10] it has been noted that veneering porcelain on the zirconia framework by the conventional manual laboratory technique resulted in significantly lower fracture strength than the conventional PFM FDPs.[7,11] Actually, porcelain chipping or fractures are the most frequently reported technical complications of zirconia ceramic FDPs.[12,13]

Recently, machine-milled ceramic bonded to zirconia plate specimens using resin cement showed significantly higher fracture strength than that of conventional porcelain-fused-to-zirconia plate specimens.[14] The same authors reported clinical application of implant-supported FDPs with a hybrid structure of CAD/CAM porcelain crowns adhered to a CAD/CAM zirconia framework (PAZ).[15–17] In addition to the high fracture strength of this system demonstrated in vitro, this system allows refabrication of the CAD/CAM porcelain crown using the recorded CAD data without making an impression when porcelain fractures occur, which is expected to minimize the associated burden for both the patient and the clinician.

The aim of this clinical report was to describe the newly developed implant-supported FDP fabrication system, which uses PAZ, and evaluate the clinical outcome after a maximum application period of 36 months.

CLINICAL REPORTS AND INITIAL TREATMENTS

Three patients with either an edentulous maxilla or mandible who requested implant prostheses and consented to participate were selected. The followings are overviews of the selected patients.

Patient 1

A 66-year-old woman presented with masticatory disturbance due to loose mandibular FDPs. Figure 30.1 shows a panoramic radiograph taken at the initial examination. The periodontal condition and appearance of the maxillary prosthesis were judged to be good. The edentulous area had insufficient bone width and height for placement of implant fixtures, and the patient was not willing to undergo sinus augmentation surgery. Clinical examination indicated that extraction of the remaining mandibular teeth was required due to severe chronic periodontitis. First, the remaining mandibular teeth were extracted, and a complete denture was immediately placed. When the extraction sockets had healed adequately, four implants were placed in the mandible based on the All-on-4 concept (Fig 30.2).[18]

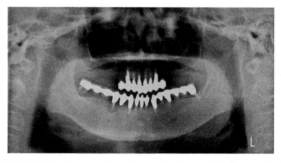

FIGURE 30.1 Panoramic radiograph taken at initial examination (patient 1).

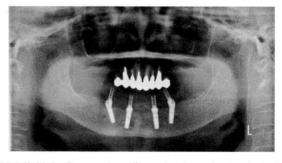

FIGURE 30.2 Panoramic radiograph taken after implant placement (patient 1).

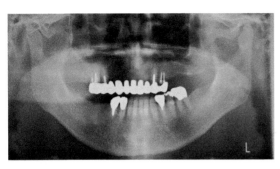

FIGURE 30.3 Panoramic radiograph taken at initial examination (patient 2).

Patient 2

A 55-year-old man presented with masticatory disturbance due to detachment of a maxillary FDP. Figure 30.3 shows the panoramic radiograph taken at the initial examination. Although the patient had a mandibular removable partial denture (RPD) fabricated by his dentist, he reported that he was not comfortable wearing it. The remaining mandibular teeth and restorations were in good condition. The patient also reported repeated detachment of the maxillary FDP. Clinical examination with radiographic assessment indicated that extraction of the remaining teeth was required due to chronic apical periodontitis, root fracture, and root caries. First, the remaining maxillary teeth were extracted, and a complete denture was immediately placed. When the extraction sockets had healed adequately, seven implants were placed in the edentulous maxilla and two implants in the mandible (Fig 30.4).

Patient 3

A 63-year-old man presented with masticatory disturbance due to multiple mobile teeth and ill-fitting RPDs. Figure 30.5 shows the panoramic radiograph taken at the initial examination. The patient was wearing RPDs in the maxilla and mandible but had difficulty chewing with the dentures. Clinical examination with radiographic assessment revealed that the quality of the dentures was not acceptable and

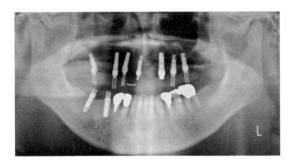

FIGURE 30.4 Panoramic radiograph taken after implant placement (patient 2).

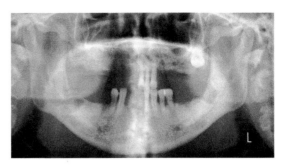

FIGURE 30.5 Panoramic radiograph taken at initial examination (patient 3).

extraction of all remaining teeth was indicated due to severe chronic periodontitis. First, six implants were placed in the maxilla immediately after extraction. Six months later, another six implants were placed in the mandible immediately after extraction (Fig 30.6).

For all patients, Branemark System® MK III implants (Nobel Biocare Services AG, Goteborg, Sweden) were used and were immediately loaded with acrylic interim prostheses.

PAZ FABRICATION

After the implant fixtures had successfully integrated with bone, final impressions were taken at the implant fixture level using the standard method, and a working model was fabricated. Then, the occlusion between the interim prosthesis and antagonistic dental arch was registered, and the interim prostheses screwed to the working models were mounted on a semiadjustable articulator using a facebow transfer technique. The diagnostic wax-up for abutment fabrication was performed on the working model attached to the articulator. Then gold–platinum alloy or zirconia custom abutments were fabricated (Figs 30.7 and 30.8). Custom abutments were connected in the oral cavity, and their position was confirmed using jigs prefabricated on the working model. Zirconia framework wax-up was performed on the custom abutments (Fig 30.9), data were input into the

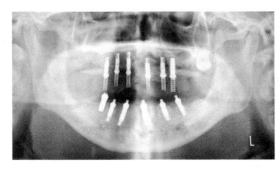

FIGURE 30.6 Panoramic radiograph taken after implant placement (patient 3).

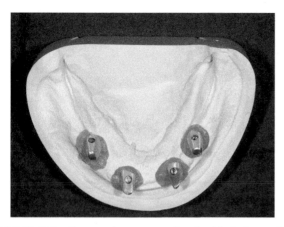

FIGURE 30.7   Custom abutments made of gold–platinum alloy.

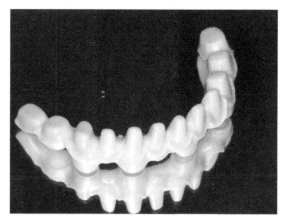

FIGURE 30.10   Completed zirconia framework.

of the CAD/CAM zirconia frameworks were taken on the models using silicone impression material, and working models for porcelain crown fabrication were made. Wax-up was performed for porcelain crowns on the models (Fig 30.11), and CAD/CAM porcelain crowns (Decsy, Digital Process Ltd, Kanagawa, Japan) were fabricated using the CAD/CAM double-scan method (Fig 30.12). After the CAD/CAM zirconia frameworks and CAD/CAM porcelain crowns were primed, they were bonded using adhesive resin cement (Panavia F2.0, Kuraray Medical, Inc., Tokyo, Japan). Finally, zirconia frameworks were primed, and the gingival area was built using gingiva-colored hybrid hard resin (Gradiagum, GC Corp., Tokyo, Japan) to complete the PAZ (Fig 30.13). After connecting the custom abutments into the oral cavity, the PAZ was cemented using temporary cement (Temporary Cement, Shofu, Inc., Kyoto, Japan).

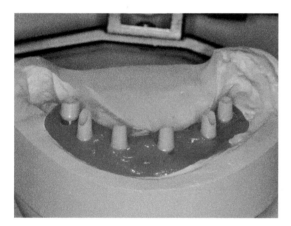

FIGURE 30.8   Custom abutments made of zirconia.

OUTCOME

Cementation of the implant superstructure improved esthetics and masticatory efficiency. In patient 1, a metal

CAD/CAM system using the double-scan technique, and CAD/CAM zirconia frameworks (Zenotec System, Wieland Dental + Technology GmbH & Co. KG, Pforzheim, Germany) were fabricated (Fig 30.10). Next, impressions

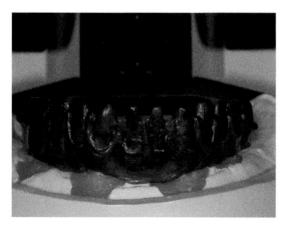

FIGURE 30.9   Zirconia framework wax-up.

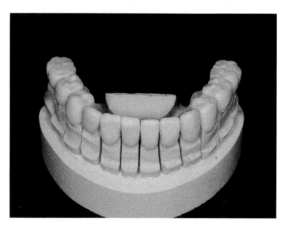

FIGURE 30.11   Porcelain crown wax-up.

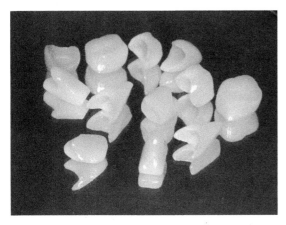

FIGURE 30.12   Completed CAD/CAM porcelain crowns.

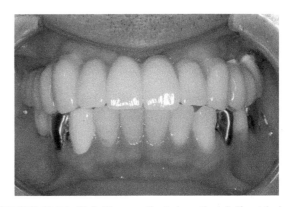

FIGURE 30.15   Definitive prosthesis in patient 2 (frontal view).

base partial denture was placed in the maxillary edentulous area. No clinical complications were reported or observed for 30 months after the PAZ was cemented to the mandible (Fig 30.14). For patient 2, as the implant fixture placed in the right posterior region of the maxilla fell out when the abutment was being connected, an additional implant fixture

was placed distally in the same area. After osseointegration, the PAZ was fabricated. No clinical complications were reported or observed for 36 months after the PAZ was cemented (Fig 30.15). In patient 3, a standard screw-retained type superstructure was fitted to the edentulous maxilla. The PAZ was attached to the edentulous mandible, and no clinical complication was reported or observed for 18 months after the placement (Fig 30.16). No undesirable outcomes, such as superstructure chipping, stomatognathic dysfunction, or peri-implant bone resorption, were observed in any of the patients.

DISCUSSION

The implant superstructures in patients 1 and 3 were implant-supported cantilever FDPs. The risk of fracture in the frame or veneering porcelain over 10 years was reported to be 3.2% in tooth-supported conventional FDPs[19] and 5.9% in tooth-supported cantilever FDPs.[20] Moreover, veneer fractures represented the most frequent technical complication in implant-supported cantilever FDPs. The estimated cumulative rate of material complications in implant-supported cantilever FDPs was reported to be 10.3% over a 5-year observation period and 19.6% over a 10-year observation period.[21] These figures suggest that

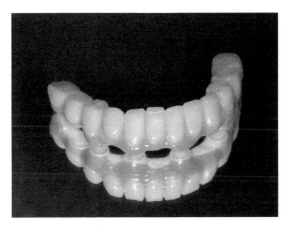

FIGURE 30.13   Completed superstructure (PAZ).

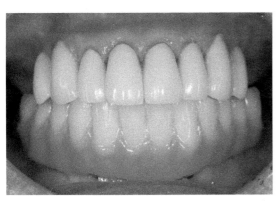

FIGURE 30.14   Definitive prosthesis in patient 1 (frontal view).

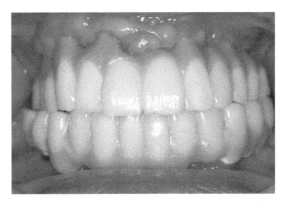

FIGURE 30.16   Definitive prosthesis in patient 3 (frontal view).

cantilever FDPs have a lower survival rate than conventional end-abutment-supported FDPs. Fortunately, no complication was found in the two cases followed up for 3 years, probably because of the high fracture strength of the PAZ system, but continued regular follow-up is necessary for a much longer period.

The 5-year prognosis based on a meta-analysis revealed that frequency of fracture was significantly higher in the veneering porcelain of implant-supported FDPs than in tooth-supported FDPs (8.8% vs. 2.9%).[22] These differences in fracture rate in implants vs. natural teeth may be because implants lack periodontal ligament and therefore lack the function of corresponding neural feedback structures.[23,24] The sensation threshold for implants is reported to be 8.75 times higher than that for natural teeth.[25] More specifically, not only is the cushioning mechanism of periodontal ligament missing, but the associated mechanoreceptors are also missing, resulting in reduced ability to adjust the bite force. Therefore, fracture of the veneering porcelain on implant-supported FDPs might be an unavoidable complication. When fracture occurs, clinicians need to replace the FDPs with temporary restorations and the FDPs have to be sent to a dental laboratory for repair. This takes time, requires technical expertise, and impairs patients' quality of life significantly. An implant superstructure that enables easy and quick repair when such complications occur, like our system, which allows easy refabrication of the CAD/CAM porcelain crown using prerecorded data, would be clinically significant. However, as no porcelain fracture was observed during the present study period, we could not demonstrate this in our patients.

It should also be noted that FDPs fabricated with our system have higher strength than FDPs with veneering porcelain on the zirconia framework prepared by the conventional manual laboratory technique.[14] Chipping and fractures of porcelain are reported to be caused by conventional porcelain layering and fusing methods, which may result in internal defects.[17] In contrast, machining of porcelain blocks using the CAD/CAM system can create crowns that maintain a high level of strength with no internal defects. In addition, advances in the adhesive material confer the advantage of better reinforcement of the ceramic. Although the study period was not very long, this might be why no mechanical complications such as chipping or fracture were observed in this study.

Lastly, this study described clinical application of the PAZ system and reported successful management of three patients using this system for 2 to 3 years. We intend to continue reviewing the present patients, increase our sample size, and optimize our fabrication techniques with the aim of improving long-term stability and prognoses. In the future, the long-term treatment outcome should be evaluated by well-designed clinical research.

CONCLUSION

Within the limitations of this clinical report, PAZ may be a potential solution for ceramic-related clinical problems, such as chipping and fracture and associated complicated repair procedures in implant-supported FDPs.

REFERENCES

1. Goodacre CJ, Bernal G, Rungcharassaeng K, et al: Clinical complications in fixed prosthodontics. *J Prosthet Dent* 2003;90:31–41.

2. Reitemeier B, Hänsel K, Kastner C, et al: Metal-ceramic failure in noble metal crowns: 7-year results of a prospective clinical trial in private practices. *Int J Prosthodont* 2006;19:397–399.

3. Sailer I, Pjetursson BE, Zwahlen M, et al: A systematic review of the survival and complication rates of all-ceramic and metal-ceramic reconstructions after an observation period of at least 3 years. Part II: fixed dental prostheses. *Clin Oral Implants Res* 2007;18(Suppl 3): 86–96.

4. Brägger U, Aeschlimann S, Bürgin W, et al: Biological and technical complications and failures with fixed partial dentures (FPD) on implants and teeth after four to five years of function. *Clin Oral Implants Res* 2001;12:26–34.

5. Gökçen-Röhlig B, Saruhanoglu A, Cifter ED, et al: Applicability of zirconia dental prostheses for metal allergy patients. *Int J Prosthodont* 2010;23:562–565.

6. Zarone F, Russo S, Sorrentino R: From porcelain-fused-to-metal to zirconia: clinical and experimental considerations. *Dent Mater* 2011;27:83–96.

7. Heintze SD, Rousson V: Survival of zirconia- and metal-supported fixed dental prostheses: a systematic review. *Int J Prosthodont* 2010;23:493–502.

8. Tinschert J, Natt G, Mautsch W, et al: Marginal fit of alumina- and zirconia-based fixed partial dentures produced by a CAD/CAM system. *Oper Dent* 2001;26:367–374.

9. Vigolo P, Fonzi F: An in vitro evaluation of fit of zirconium-oxide-based ceramic four-unit fixed partial dentures, generated with three different CAD/CAM systems, before and after porcelain firing cycles and after glaze cycles. *J Prosthodont* 2008;17:621–626.

10. Sailer I, Gottnerb J, Kanelb S, et al: Randomized controlled clinical trial of zirconia-ceramic and metal-ceramic posterior fixed dental prostheses: a 3-year follow-up. *Int J Prosthodont* 2009;22:553–560.

11. Ashkanani HM, Raigrodski AJ, Flinn BD, et al: Flexural and shear strengths of ZrO_2 and a high-noble alloy bonded to their corresponding porcelains. *J Prosthet Dent* 2008;100:274–284.

12. Vigolo P, Mutinelli S: Evaluation of zirconium-oxide-based ceramic single-unit posterior fixed dental prostheses (FDPs) generated with two CAD/CAM systems compared to porcelain-fused-to-metal single-unit posterior FDPs: a 5-year clinical prospective study. *J Prosthodont* 2012;21:265–269.

13. Hatta M, Shinya A, Yokoyama D, et al: The effect of surface treatment on bond strength of layering porcelain and hybrid composite bonded to zirconium dioxide ceramics. *J Prosthodont Res* 2011;55:146–153.

14. Kuriyama S, Terui Y, Higuchi D, et al: Novel fabrication method for zirconia restorations: bonding strength of machinable ceramic to zirconia with resin cements. *Dent Mater J* 2011;30:419–424.

15. Kunii J, Hotta Y, Tamaki Y, et al: Effect of sintering on the marginal and internal fit of CAD/CAM-fabricated zirconia frameworks. *Dent Mater J* 2007;26:820–826.

16. Takeuchi K, Fujishima A, Manabe A, et al: Combination treatment of tribochemical treatment and phosphoric acid ester monomer of zirconia ceramics enhances the bonding durability of resin-based luting cements. *Dent Mater J* 2010;29:316–323.

17. Miyazaki T, Hotta Y: CAD/CAM systems available for the fabrication of crown and bridge restorations. *Aust Dent J* 2011;56(Suppl 1): 97–106.

18. Maló P, Rangert B, Nobre M: "All-on-Four" immediate-function concept with Brånemark System implants for completely edentulous mandibles: a retrospective clinical study. *Clin Implant Dent Relat Res* 2003;5(Suppl 1): 2–9.

19. Tan K, Pjetursson BE, Lang NP, et al: A systematic review of the survival and complication rates of fixed partial dentures (FPDs) after an observation period of at least 5 years. *Clin Oral Implants Res* 2004;15:654–666.

20. Pjetursson BE, Tan K, Lang NP, et al: A systematic review of the survival and complication rates of fixed partial dentures (FPDs) after an observation period of at least 5 years. *Clin Oral Implants Res* 2004;15:667–676.

21. Aglietta M, Siciliano VI, Zwahlen M, et al: A systematic review of the survival and complication rates of implant supported fixed dental prostheses with cantilever extensions after an observation period of at least 5 years. *Clin Oral Implants Res* 2009;20:441–451.

22. Pjetursson BE, Brägger U, Lang NP, et al: Comparison of survival and complication rates of tooth-supported fixed dental prostheses (FDPs) and implant-supported FDPs and single crowns (SCs). *Clin Oral Implants Res* 2007;18(Suppl 3): 97–113.

23. Jacobs R, van Steenberghe D: Role of periodontal ligament receptors in the tactile function of teeth: a review. *J Periodontal Res* 1994;29:153–167.

24. Schulte W: Implants and the periodontium. *Int Dent J* 1995;45:16–26.

25. Hämmerle CH, Wagner D, Brägger U, et al: Threshold of tactile sensitivity perceived with dental endosseous implants and natural teeth. *Clin Oral Implants Res* 1995;6:83–90.

31

FULL ZIRCONIA FIXED DETACHABLE IMPLANT-RETAINED RESTORATIONS MANUFACTURED FROM MONOLITHIC ZIRCONIA: CLINICAL REPORT AFTER TWO YEARS IN SERVICE

Fernando Rojas-Vizcaya, DDS, MS[1,2]

[1]Mediterranean Prosthodontic Institute, Implant Prosthodontics, Castellon, Spain
[2]Adjunct Assistant Professor, Department of Prosthodontics, UNC School of Dentistry, Chapel Hill, NC

Keywords

Dental implants; zirconia frameworks; monolithic zirconia; fixed detachable restoration; full arch; full zirconia; screw-retained restoration.

Correspondence

Fernando Rojas-Vizcaya, Mediterranean Prosthodontic Institute, Avenida Rey Don Jaime, 5, Entresuelo, Castellon 12001, Spain. E-mail: frojasv@prosthodontics.es, rojasf@dentistry.unc.edu

Accepted July 17, 2011

Published in *Journal of Prosthodontics* October 2011; Vol. 20, Issue 7

doi: 10.1111/j.1532-849X.2011.00784.x

ABSTRACT

The most frequently encountered problem with fixed detachable dental prostheses is loosening or fracture of the prosthetic screws. Other problems include wear, separation, or fracture of the resin teeth from the metal/acrylic prosthesis, chipping or fracture of porcelain from the metal/ceramic or zirconia/ceramic prosthesis, and fracture of the framework in some free-end prostheses. For this type of prosthesis, it is necessary to place the implants in a position that enables occlusal or lingual access so as not to impair the esthetics. This clinical report describes the restoration of a patient with complete fixed detachable maxillary and mandibular prostheses made of monolithic zirconia with angled dental implants with buccal access. The prostheses were esthetically pleasing, and no clinical complications have been reported after 2 years.

Full-mouth reconstruction of a patient using dental implants is a challenge if there is vertical and horizontal bone resorption, since this includes the gingival area and restricts the position of the implants; however, hard- and soft-tissue grafting may allow the implants to be placed into the desired position. Although it is possible to regenerate lost tissues, an alternative is to use fixed detachable prostheses that restore the function and the esthetics of the gingiva and teeth. Various material combinations, including metal/acrylic, metal/ceramic, and zirconia/ceramic, have been used for constructing this type of restoration.[1–11]

Fixed detachable dental prostheses made of metal/acrylic may pose the following problems: loosening of the acrylic teeth, lack of natural color primarily in the prosthetic gingiva area, and wear of the occluding surfaces over time. Consequently replacement of teeth and maintenance of the prosthesis are required.[3–8] Prostheses made of metal/porcelain offer an excellent esthetic result; however, a major disadvantage of metal/porcelain prostheses is that the porcelain can break, endangering the entire restoration.[12–16] In zirconia/ceramic prostheses, ceramic chipping[17–19] or breakage of the zirconia framework can make the repair impossible.[20,21] Additionally, if the implant is in an angled position because of the anatomy of the bone, it may be necessary to use an angled abutment to avoid buccal access through the prosthesis in the esthetic area. Additionally, for patients with a high smile line, the treatment of the prosthetic gingiva with acrylic or ceramic is important.[22,23]

The zirconium oxide (yttrium-partially stabilized with tetragonal polycrystalline structure)[24] used to fabricate the prostheses described in this clinical report has been used successfully since the 1970s for orthopedic purposes.[25] It is made of raw mineral materials, such as chemically manufactured zirconium sand, partially stabilized with yttrium, and converted by mechanical procedures into zirconia blocks.[24–28] Zirconium is used in the manufacture of many types of dental restorations[26] and may be a more suitable prosthetic material due to its capability for limiting bacterial colonization,[27,28] and because it produces less wear to antagonistic teeth than does feldspathic dental porcelain.[29]

This clinical report describes a complete restoration using monolithic zirconia-fixed detachable maxillary and mandibular prostheses. The incisal edges and occluding surfaces were made of monolithic zirconia (Prettau Zirconia, Zirkonzahn, Gais, Italy) to decrease the risk of chipping or fracture.

CLINICAL REPORT

A 52-year-old man presented to the Mediterranean Prosthodontic Institute (MPI) in Castellon, Spain with a request to have "fixed teeth." A comprehensive clinical and radiographic examination revealed advanced bone loss due to advanced periodontal disease (Fig 31.1). His general health was not impaired.

According to the Prosthodontic Diagnostic Index (PDI) for classification of partial edentulism, the patient was characterized as class IV.[30] A panoramic radiograph was made, and the possibility of inserting dental implants in the remaining bone was considered, although not in the lower posterior region on both sides. A complete restoration of the entire

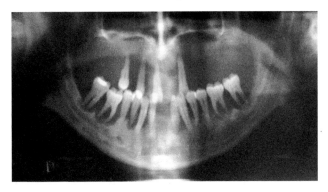

FIGURE 31.1 Residual dentition and bone loss due to advanced periodontal disease.

mouth was planned by using fixed detachable prostheses supported by dental implants.

The treatment was divided into stages in order to control the patient's function and esthetic appearance. In the first stage, teeth were extracted without alveolectomy or ridge preservation. Insertion of the immediate interim complete denture was made, so as to restore the occlusal vertical dimension (OVD)[31] and to determine some aspects of the esthetics.

Eight maxillary and six mandibular fluoride-modified implant surfaces (OsseoSpeed, AstraTech AB, Mölndal, Sweden) were placed in the 8th and 12th week, respectively (Figs 31.2 and 31.3) (Table 31.1). A duplicate of the interim prosthesis was used as a surgical drilling template.

Insertion of straight healing abutments (Healing Abutment, AstraTech AB) clearly showed the angulations of the implants and the future emergence profile in the buccal areas. After suturing, the interim complete dentures were adapted, and acrylic was reduced in the healing abutment areas so that the dentures did not touch the healing abutments during the osseointegration period. No soft liner was used.

After 8 weeks of osseointegration, the healing abutments were replaced by solid titanium abutments (3 mm high) for screw-retained restorations (20° UniAbutments, AstraTech AB) in each implant site (Fig 31.4). An open tray definitive abutment level impression was made with a polysiloxane impression material (Coltoflax; Colte'ne/Whaledent AG, Altstätten, Switzerland). Closing copings (20° ProHeal Cap, AstraTech AB) were placed on the abutments. Soft tissue was reproduced in the impression using vinylpolysiloxane (Gingifast Rigid; Zhermack, Rovigo, Italy), and maxillary and mandibular definitive casts were poured with type IV stone (T.C. 15; Techim Group, Milan, Italy).

The maxillary relation was taken with an arbitrary ear face-bow (Denar Slidematic Facebow; Waterpik Technologies, Inc., Ft. Collins, CO). The infraorbital margin was used as a third point of reference. The OVD and an interocclusal centric relation were transferred to a semiadjustable articulator (Hanau Modular Articulator System 190; Waterpik

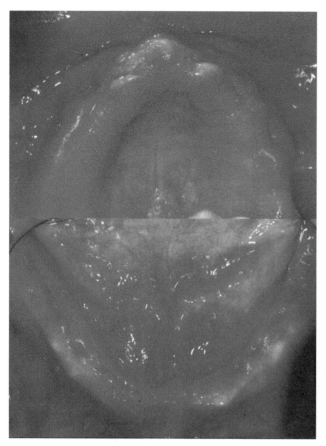

FIGURE 31.2 Twelve weeks after extractions.

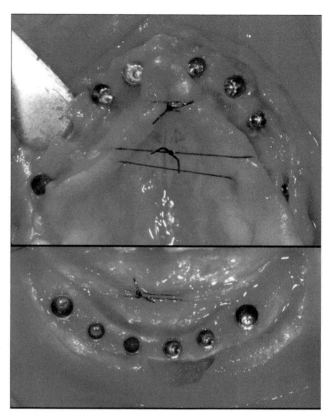

FIGURE 31.3 Implant placement in maxilla and mandible for conventional loading.

Technologies, Inc.) using occlusal rims. Average setting of the condylar inclination on the articulator was 33° for the sagittal and 15° for the lateral condyle path inclination.[32] Afterward, a verification device was fabricated intraorally to evaluate the accuracy of the definitive cast. Impression copings were connected to the abutments and splinted to each other with acrylic resin (Duralay, Reliance, Dental Mfg. Co. Worth, IL). The verification jig was sectioned and reconnected, unscrewed, and transferred to the definitive cast. Passive fit of the index on the definitive cast was confirmed, and the accuracy of the definitive cast was verified.

Afterward, two fixed detachable interim maxillary and mandibular prostheses were manufactured in self-curing acrylic resin (Palapress Vario; Heraeus Kulzer, Hanau, Germany), using acrylic denture teeth, mold T46 for anterior and PU31 for posterior teeth (Vita MFT; VITA Zahnfabrik, Bad Säckingen, Germany), and color A2 (VITAPAN classical shade guide; VITA Zahnfabrik). A metal framework and temporary cylinders (Temporary Cylinder, Uni 20°, Astra-Tech AB) were built onto the lower fixed detachable prosthesis. This design was used to provide an increased resistance to deformation in the area of the free-end prostheses. The passive fit of the maxillary and mandibular fixed

detachable interim prostheses on the abutments was evaluated in different ways. First, pressure was applied first on one end abutment and then on the other side[33] to look for movement of the prostheses. A visual check was then carried out, and fit was evaluated with an explorer.[34] Passivity was

TABLE 31.1 **Implant Distribution, Diameters, and Lengths**

Implant Distribution	Implant Diameter (mm)	Implant Length (mm)
3	3.5	11
4	3.5	11
5	4.5	11
7	4.0	8
9	4.5	11
11	4.5	9
12	4.5	13
14	4.5	11
22	4.5	11
23	3.5	11
24	3.5	11
26	3.5	11
27	3.5	11
28	4.5	9

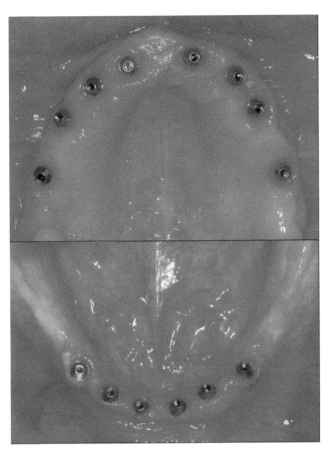

FIGURE 31.4   Solid titanium abutments for screw-retained fixed detachable restorations.

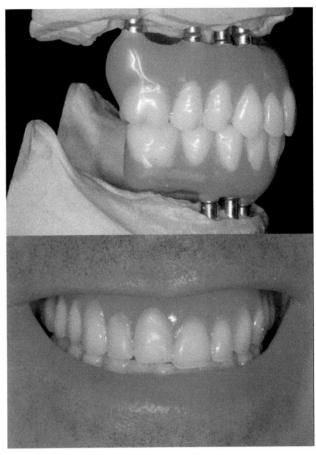

FIGURE 31.5   Fixed detachable interim prosthesis for determination of standard esthetic parameters.

verified with an individual screw[35] in one of the end abutments. No movement of the restoration was noticed, and the restoration remained in its position at the opposite end abutment. The fit between the prostheses and all abutments was clinically verified in three dimensions, and was confirmed in two dimensions via periapical radiographs.[36]

Through these fixed detachable interim prostheses, the parameters of esthetics and function were determined (Fig 31.5). Analysis of the patient's smile showed that the commissural line was not parallel to the interpupillary line, and the lip showed some asymmetries when relaxed. Also, there were asymmetrical movements of the lips at different moments during smiling, making the analysis difficult. These modifications were made in the interim fixed detachable prostheses: the length of the maxillary central incisors was reduced intraorally using a high-speed diamond bur (Komet 5850.314.016; Komet USA LLC, Rock Hill, SC), and the patient's smile line was drawn in relation to the lower lip. The cervical contour of the maxillary anterior teeth was lengthened in an apical direction by adding light-cured composites (Z100 Restorative, 3M ESPE, St. Paul, MN) to compensate for the incisal reduction and to reduce the gingival area visible when smiling (Fig 31.5).

When all esthetic and functional parameters for the patient were satisfied, maxillary and mandibular impressions of the prostheses were made with irreversible hydrocolloid (Cavex CA37; Cavex, Haarlem, The Netherlands), and poured with type III stone (Elite model; Zhermack), copying the interim fixed detachable prostheses. Afterward, the patient's fixed detachable interim prostheses were removed, and the maxillary prosthesis was screwed into the previously articulated definitive cast. Afterward, the cast of the mandibular interim prosthesis was articulated at the same OVD against the maxillary definitive cast and interim prosthesis. Then, the maxillary cast was articulated against the previously mounted mandibular cast. By this method of cross-mounted casts, the dental technician manufactured the maxillary fixed detachable white resin prosthesis (Frame, Zirkonzahn) by using the mandibular cast as an antagonist to control the occlusal plane, the midline, and the smile line. As soon as the two prostheses made of white resin (Frame) were manufactured, they were screwed in the patient's mouth to evaluate occlusion and esthetics (Fig 31.6). The passive fit of the maxillary and mandibular white resin prostheses (Frame) on the abutments was evaluated in the same way as for the

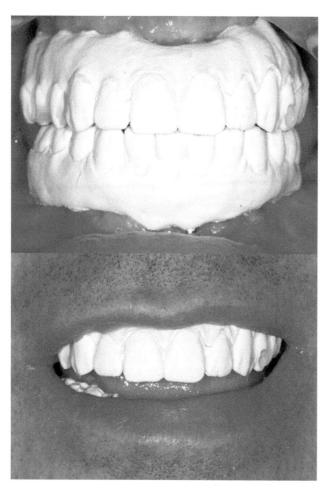

FIGURE 31.6   White resin frame to evaluate the final esthetics and occlusion intraorally.

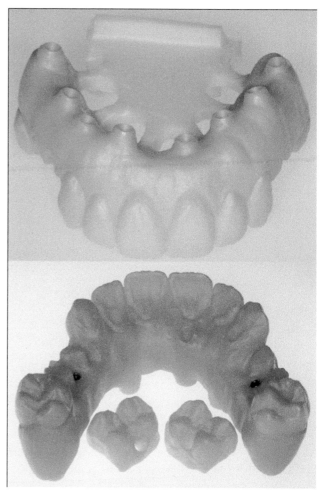

FIGURE 31.7   Full zirconia prosthesis from a monolithic zirconia before being colored.

interim prostheses. No adjustments to the white resin prostheses were required.

The white acrylic prostheses were copied into full zirconia prostheses (Prettau, Zirkonzahn) from a 40 mm high block of zirconium oxide (Ytrium-partially stabilized with tetragonal polycrystalline structure) (Prettau Zirconia 16er XH40, Zirkonzahn) using a copy-milling unit (Zirkograph 025 ECO, Zirkonzahn) (Fig 31.7). The milled units were colored as appropriate for teeth and gingiva (Color Liquid, Zirkonzahn). The gingival color was selected for the patient by means of a color guide for the pink-colored ceramic (Ceramic Tissue, Zirkonzahn). Finally the prostheses were dried and then sintered (Fig 31.8).

The passive fit of the maxillary and mandibular restorations on the abutments was evaluated in the same way as for the interim fixed detachable prostheses and white resin prostheses (Frame), and the fit was confirmed in two dimensions via periapical radiographs (Fig 31.9). The lower fixed detachable prosthesis was screwed and tightened with a 15 N cm torque. In the maxilla, first the macro structure was screwed, and then the substructures were screwed with 15 N cm torque (Fig 31.10). Afterward, the access holes were covered with

gutta-percha (Gutta Percha; Henry Schein, Inc, Melville, NY) and light-cured composite (Z100 Restorative).

The initial periapical radiograph (Fig 31.9) shows the fitting of the fixed detachable restorations on the abutments and the bone at the level of the implants. After 2 years, the periapical radiograph showed no changes to the bone level (Fig 31.11) when compared with the initial periapical radiographs. The soft tissue remained stable, with no inflammation or bleeding in any region. There was no presence of tartar. No change could be seen in the restorations, with no fractures within the occlusal or incisal areas or any wear. The patient reported no problems (Fig 31.12). The prosthesis made of monolithic zirconia improved the patient's oral function and esthetic appearance.

DISCUSSION

There have been previous reports on the use of fixed detachable prostheses made of metal/acrylic, metal/ceramic, or

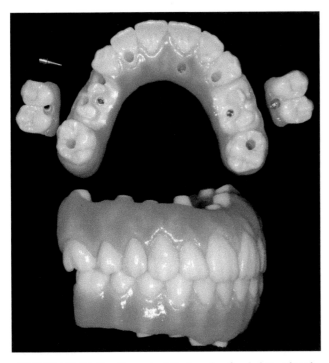

FIGURE 31.8 Prostheses in full zirconia after being colored.

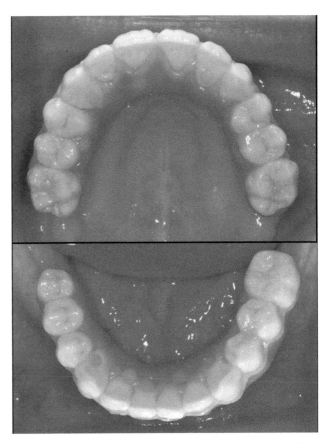

FIGURE 31.10 Restorations screwed into the abutments. Note the full-zirconia occlusal surface and no evidence of chipping after more than 2 years.

zirconia/ceramic. In studies of hybrid prostheses using frameworks of various materials, several different complications arose. In 1999, Bergendal et al compared titanium frameworks and gold alloys over 5 years,[3] and reported slightly more fractures of Ti frameworks than gold alloy frameworks and more fractures of artificial teeth in the Ti frameworks. Most fractures were related to the welding joints at the distal abutments. In 2000, Örtorp et al reported no mechanical complications except for some fractures of the resin facing[4] in a 1-year prospective study. In 2003, Duncan et al, in another prospective study regarding a clinical test over a period of 36 months, reported that 68% of patients provided with fixed detachable prostheses had complications.[5] For the majority of patients, this concerned fracture of the resin teeth. This occurred more frequently in the anterior than posterior area and with a greater frequency after 1 year of use.

In 2009, Örtorp and Jemt conducted a comparative follow-up study on a supervised period of 15 years, in which laser-welded Ti frameworks were compared with gold alloy frameworks.[6] In that study, the fracture of the resin or acrylic teeth and the inflammation of the soft tissue were the most common complications with hybrid prostheses fabricated with Ti frameworks. Fractures in the Ti framework were detected in 15.5% of the patients. More fractures were detected in Ti frameworks than in gold alloy frameworks.[6]

The most common complication with metal/acrylic restorations is the need to replace the acrylic resin prosthetic teeth

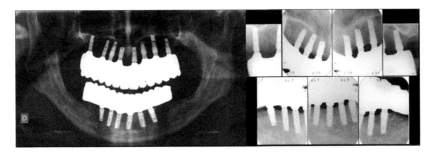

FIGURE 31.9 Initial X-ray of the full-zirconia fixed detachable restorations. Note the marginal bone at the level of the implants and the fit of the restorations.

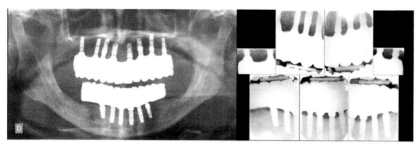

FIGURE 31.11   Radiographic control after 2 years in use showing stable marginal bone at the level of the implants.

due to wear or fracture of the acrylic teeth. Fracture of the resin tooth is due to different factors, including poor bonding of the tooth to the acrylic resin, trauma, and insufficient support from the framework. Resin tooth wear could be a result of increased occlusal forces using fixed prostheses, or in some cases, due to parafunctional activities.[7,8] In ceramometal restorations, the chipping or fracture of the ceramic is due to different factors: impact and fatigue load, occlusal forces, differences in thermal expansion coefficients, low-elastic modulus of the metal, improper design, microdefects, and trauma.[13–16]

Some clinical reports on the use of porcelain-veneered zirconia prostheses reported fractures in veneering porcelain[9,17,18] and in all-ceramic cantilever FPDs.[20,21] Ina 2008 review, Denry and Kelly found 15 major studies of zirconia prostheses where fractures were uncommon, but chipping with the porcelain veneer was present in all studies.[26] The difference in the coefficients of thermal expansion that may produce residual stresses during the fabrication of all-ceramic crowns and fixed partial dentures (FPDs), and the interface between the veneering porcelain and the zirconia substructure are the origin of the chipping in these type of restorations.[17,18]

There are only a few reports on hybrid prosthetic restorations with zirconia frameworks. Those regarding FPDs have shown that fracture of the porcelain facing is caused by the strain in the framework, since most of the breakages arose in the interface between the framework and porcelain layer.[37,38] In a 2007 prospective clinical cohort study, Sailer et al reported a 97.8% success rate of zirconia frameworks, and chipping of the veneering ceramic in 15.2% after 5 years of clinical observation.[39] Moreover, there are some positive reports concerning cases with zirconia frameworks on natural teeth[40] and others concerning hybrid prostheses on implants using zirconia frameworks without any complication during a monitoring period of 6 months.[10,11] Long-term studies must be carried out using zircoina/ceramic implant-supported, full-arch fixed restorations.

As far as this author's knowledge, no clinical report has yet been published on a monolithic zirconia complete fixed detachable restoration. In the future, long-term studies must be carried out using this type of restoration, to compare this kind of material with the materials existing on the market, and to determine the advantages discussed in this clinical report.

ACKNOWLEDGMENTS

The author would like to acknowledge George Walcher, DT, from the dental laboratory of Enrico Steger in Bruneck, Italy, for the final work in the case; and Jorge Cid Yañez, DT, from the laboratory of the Mediterranean Prosthodontic Institute in Castellon, Spain for the provisional fixed detachable prostheses.

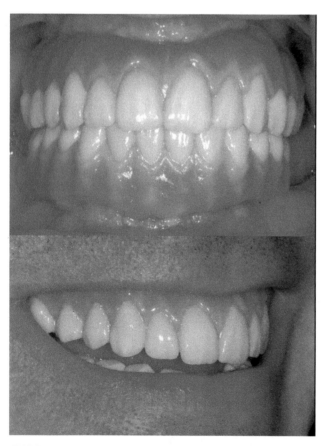

FIGURE 31.12   Esthetics and function were restored with the full-zirconia restorations.

REFERENCES

1. Sjögren G, Andersson M, Bergman M: Laser welding of titanium in dentistry. *Acta Odontol Scand* 1988;46:247–253.

2. Örtorp A, Linden B, Jemt T: Clinical experiences of laser-welded titanium frameworks supported by implants in the edentulous mandible. A 5-year follow-up study. *Int J Prosthodont* 1999;12:65–72.

3. Bergendal B, Palmqvist S: Laser-welded titanium framework for implant-supported fixed prostheses: a 5-year report. *Int J Oral Maxillofac Implants* 1999;14:69–71.

4. Örtorp A, Jemt T: Clinical experiences of computer numeric control-milled titanium frameworks supported by implants in the edentulous jaw: a 5-year prospective study. *Clin Implant Dent Relat Res* 2000;2:2–9.

5. Duncan JP, Nazarova E, Vogiatzi T, et al: Prosthodontic complications in a prospective clinical trial of single-stage implants at 36 months. *Int J Oral Maxillofac Implants* 2003;18:561–565.

6. Örtorp A, Jemt T: Early laser-welded titanium frameworks supported by implants in the edentulous mandible: a 15-year comparative follow-up study. *Clin Implant Dent Relat Res* 2009;11:311–322.

7. Purcell BA, McGlumphy EA, Holloway JA, et al: Prosthetic complications in mandibular metal-resin implant-fixed complete dental prostheses: a 5- to 9-year analysis. *Int J Oral Maxillofac Implants* 2008;23:847–857.

8. Bozini T, Petridis H, Garefis K: A meta-analysis of prosthodontic complication rates of implant-supported fixed dental prostheses in edentulous patients after an observation period of at least 5 years. *Int J Oral Maxillofac Implants* 2011;26:304–318.

9. Larsson C, Vult von Steyern P, Nilner K: A prospective study of implant-supported full-arch yttria-stabilized tetragonal zirconia polycrystal mandibular fixed dental prostheses: three-year results. *Int J Prosthodont* 2010;23:364–369.

10. Papaspyridakos P, Lal K: Complete arch implant rehabilitation using subtractive rapid prototyping and porcelain fused to zirconia prosthesis: a clinical report. *J Prosthet Dent* 2008;100:165–172.

11. Hassel AJ, Shahin R, Kreuter A, et al: Rehabilitation of an edentulous mandible with an implant-supported fixed prosthesis using an all-ceramic framework: a case report. *Quintessence Int* 2008;39:421–426.

12. Linkevicius T, Vladimirovas E, Grybauskas S, et al: Veneer fracture in implant-supported metal-ceramic restorations. Part I: overall success rate and impact of occlusal guidance. *Stomatologija* 2008;10:133–139.

13. Roberts DH: The failure of retainers in bridge prostheses. An analysis of 2,000 retainers. *Br Dent J* 1970;128:117–124.

14. Jacobi R, Shillingburg HT Jr, Duncanson MG Jr: Effect of abutment mobility, site, and angle of impact on retention of fixed partial dentures. *J Prosthet Dent* 1985;54:178–183.

15. Reuter JE, Brose MO: Failures in full crown retained dental bridges. *Br Dent J* 1984;157:61–63.

16. Llobell A, Nicholls JI, Kois JC, et al: Fatigue life of porcelain repair systems. *Int J Prosthodont* 1992;5:205–213.

17. Guess PC, Att W, Strub JR: Zirconia in fixed implant prosthodontics. *Clin Implant Dent Relat Res* 2010 Dec 22 [Epub ahead of print].

18. Swain MV: Unstable cracking (chipping) of veneering porcelain on all-ceramic dental crowns and fixed partial dentures. *Acta Biomater* 2009;5:1668–1677.

19. Larsson C, Vult von Steyern P, Nilner K: A prospective study of implant-supported full-arch yttria-stabilized tetragonal zirconia polycrystal mandibular fixed dental prostheses: three-year results. *Int J Prosthodont* 2010;23:364–369.

20. Ohlmann B, Marienburg K, Gabbert O, et al: Fracture-load values of all-ceramic cantilevered FPDs with different framework designs. *Int J Prosthodont* 2009;22:49–52.

21. Al-Amleh B, Lyons K, Swain M: Clinical trials in zirconia: a systematic review. *J Oral Rehabil* 2010;37:641–652.

22. Zitzmann NU, Marinello CP: Treatment plan for restoring the edentulous maxilla with implant-supported restorations: removable overdenture versus fixed partial denture design. *J Prosthet Dent* 1999;82:188–196.

23. Bidra AS, Agar JR: A classification system of patients for esthetic fixed implant-supported prostheses in the edentulous maxilla. *Compend Contin Educ Dent* 2010;31:366–374.

24. Kelly JR, Denry I: Stabilized zirconia as a structural ceramic: an overview. *Dent Mater* 2008;24:289–298.

25. Chevalier J, Gremillar L: Ceramics for medical applications: a picture for the next 20 years. *J Eur Ceramic Soc* 2009;29:1245–1255.

26. Denry I, Kelly JR: State of the art of zirconia for dental applications. *Dent Mater* 2008;24:299–307.

27. Rimondini L, Cerroni L, Carrassi A, et al: Bacterial colonization of zirconia ceramic surfaces: an in vitro and in vivo study. *Int J Oral Maxillofac Implants* 2002;17:793–798.

28. Scarano A, Piattelli M, Caputi S, et al: Bacterial adhesion on commercially pure titanium and zirconium oxide disks: an in vivo human study. *J Periodontol* 2004;75:292–296.

29. Jung YS, Lee JW, Choi YJ, et al: A study on the in-vitro wear of the natural tooth structure by opposing zirconia or dental porcelain. *J Adv Prosthodont* 2010;2:111–115.

30. McGarry TJ, Nimmo A, Skiba JF, et al: Classification system for partial edentulism. *J Prosthodont* 2002;11:181–193.

31. Turrel AJ: Clinical assessment of vertical dimension. *J Prosthet Dent* 1972;28:238–246.

32. Zarb GA, Carlsson GE, Bolender CL: *Boucher's Prosthodontic Treatment for Edentulous Patients* (ed 11) St. Louis, Mosby, 1997, pp 218–229.

33. Henry PJ: An alternate method for the production of accurate cast and occlusal records in the osseointegrated implant rehabilitation. *J Prosthet Dent* 1987;58:694–697.

34. Yanase RT, Binon PP, Jemt T, et al: Current issue form. How do you test a cast framework for a full arch fixed implant supported prosthesis? *Int J Oral Maxillofac Implants* 1994;9:471–474.

35. Tan KB, Rubenstein JE, Nicholls JI, et al: Three-dimensional analysis of the casting accuracy of one piece, osseointegrated implant retained prostheses. *Int J Prosthodont* 1993;6:346–363.

36. Hollender L, Rockler B: Radiographic evaluation of osseointegrated implants of the jaws. Experimental study of the influence of radiographic techniques on the measurement of the relation between implant and bone. *Dentomaxillofac Radiol* 1980;9:91–95.

37. Flemming GJ, Dickens M, Thomas LJ, et al: The in vitro failure of all ceramic crowns and the connector area of fixed partial dentures using bilayered ceramic specimens: the influence of core to dentin thickness ratio. *Dent Mater* 2006;22:771–777.

38. Tsumita M, Kokubo Y, Vult von Steyern P, et al: Effect of framework shape on the fracture strength of implant-supported all-ceramic fixed partial dentures in the molar region. *J Prosthodont* 2008;17:274–285.

39. Sailer I, Fehér A, Filser F, et al: Five-year clinical results of zirconia frameworks for posterior fixed partial dentures. *Int J Prosthodont* 2007;20:383–388.

40. Keough BE, Kay HB, Sager RD: A ten-unit all-ceramic anterior fixed partial denture using Y-TZP zirconia. *Pract Proced Aesthet Dent* 2006;18:37–43.

32

MAXILLARY FULL-ARCH IMMEDIATELY LOADED IMPLANT-SUPPORTED FIXED PROSTHESIS DESIGNED AND PRODUCED BY PHOTOGRAMMETRY AND DIGITAL PRINTING: A CLINICAL REPORT

DAVID PENARROCHA-OLTRA, DDS, MSC, PHD,[1] RUBEN AGUSTIN-PANADERO, DMD, PHD,[2] GUILLERMO PRADIES, DMD,[3] SONIA GOMAR-VERCHER, PHD,[4] AND MIGUEL PENARROCHA-DIAGO, MD, DDS, PHD[1]

[1]Department of Oral Surgery and Implant Dentistry, Valencia University Medical and Dental School, Valencia, Spain
[2]Department of Stomatology, Valencia University Medical and Dental School, Valencia, Spain
[3]Department of Buccofacial Prostheses, Complutense University Dental School, Madrid, Spain
[4]Private Dental Practice, Valencia, Spain

Keywords

Dental implants; photogrammetry; dental impression technique; CAD/CAM.

Correspondence

Miguel Peñarrocha-Diago, Clínicas Odontológicas, Gascó Oliag 1, 46021 Valencia, Spain. E-mail: miguel.penarrocha@uv.es.

The authors deny any conflicts of interest.

Accepted March 25, 2015

Published in *Journal of Prosthodontics* December 2015

doi: 10.1111/jopr.12364

ABSTRACT

The present clinical report describes the use of a photogrammetry system (PICcamera) for obtaining impressions and designing and producing an immediately loaded CAD/CAM provisional fixed prosthesis delivered in the mouth within 24 hours after implant placement in the maxilla. The stereo camera was used to capture the implant positions, automatically taking 350 images in less than 2 minutes. This photogrammetry system takes 10 pictures per second with a margin of error of under $10\,\mu m$ between two scan bodies, and identifies the spatial position of each implant without physical contact. The three-dimensional data for each implant are registered in vector format, together with all interrelated implant angles and distances. The information is stored in an STL file (PICfile). Information on soft tissues was obtained from an irreversible hydrocolloid impression that was poured in stone and scanned. An immediately loaded screw-retained fixed prosthesis was made from acetalic resin using CAD/CAM, and its passive fit was evaluated in the mouth using the Sheffield test and screw resistance test.

The conventional method of producing an implant-fixed prosthesis supported by multiple implants consists of taking impressions of implants and soft tissues with impression copings and impression materials and then producing the prosthesis using a master cast acquired from the impression.[1] More recently, intraoral scanners have been used for impression procedures in cases involving multiple implants for rehabilitating edentulous areas of a limited span.[1] However, the reliability of intraoral scanners remains questionable when they are used for the prosthetic rehabilitation of a complete arch.[1]

Photogrammetry is an option for direct and reliable recording of the position of intraoral implants. It registers the geometrical properties of three-dimensional (3D) objects and their interrelated spatial positions from photographic images. Photogrammetry was introduced in dentistry by Jemt and Lie in 1994 to analyze the distortion of implant frameworks.[2] The technique can also be used as a novel option for reliable, direct intraoral registration of the positions of multiple implants. So far, the technique has been used in laboratory studies to measure implant positions and to ensure the fit of prostheses, as well as for assessing framework deformations and mucosal recession.[3]

Jemt et al[4] described the use of photogrammetry for registering the positions of dental implants intraorally. They compared this technique with conventional impression taking, and concluded that photogrammetry constitutes a valid alternative. Since then, the technical advances have been considerable but have not been accompanied by developments in the application of photogrammetry to implant dentistry. In 2005, Ortrop et al demonstrated that under laboratory conditions, the 3D precision of implant center-point measurements with this technique averaged a 12 μm margin of error. Three-dimensional information can also be transferred to a computer for further analysis and verification.[5]

Photogrammetry has also been proposed as a technique for generating a 3D model of the patient's face and dental arch, for occlusion registration, and for treatment planning and documentation.[6] However, to date photogrammetry has not been proposed or even suggested as a technique for producing a complete-arch implant-fixed prosthesis in combination with digital printing technology. This clinical report describes a photogrammetry (stereo camera) system used to record the positions of multiple dental implants for rehabilitating patients with implant-supported fixed prostheses.

CLINICAL REPORT

A 60-year-old man reported to the Oral Surgery Unit of the University of Valencia (Valencia, Spain) requesting rehabilitation of the maxilla with an implant-supported complete-arch fixed prosthesis. He presented with a defective maxillary fixed partial denture, with the maxillary right lateral incisor, left central incisor, and left canine as abutments. All of the abutments presented caries secondary to inadequate marginal fit. The maxillary left second premolar was devitalized, and showed moderate periodontal involvement with grade II mobility, whereas the maxillary right second molar showed severe periodontal involvement with grade III mobility (Fig 32.1).

The treatment plan consisted of the extraction of all the maxillary teeth, with implant placement and immediate loading of a fixed prosthesis. First, impressions of the upper and lower arches were made in irreversible hydrocolloid impression material to obtain the soft tissues from the diagnostic casts before implant surgery (Fig 32.2). Diagnostic waxing was done to determine implant positions. Based on the diagnostic waxing study, an implant surgical guide was prepared, planning implant placements in the maxillary right first molar, right first and second premolar, right central incisor, left lateral incisor, left first premolar, and left first and second molar positions. The presence of enough residual alveolar bone height was confirmed by means of a panoramic radiograph and computerized axial tomography.

Eight implants were placed as planned (Mozo-Grau®, Valladolid, Spain; Fig 32.3A). During implant surgery the maxillary right second molar was maintained in order to facilitate spatial capture of the implant positions. To this effect, the stereo camera was used to register the prosthetic data. First, patient demographic and medical data were entered into the system. Then, the positions and the references of the implants (manufacturer, model, platform diameter, and diameter and height of the healing abutments) and

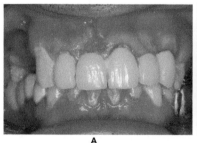
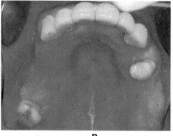
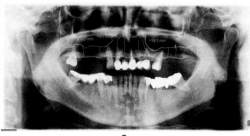

FIGURE 32.1   (A) Pretreatment frontal view of maximum intercuspation; (B) pretreatment occlusal view of the maxilla; and (C) pretreatment panoramic radiograph.

A

B

D

C

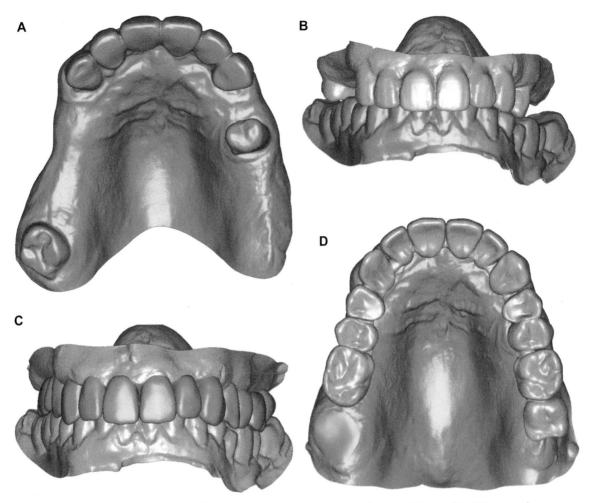

FIGURE 32.2   (A) Scanned image of the pretreatment occlusal view of the maxilla; (B) scanned image of the pretreatment frontal view of maximum intercuspation; (C) virtual image of the frontal view of the diagnostic wax-up; and (D) virtual image of the occlusal view of the diagnostic wax-up.

the code of each scan body were entered. The stereo camera was located 15 to 30 cm from the mouth of the patient at a maximum angle of 45° to the scan bodies. The camera took 50 to 60 3D photographs of each pair of PICabutments (PICdental, Majadahonda, Spain). The PICcamera was mounted on a tripod to ensure stability, and the patient's head was moved into the correct position for capturing all the scan bodies. Data registered with the PICcamera for each abutment appeared onscreen. When the computer was registering data, a red bar appeared that turned green when the registration process was completed (Figs 32.3B and 32.3E). In this way, the photogrammetry device was used to identify the spatial position of each implant without physical contact. A total of 350 images were captured in less than 2 minutes to determine the relative position of each implant (angle and distance) in vector format. The final information was then stored in the system as an STL file (PICfile®; Fig 32.4A).

Photogrammetry does not register the patient's peri-implant soft tissues, only the vectorial relationship between

the implant prosthetic platforms. Healing abutments were placed, and an irreversible hydrocolloid impression of the upper maxilla was made. The stone cast was scanned with an extraoral 3D scanner PICscan in open STL format to obtain soft-tissue information. These data were then entered in the CAD software together with the PICfile.

The PICfile and the digitized cast were aligned using PICpro® (PICdental), dental CAD software based on Exocad (Exocad GmbH, Darmstadt, Germany) with three-point registration, and subsequent enhancement using best-fit alignment. This process transferred the relative implant positions to the digital cast, including the shape of the soft tissues, which could then be used to determine the interfaces of the future prosthesis in relation to the patient's gingiva (Fig 32.4B).

The initial pretreatment diagnostic casts, including both upper and lower arches and their occlusion, were scanned in order to design and produce the interim prosthesis in proper occlusion (using CAD software). After surgery, STL files of the pretreatment diagnostic casts and the scanned implant

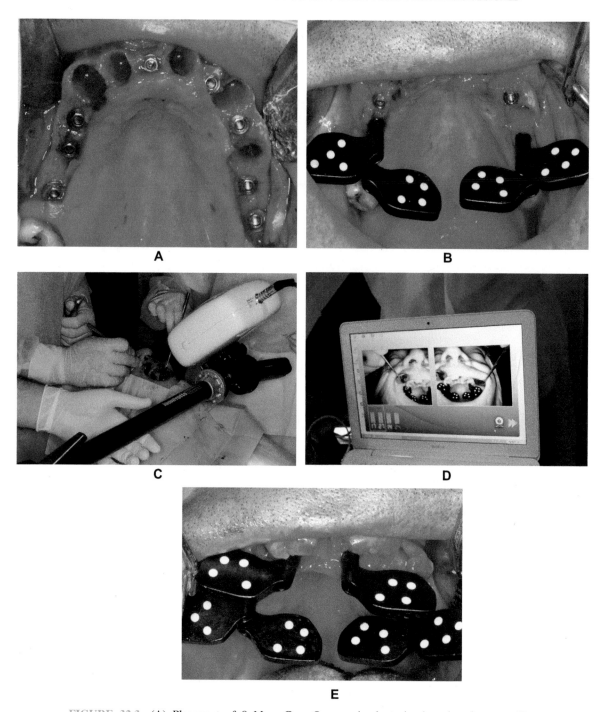

FIGURE 32.3   (A) Placement of 8 Mozo-Grau Osseous implants in the edentulous maxilla; (B) placement of PICabutments on posterior implants; (C) intraoral scan performed with the stereo camera; (D) data processing with the stereo camera software; and (E) placement and image capture of Picabutments® on anterior implants

master cast were superimposed. This was done using the palatine, retrotuberosity areas and the remaining maxillary right second molars of the two images as references.

The fixed interim prosthesis was designed using Exocad in STL format (Figs 32.4C and 32.4D). A computer numeric-controlled milling machine with 5 degrees of freedom (Hermle C20; Maschinenfabrik Berthold Hermle AG, Gosheim, Germany) was used to produce the prosthesis in acetalic resin (TSM Acetal Dental; Pressing Dental Srl, Falciano, Republic of San Marino).

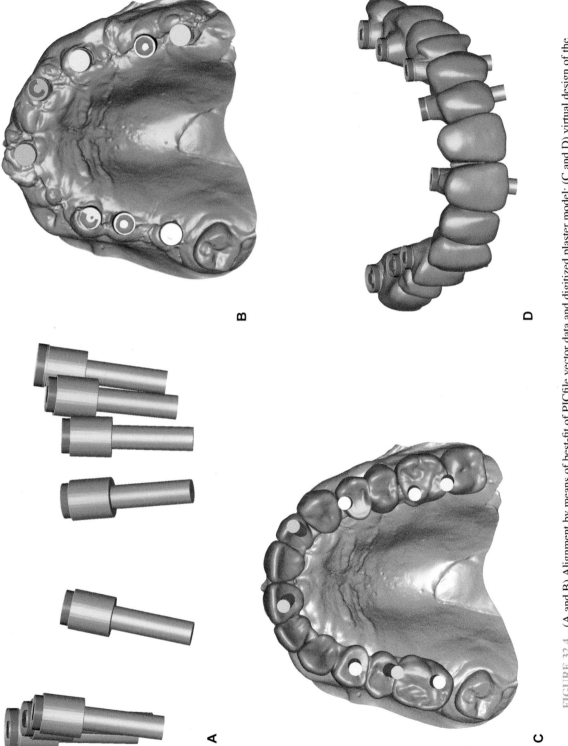

FIGURE 32.4 (A and B) Alignment by means of best-fit of PICfile vector data and digitized plaster model; (C and D) virtual design of the prosthesis for immediate loading, showing the emergence profile.

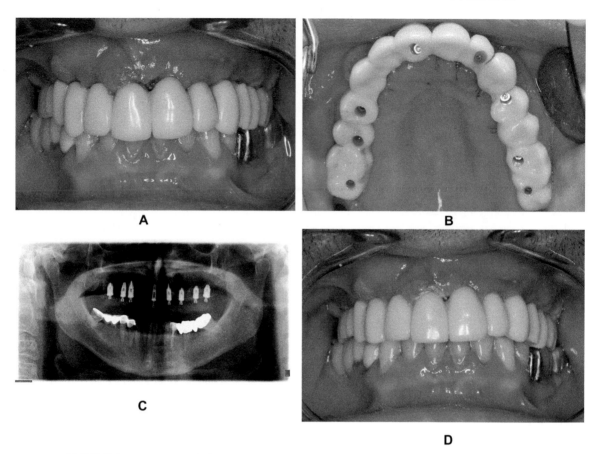

FIGURE 32.5 (A) Frontal view of the immediately loaded fixed interim prosthesis; (B) occlusal view of the immediately loaded fixed interim prosthesis; (C) panoramic radiograph of the immediately loaded fixed interim prosthesis; and (D) frontal view of the interim prosthesis 1 week after delivery.

The interim fixed implant-supported prosthesis was evaluated in the patient's mouth. Passive fit between the framework and the implants was tested using the Sheffield test (one-screw test), the screw resistance test, and the digital pressure test. In addition, panoramic X-rays were taken. After the fit was confirmed, the prosthesis was screwed in place applying 25 N cm torque (Figs 32.5A–C). The two operators noted no tension, misfit, or lack of adaptation at the time of screwing the framework in place.

The maxillary right second molar was then removed after fitting the interim prosthesis. The patient was advised to stay on a soft diet for the first 3 months and to avoid chewing movements that would generate excessive forces. He returned for checkups 1 week, 1 month, and 3 months after implant placement, and showed no biological or prosthetic complications (Figs 32.5D and 32.6A).

After 3 months, the final maxillary implant fixed prosthesis was produced and delivered. An STL file (PICfile) obtained by photogrammetry on the day of implant surgery was used for producing the prosthesis. Only a new irreversible hydrocolloid impression for reproducing the current state of the soft tissue was required. Then, best-fit alignment (PICpro) was performed using the soft-tissue scan and the implant vectorial positions. With this new file, the model cast was then produced by stereolithography on which the final prosthesis was performed. To build the master model, the digital model was processed, providing the specific geometries of the implant connections, and then produced by stereolithography using a 3D printer (Objet 250® Eden; Stratasys, Rehovot, Israel). The model was processed in a manner that would allow for the addition of false gum at a later stage in the laboratory. The metal structure was reduced from the immediately loaded prosthesis shape and screw retained in the printed master model for finishing of the fixed prosthesis. Three months after placement of the fixed prosthesis, the definitive prosthesis was produced; the peri-implant mucosa and implant osseointegration were found to be normal (Figs 32.6B and 32.6C).

DISCUSSION

The literature has warranted immediate loading protocols. As long ago as 1997, Tarnow et al[3] described an immediate

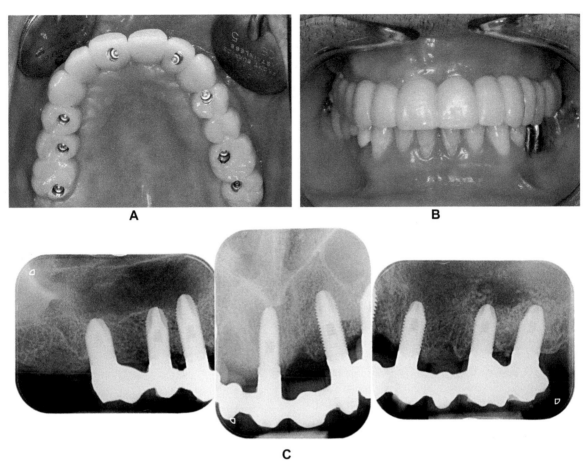

FIGURE 32.6   (A) Frontal view of the definitive maxillary fixed metal-ceramic prosthesis; (B) occlusal view of the definitive maxillary fixed metal ceramic prosthesis; and (C) periapical radiographs of the completed definitive prosthesis.

loading protocol for edentulous maxillae that aimed to stabilize intraosseous dental implants. The same author and several other investigators[3,7] have described the clinical factors to be considered when deciding whether to opt for immediate loading. Factors that allow immediate loading in the maxilla are (1) primary stability of the implants; (2) adequate splinting of the implants; (3) interim prostheses that promote implant splinting and reduce the mechanical forces to which implants are subjected; and (4) prevention of restoration movement during the healing period.

Primary implant stability must be achieved for immediate loading. It is advisable for the implant insertion torque to be greater than 35 N cm, with an implant stability quotient of over 60, as measured by resonance frequency (Osstell®, Gothenburg, Sweden).[8] This is only possible when the patient presents adequate bone quantity and quality. The implants (surface characteristics and dimensions) and clinical techniques should be selected to maximize and maintain bone-to-implant contact.[9]

In this report, the acetalic resin used as immediate loading prosthetic material was sufficiently resistant, as it offers a resistance of 123.5 ± 4.08 N (in response to thermocycling and cyclic loading), according to Arıkan et al.[10] This material is a semicrystalline polymer (75–85% crystalline) and has a number of additional advantages for applications of this kind, such as high abrasion resistance, a low friction coefficient, high thermal resistance, good electrical and dielectric properties, low water absorption, a lack of toxicity or allergenicity, and good esthetic effects.[10]

Intraoral photographic and video scanners share some of the advantages of photogrammetry. Scanners generate 3D images on the basis of a cloud of points that are able to reproduce surfaces. To join the points, they use a so-called best-fit algorithm, which causes as many points as possible to coincide. Although practical evidence is limited, theoretically such successive joining of clouds of points could lead to the accumulation of error. For this reason, reliability decreases progressively with an increasing number of analyzed implants.[11,12] However, photogrammetry, in contrast to intraoral scanners, takes all measured data in each picture without matching needs, and generates director vectors of the exact positions of the implants in relation to each other. The information that makes it possible to calculate the positions of the implants is obtained without superimposing photos, which potentially ensures greater precision and a better prosthetic fit.

To digitize implants with intraoral scanners, it is still necessary to use the so-called scan bodies, which must have specific design, geometry, and reflection characteristics to obtain an accurate impression. Although they have been used in indirect scanning for years, there is practically no experience with their use in intraoral scanning. Commercial intraoral scan bodies for different implants are available, but no clinical studies other than clinical reports have been published. A recent study found conventional impression taking and white-light scanning of stone casts to yield a more accurate fit of an implant-supported prosthesis than scanning scan bodies intraorally.[13] In another study, a digitally coded healing abutment (Encode™; Biomet 3i, Palm Beach Gardens, FL) was proposed as an alternative solution to the direct and indirect implant scanning techniques.[2] With this system, an encoded abutment is screwed into the implant, an irreversible hydrocolloid impression is made, and the plaster print left by the abutment is directly scanned and digitally interpreted using a CAD/CAM system. To date, this technique has been tested in vivo for single implants and in vitro for up to six implants.[2] In summary, the technical features of the intraoral scanner system are undergoing rapid development; however, with the exception of experimental protocols,[14] intraoral scanning devices are currently not predictable in obtaining accurate impressions of more than three or four implants over the complete arch of the maxilla or mandible.[1]

Photogrammetry avoids the inconveniences of conventional impression techniques. There is no need for impression abutments, implant body analogs, trays, or impression materials. The PICcamera measures angles and distances between prosthetic attachments placed on the implants, allowing the patient total freedom of movement, and the presence of blood, saliva, or any other organic or inorganic residues does not affect measurement precision.[6] Avoiding the use of impression materials to register implant positions potentially reduces the possibility of error due to dimensional changes of the materials. In the opinion of the authors, the described technique also offers other advantages such as reduced chairside time, less economic costs over the long term, and greater patient comfort.

A limitation of this photogrammetric technology is the fact that it does not register the soft tissues. The PICfile only contains the information on position and angulation of the implants. This inconvenience is easily solved by scanning the patient cast, which provides the missing information. The two sets of data (PICfile and scanned cast) are aligned by best-fit, which allows virtual relation of the implants to the soft tissues. With implant positions determined by the stereo camera, and using an irreversible hydrocolloid impression of the soft tissues, the laboratory can produce multiple implant prosthetic structures using CAD/CAM, without the need for casting or milling procedures.[12]

CONCLUSIONS

Photogrammetry allows precise registry of the position and angulation of multiple implants in the three dimensions, converting all the clinically relevant information directly from the patient to a digital file, and eliminating the need for impression posts, implant analogs, trays, and impression materials. Further studies with control groups are needed to compare the accuracy of photogrammetry with the other available techniques for digitizing implant positions.

REFERENCES

1. Eliasson A, Ortorp A: The accuracy of an implant impression technique using digitally coded healing abutment. *Clin Implant Dent Relat Res* 2012;14(Suppl 1): 30–38.

2. Jemt T, Lie A: Accuracy of implant-supported prostheses in the edentulous jaw: analysis of precision of fit between cast gold-alloy frameworks and master casts by means of a three-dimensional photogrammetric technique. *Clin Oral Implants Res* 1995;6:172–180.

3. Tarnow DP, Emtiaz S, Classi A: Immediate loading of threaded implants at stage 1 surgery in edentulous arches. Ten consecutive case reports with 1 to 5 year data. *Int J Oral Maxillofac Implants* 1997;12:319–324.

4. Jemt T, Bäck T, Petersson A: Photogrammetry—an alternative to conventional impressions in implant dentistry? A clinical pilot study. *Int J Prosthodont* 1999;12:363–368.

5. Ortorp A, Jemt T, Bäck T: Photogrammetry and conventional impressions for recording implant positions: a comparative laboratory study. *Clin Implant Dent Relat Res* 2005;7:43–50.

6. Pradíes G, Ferreiroa A, Ozcan M, et al: Using stereophotogrammetric technology for obtaining intraoral digital impressions of implants. *J Am Dent Assoc* 2014;145:338–344.

7. Uribe R, Peñarrocha M, Balaguer J, et al: Immediate loading in implantology. *Med Oral Patol Oral Cir Bucal* 2005;10(Suppl 2): E143–E153.

8. Peñarrocha-Oltra D, Covani U, Aparicio A, et al: Immediate versus conventional loading for the maxilla with implants placed into fresh and healed extraction sites to support a full-arch fixed prosthesis: nonrandomized controlled clinical study. *Int J Oral Maxillofac Implants* 2013;28:1116–1124.

9. Degidi M, Piattelli A: Comparative analysis study of 702 dental implants subjected to immediate functional loading and immediate non-functional loading to traditional healing periods with a follow up of up to 24 months. *Int J Oral Maxillofac Implants* 2005;20:99–107.

10. Arikan A, Ozkan YK, Arda T, et al: Effect of 180 days of water storage on the transverse strength of acetal resin denture base material. *J Prosthodont* 2010;19:47–51.

11. Eliasson A, Ortorp A: The accuracy of an implant impression technique using digitally coded healing abutments. *Clin Implant Dent Relat Res* 2012;14(Suppl 1): e30–e38.

12. Fuster-Torres MA, Albalat-Estela S, Alcañiz-Raya M, et al: CAD/CAM dental systems in implant dentistry: update. *Med Oral Patol Oral Cir Bucal* 2009;14:E141–E145.

13. Stimmelmayr M, Güth JF, Erdelt K, et al: Digital evaluation of the reproducibility of implant scanbody fit—an in vitro study. *Clin Oral Investig* 2012;16:851–856.

14. Moreno A, Giménez B, Ozcan M, et al: A clinical protocol for intraoral digital impression of screw-retained CAD/CAM framework on multiple implants based on wave front sampling technology. *Implant Dent* 2013;22:320–325.

33

FULL-ARCH, IMPLANT-SUPPORTED MONOLITHIC ZIRCONIA REHABILITATIONS: PILOT CLINICAL EVALUATION OF WEAR AGAINST NATURAL OR COMPOSITE TEETH

Paolo Cardelli, dds,[1] Francesco Pio Manobianco, dds,[1] Nicola Serafini, dds,[1] Giovanna Murmura, md, dds, phd,[1] and Florian Beuer, dmd, phd[2]

[1]Department of Medical, Oral and Biotechnological Sciences, University "G. d'Annunzio" of Chieti-Pescara, Chieti, Italy
[2]Department of Prosthodontics, Geriatic Dentistry and Craniomandibular Disorders, Charité – Universitätsmedizin Berlin, Berlin, Germany

Keywords

Y-TZP; attrition; contact; replica; screw-retained; dental implant; 3D scanner; prosthesis.

Correspondence

Dr. Paolo Cardelli, Department of Medical, Oral and Biotechnological Sciences, University "G. d'Annunzio" of Chieti-Pescara, Via dei Vestini, 31, 66100 Chieti – CH, Italy. E-mail: paolo.cardelli@unich.it

The authors declare that they have no conflict of interest.

Accepted April 11, 2015

Published in Journal of Prosthodontics October 2015

doi: 10.1111/jopr.12374

ABSTRACT

Purpose: To clinically evaluate the amount of contact wear generated between full-arch monolithic zirconia implant-supported restorations and natural or composite antagonists, over a 1-year period.

Materials and Methods: Forty-seven teeth from clinically functional, full-arch monolithic zirconia screw-retained implant prostheses (FDPs) and their antagonists were investigated. The first group ("Zirconia-E") was opposed to natural teeth ("Enamel"), whereas the other one ("Zirconia-CR") was opposed to nanohybrid composite teeth ("Composite Resin"). Replicas of the restorations and their antagonists were obtained immediately after delivery (T_0) and after 1 year of clinical service (T_1). Each tooth surface was individually evaluated three-dimensionally by software to quantify the vertical distance between the two scans (Hausdorff distance), which was considered as contact wear. Data obtained for each arch were subjected to one-way ANOVA test and a post hoc analysis (Tukey's test) at a 5% level of significance. Furthermore, the influence of the location of the teeth (anterior or posterior) was analyzed. Minimum post hoc statistical power between statistically different groups was 99.6%.

Results: Mean values were $63 \pm 23 \, \mu m$ for Zirconia-E, $76 \pm 29 \, \mu m$ for enamel, $70 \pm 38 \, \mu m$ for composite resin; Zirconia-CR had a mean value of $19 \pm 4 \, \mu m$ and significantly differed from the other groups. Contact wear between anterior and posterior teeth differed significantly only in the composite resin arch, with a mean of $39 \pm 22 \, \mu m$ for anterior teeth versus $101 \pm 19 \, \mu m$ for posterior ones.

Conclusions: Within the limitations of this preliminary evaluation, monolithic zirconia full-arch rehabilitations induced a clinically acceptable wear on natural and composite antagonists over a 1-year period; they might be considered a viable solution for implant-supported rehabilitations.

Within the different metal-free materials for prosthetic rehabilitations, zirconia-based ceramics have been successfully used as frameworks for single crowns and fixed dental prostheses (FDPs), thanks to the absence of a metal framework, while retaining adequate mechanical properties.[1,2] However, chipping and delamination of the veneering ceramic have been reported as the most frequent clinical complications due to different factors.[3–6] To overcome this problem, increased translucency zirconia blanks were introduced for full contour restorations. The abrasive pattern of monolithic zirconia versus natural enamel has been argued and investigated in different in vitro studies;[7–9] the results showed less antagonist wear compared to veneered restorations.[10,11] The treatment of the zirconia surface, such as glazing or polishing, can also affect the contact wear.[12,13] A polished zirconia surface significantly reduced the wear of the restoration and opposing natural teeth in an in vitro model.[14,15] In clinical conditions, however, many other factors influence the complex interaction between dental enamel and opposing substrates: patient-related factors such as dietary habits, dysfunctional occlusion, masticatory forces, and bruxism contribute to accelerated enamel loss of antagonist teeth.[16] The physiological wear of the enamel in vivo is considered to be between 30 and 40 μm/year.[17] Therefore, contact wear is a complex process, dependent on time and involving mechanical and chemical wear. When dental restorations are supported by dental implants a more than eight times higher threshold of perception has been recorded compared to natural teeth.[18] Only clinical investigations are suitable to illuminate and understand the wear process of dental materials; however, clinical data on monolithic zirconia wear patterns after more than 6 months of clinical service time are not available to the authors' best knowledge.

The aim of the study is to clinically evaluate the amount of contact wear generated between full-arch monolithic zirconia implant-supported restorations and natural or composite antagonists, over a 1-year period. The working hypothesis is that zirconia will cause different wear patterns on enamel and restorative materials.

MATERIALS AND METHODS

Two patients with four implants each in edentulous upper or lower jaws were scheduled to support full-arch monolithic zirconia screw-retained FDPs. Both patients, one male and one female, were 65 years old and without parafunctional habits. After a pick-up impression with type 1 plaster (BF Plaster; Dental Torino, Italy), a bite registration was made with wax on a screw-retained resin base, recording the centric relation: anterior and posterior teeth were then tried in on the same screw-retained resin base. A double-scan of the master model with cylinders and with a mock-up led to the restoration project. After design refinement, the full-arch restorations were milled in presintered, yttria-stabilized zirconia (Y-TZP; NexxZr; Sagemax, Federal Way, WA) and color infiltrated before sintering. Minor veneering was performed in the buccal areas by means of single porcelain firing with adequate coefficient of thermal expansion (CTE; Lava Ceram; 3M ESPE, Seefeld, Germany). After try-in and glazing, the prostheses were luted to the screwed titanium cylinders with a composite material (Nimetic Cem; 3M ESPE) and delivered with the recommended torque. Access holes were sealed with composite resin.

The first monolithic zirconia rehabilitation ("Zirconia-E"— 11 teeth) in the upper jaw was opposed to natural teeth ("Enamel"—12 teeth; Fig 33.1), whereas the other one

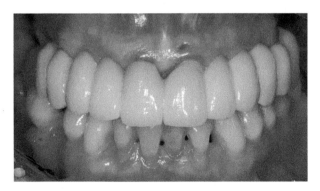

FIGURE 33.1   Full-arch "Zirconia-E" maxillary monolithic zirconia rehabilitation opposed to "Enamel" mandibular natural teeth.

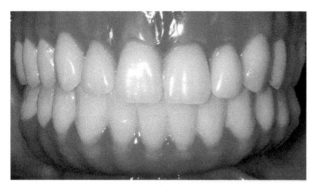

FIGURE 33.2 "Composite" maxillary rehabilitation opposed to full-arch "Zirconia-CR" mandibular monolithic zirconia rehabilitation.

("Zirconia-CR"—12 teeth) in the lower jaw was opposed to nanohybrid composite teeth ("Composite Resin"—12 teeth; Fig 33.2). Both rehabilitations were built with a group function occlusal scheme, where canines and premolars lead the laterotrusion. No dynamic contacts were present at the mediotrusion side. Before experimental steps, Internal Review Board (IRB) approval was secured, and patient informed consent was obtained.

After 2 weeks to allow occlusal correction if needed, two-phase one-step impressions were acquired on zirconia restoration and their opposing arches with hydrophilic poly(vinyl siloxane) in metal stock trays (Virtual Putty and Light; Ivoclar Vivadent, Schaan, Liechtenstein).

Polyurethane resin (KW New; Techim srl, Arese, Italy) was used to obtain replicas of restorations and their antagonists after delivery and occlusal check (T_0); the impression and the replicas were performed again after 1 year of function (T_1) (Figs 33.3 and 33.4).

The resin replicas were acquired with a 3D scanner (Echo2 Scanner; Sweden & Martina, Due Carrare, Italy), and each couple of meshes (T_0 and T_1) was superimposed with appropriate software (MeshLab v. 1.3.2, ISTI-CNR, University of Pisa, Italy) (Fig 33.5). For every single arch, the occlusal tooth surfaces were individually evaluated to quantify the vertical distance between the two scans (Hausdorff distance) at each point, which could indicate the extent of wear that occurred. The mean vertical distance for each tooth was considered the wear value. Each arch constituted an experimental group, in a case-control design.

The data obtained for each arch were subjected to one-way ANOVA test and, as post hoc analysis, Tukey's test. The same type of analysis was performed again after splitting the data obtained for each arch between anterior (incisors and canines) and posterior teeth (premolars and molars).

RESULTS

Zirconia-CR group showed a significantly lower mean wear compared to the other groups (Table 33.1). Statistical analysis of anterior versus posterior values for each group showed

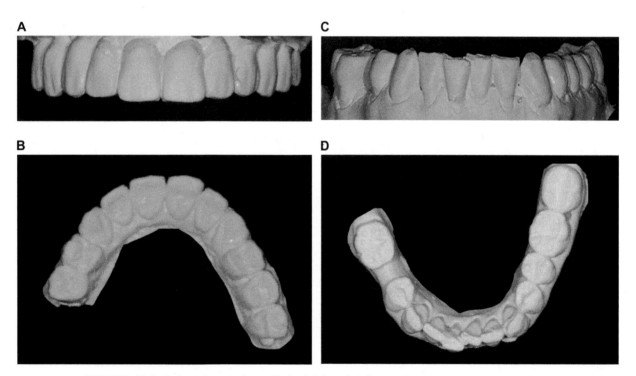

FIGURE 33.3 Polyurethane resin replicas of "Zirconia-E" (A and B) and "Enamel" (C and D) arches after 1 year of function.

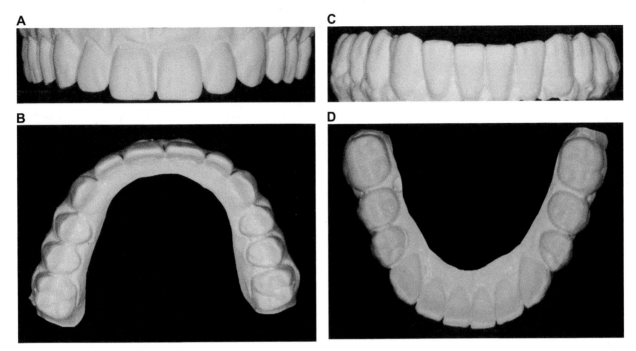

FIGURE 33.4 Polyurethane resin replicas of "Composite Resin" (A and B) and "Zirconia-CR" (C and D) arches after 1 year of function.

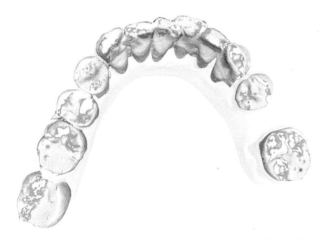

FIGURE 33.5 Three-dimensional superimposition of the replicas obtained at the time of restoration delivery and after 1 year of function, for the "Enamel" arch.

TABLE 33.1 **Mean Wear (µm) and Standard Deviation of the Four Arches**

Group	Mean Wear
Zirconia-E	63 ± 23[a]
Enamel	76 ± 29[a]
Composite resin	70 ± 38[a]
Zirconia-CR	19 ± 4[b]

Note: The different superscript letters identify statistically different values between the analyzed groups.

a statistically significant difference in mean wear of the composite resin arch: 39 ± 22 µm for anterior teeth versus 101 ± 19 µm for posterior teeth. Minimum post hoc statistical power between statistically different groups was 99.6%.

DISCUSSION

The wear induced by monolithic zirconia on natural antagonists has already been studied in vitro;[7–9] the effects on composite resin have also been investigated.[19–21] Furthermore, only one study investigated the wear caused by full-contour zirconia restorations in vivo, with a 6-month follow-up.[22] The present clinical investigation evaluated the contact wear induced by full-arch implant-supported monolithic zirconia, with a 1-year follow-up. The location of the restoration on different arches (maxilla vs. mandible) was not considered as a limiting factor, because the position of the natural antagonist teeth is not considered as a factor affecting wear.[23]

The wear was evaluated by processing of three-dimensional images obtained with an optical scanner and superimposition software with adequate accuracy (10 µm).[24] This method has already been used in dentistry and has been reported in the literature for detecting the wear of materials and evaluating the accuracy of techniques for taking impressions on implants.[25,26] Possible inaccuracies caused by the transfer to the laboratory and the fabrication of the replicas have to be considered as a limiting factor of this study; however, this represents the only opportunity to evaluate the wear. In the future, intraoral scanning devices might be more accurate than the presented indirect way via fabricating replicas.

The collected data revealed that mean wear occurring on monolithic zirconia in 1 year is comparable to that occurring on its enamel antagonist, confirming previous in vitro findings.[8] Moreover, previous clinical studies reported that ceramics veneered over different cores induced an enamel wear of about 60 μm/year,[27] whereas monolithic zirconia induced 33 μm of enamel wear over 6 months of function.[21] Both values are comparable to the mean enamel wear of 75 μm recorded in the present investigation. The zirconia restorations monitored in this study were glazed before delivery; previous in vitro findings reported higher wear of glazed zirconia specimens over polished ones.[14,15] Additional clinical evaluations will clarify the eventual differences between the two surface treatments.

The mean wear of the zirconia arch was significantly lower compared to its composite antagonist; the composite mean wear, however, is comparable to natural enamel. Having similar wear behavior as natural tooth structure has been defined as a major objective for restorative materials.[28] However, showing slightly more wear than enamel might even preserve natural structure.[7] The statistical analysis was performed again after splitting anterior and posterior data of each group. Zirconia and enamel exhibited homogeneous wear, while the opposing composite arch wear is focused on the posterior region. These results represent data from a pilot study with only two patients. Patient-related factors like biting forces, chewing behavior, or occlusal habits might be better balanced when more patients are involved. Because there are no previous clinical investigations on zirconia-to-composite wear, further studies are needed to clarify the overall wear ratio and its eventual concentration pattern.

CONCLUSION

Within the limitations of this preliminary evaluation, monolithic zirconia full-arch rehabilitations induced a clinically acceptable wear on natural and composite antagonists over a 1-year period; they could be considered a viable solution for implant-supported rehabilitations.

REFERENCES

1. Zarone F, Russo S, Sorrentino R: From porcelain-fused-to-metal to zirconia: clinical and experimental considerations. *Dent Mater* 2011;27:83–96.

2. Bachhav VC, Aras MA: Zirconia-based fixed partial dentures: a clinical review. *Quintessence Int* 2011;42:173–182.

3. Heintze SD, Rousson V: Survival of zirconia- and metal-supported fixed dental prostheses: a systematic review. *Int J Prosthodont* 2010;23:493–502.

4. Larsson C, Wennerberg A: The clinical success of zirconia-based crowns: a systematic review. *Int J Prosthodont* 2014;27:33–43.

5. Sailer I, Pjetursson BE, Zwahlen M, et al: A systematic review of the survival and complication rates of all-ceramic and metal-ceramic reconstructions after an observation period of at least 3 years. Part II: fixed dental prostheses. *Clin Oral Implants Res* 2007;18:86–96.

6. Raigrodski AJ, Hillstead MB, Meng GK, et al: Survival and complications of zirconia-based fixed dental prostheses: a systematic review. *J Prosthet Dent* 2012;107:170–177.

7. Sripetchdanond J, Leevailoj C: Wear of human enamel opposing monolithic zirconia, glass ceramic, and composite resin: an in vitro study. *J Prosthet Dent* 2014;112:1141–1150.

8. Passos SP, Torrealba Y, Major P, et al: In vitro wear behavior of zirconia opposing enamel: a systematic review. *J Prosthodont* 2014;23:593–601.

9. Park JH, Park S, Lee K, et al: Antagonist wear of three CAD/CAM anatomic contour zirconia ceramics. *J Prosthet Dent* 2014;111:20–29.

10. Kim MJ, Oh SH, Kim JH, et al: Wear evaluation of the human enamel opposing different Y-TZP dental ceramics and other porcelains. *J Dent* 2012;40:979–988.

11. Preis V, Behr M, Kolbeck C, et al: Wear performance of substructure ceramics and veneering porcelains. *Dent Mater* 2011;27:796–804.

12. Mitov G, Heintze SD, Walz S, et al: Wear behavior of dental Y-TZP ceramic against natural enamel after different finishing procedures. *Dent Mater* 2012;28:909–918.

13. Preis V, Weiser F, Handel G, et al: Wear performance of monolithic dental ceramics with different surface treatments. *Quintessence Int* 2013;44:393–405.

14. Janyavula S, Lawson N, Cakir D, et al: The wear of polished and glazed zirconia against enamel. *J Prosthet Dent* 2013;109:22–29.

15. Amer R, Kürklü D, Kateeb E, et al: Three-body wear potential of dental yttrium-stabilized zirconia ceramic after grinding, polishing, and glazing treatments. *J Prosthet Dent* 2014;112:1151–1155.

16. Oh WS, Delong R, Anusavice KJ: Factors affecting enamel and ceramic wear: a literature review. *J Prosthet Dent* 2002;87:451–459.

17. Xu HH, Smith DT, Jahanmir S, et al: Indentation damage and mechanical properties of human enamel and dentin. *J Dent Res* 1998;77:472–480.

18. Hämmerle CH, Wagner D, Brägger U, et al: Threshold of tactile sensitivity perceived with dental endosseous implants and natural teeth. *Clin Oral Implants Res* 1995;6:83–90.

19. Ghazal M, Kern M: The influence of antagonistic surface roughness on the wear of human enamel and nanofilled

composite resin artificial teeth. *J Prosthet Dent* 2009;101: 342–349.

20. Ghazal M, Kern M: Wear of human enamel and nano-filled composite resin denture teeth under different loading forces. *J Oral Rehabil* 2009;36:58–64.

21. Ghazal M, Albashaireh ZS, Kern M: Wear resistance of nano-filled composite resin and feldspathic ceramic artificial teeth. *J Prosthet Dent* 2008;100:441–448.

22. Stober T, Bermejo JL, Rammelsberg P, et al: Enamel wear caused by monolithic zirconia crowns after 6 months of clinical use. *J Oral Rehabil* 2014;41:314–322.

23. Hmaidouch R, Weigl P: Tooth wear against ceramic crowns in posterior region: a systematic literature review. *Int J Oral Sci* 2013;5:183–190.

24. Echo2 Technical Data 2014, Sweden & Martina, Italy.

25. Mehl A, Gloger W, Kunzelmann KH, et al: A new optical 3D device for the detection of wear. *J Dent Res* 1997;76:1799–1807.

26. Calesini G, Zarone F, Sorrentino R, et al: Effect of 2 impression techniques on the dimensional accuracy of working implant prosthesis models: an in vitro study. *J Craniofac Surg* 2014;25:822–827.

27. Esquivel-Upshaw JF, Rose WF, Jr, Barrett AA, et al: Three years in vivo wear: core-ceramic, veneers, and enamel antagonists. *Dent Mater* 2012;28:615–621.

28. Lee A, Swain M, He L, et al: Wear behavior of human enamel against lithium disilicate glass ceramic and type III gold. *J Prosthet Dent* 2014;112:1399–1405.

34

DOUBLE FULL-ARCH VERSUS SINGLE FULL-ARCH, FOUR IMPLANT-SUPPORTED REHABILITATIONS: A RETROSPECTIVE, 5-YEAR COHORT STUDY

PAULO MALÓ, DDS, PHD,[1] MIGUEL DE ARAÚJO NOBRE, RDH, MSC EPI,[2] ARMANDO LOPES, DDS, MSC,[1] AND ROLANDO RODRIGUES, DDS[3]

[1]Oral Surgery Department, Maló Clinic, Lisbon, Portugal
[2]Research and Development Department, Maló Clinic, Lisbon, Portugal
[3]Prosthodontics Department, Maló Clinic, Lisbon, Portugal

Keywords
Dental implants; immediate function; All-on-4.

Correspondence
Paulo Maló, Maló Clinic, Avenida dos Combatentes, 43, 9° C, Ed. Green Park, 1600-042 Lisboa, Portugal. E-mail: research@maloclinics.com

This study was funded by a grant from Nobel Biocare Services AG (grant no. 2012–1103). Professor Paulo Maló is currently a consultant for Nobel Biocare AB.

Accepted June 10, 2014

Published in *Journal of Prosthodontics* June 2015; Vol. 24, Issue 4

doi: 10.1111/jopr.12228

ABSTRACT

Purpose: To report the 5-year outcome of the All-on-4 treatment concept comparing double full-arch (G1) and single-arch (G2) groups.

Materials and Methods: This retrospective cohort study included 110 patients (68 women and 42 men, average age of 55.5 years) with 440 NobelSpeedy groovy implants. One hundred sixty-five full-arch, fixed, immediately loaded prostheses in both jaws were followed for 5 years. G1 consisted of 55 patients with double-arch rehabilitations occluded with implant-supported fixed prostheses, and G2 consisted of 55 patients with maxillary single-arch rehabilitations or mandibular single-arch rehabilitations occluded with natural teeth or removable prostheses. The groups were matched for age (± 6 years) and gender. Primary outcome measures were cumulative prosthetic (both interim and definitive) and implant survival (Kaplan–Meier product limit estimator). Secondary outcome measures were marginal bone levels at 5 years (through periapical radiographs and using the patient as unit of analysis) and the incidence of mechanical and biological complications. Differences in survival curves (log-rank test), marginal bone level (Mann–Whitney U test), and complications (chi-square test) were compared inferentially between the two groups using the patient as unit of analysis with significance level set at $p < 0.05$.

Results: No dropouts occurred. Prosthetic survival was 100%. Five patients lost 5 implants (G1: $n = 3$; G2: $n = 2$) before 1 year, rendering an estimated cumulative survival rate of 95.5% (G1: 94.5%; G2: 96.4%; Kaplan–Meier, $p = 0.645$, nonsignificant). The average (SD) marginal bone level was 1.56 mm (0.89) at 5 years [G1: 1.45 mm (0.77); G2: 1.67 mm (0.99); $p = 0.414$]. The incidence rate of mechanical complications (in both interim and definitive prostheses) was 0.16 and 0.13 for G1 and G2, respectively ($p = 0.032$). The incidence rate of biological complications was 0.06 and 0.05 for G1 and G2, respectively ($p = 0.669$).

Conclusions: Based on the results, rehabilitating double- or single-arch edentulous patients did not yield significant differences on survival curves. The incidence of mechanical complications was significantly higher for double-arch rehabilitated patients but nevertheless, these mechanical complications did not affect the long-term survival of either the prostheses or the implants.

The success of an edentulous rehabilitation is dependent on the development of shared goals for both the patient and the clinical team. New and improved treatment procedures, such as the continuous development of dental implant therapies, the evaluation of issues concerning prosthetic function, and prosthesis quality, are necessary to successfully rehabilitate the edentulous patient.[1] The use of removable prosthetics frequently leads to mucosal irritation, under-extension of the denture bases, incorrect jaw relationships, incorrect occlusal vertical dimension, and inadequate posterior palatal seal.[2] Some pathological manifestations of denture use include stomatitis, traumatic ulcers, irritation-induced hyperplasia, altered taste perception, burning mouth syndrome, and gagging. Some rehabilitation therapies do not replace dimensional changes of the lower third of the face caused by continued resorption of the mandibular alveolar bone, which causes greater difficulties for denture construction; overall, removable dentures do not obtain the physiological, psychological, and social complete satisfaction of the individual who needs full-arch rehabilitation.[3] Oral implant placement may prevent the continued resorption of bone and has been associated with increased mandibular bone height distal to the implant location.[4,5] High success rates have been reported when rehabilitating completely edentulous patients using four or more implants, and in the late 1990s, various authors published clinical reports regarding the possibility of early or immediate loading of implants with fixed provisional full-arch restorations.[6–8]

In 2003, Maló et al[9] introduced the All-on-4 treatment concept. This protocol requires the placement of four interforaminal implants in the mandible, with the distal implants tilted distally by 30° to achieve a more favorable distribution of implants, thereby minimizing cantilever extensions that could jeopardize osseointegration of the distal implants.[10]

Immediate loading in the edentulous maxilla is perceived as a greater challenge than in the mandible, mostly due to the lower bone density in this jaw. Furthermore, implant anchorage in the totally edentulous maxilla is often restricted because of bone resorption, a frequent condition in the posterior regions of the jaws where bone grafting is often indicated. Implant tilting has been shown to be a good alternative to bone grafting in the maxilla, as indicated in the clinical results of several studies.[11–13] By tilting the posterior implant, a more posterior implant position can be reached, reducing the cantilever compared to axially placed implants. Cantilever extensions seem to be associated with a decreased prosthetic survival rate.[14–16] Tilting the posterior implant can also provide improved implant anchorage by engaging the apex of the implants with the cortical bone of the anterior wall of the sinus and the nasal fossae.[17]

The use of four implants in the maxilla is supported by results from short- and long-term clinical studies.[12,13,17–19] Good clinical outcomes from studies using protocols in which four implants were placed to support a full-arch prosthesis indicate that the placement of additional implants may not be necessary for successful implant treatment of edentulous jaws.[19,20]

More recently, several authors have noted that the use of the All-on-4 treatment concept with a 30° inclination of the distal implants reduced the maximum stress in the distal crestal bone,[21,22] with no difference in marginal bone resorption between tilted and straight implants.[23] Furthermore, other authors[24] reported no significant differences in loading parameters when comparing the use of more implants, demonstrating the importance of conceding enough space between implants.

The implant surgical protocol may influence the outcome of full-arch rehabilitation in the long-term, as can the size of cantilever, bar material, and type of bone.[25] A recent systematic review[26] stated that biologic and technical complications occur continuously over time as a result of fatigue and stress.

Fazi et al[10] reported that when comparing several implant numbers and positions, the use of the All-on-4 treatment concept not only reduced load bearing from bone, but also from implants and frameworks. Rehabilitating the completely edentulous patient is still a challenge. The rate for absence of complications in prosthetic full-arch rehabilitations is less than 30% at 5 years and 8% at 10 years,[26] with the most common complications being periimplant bone loss, screw fracture, hypertrophy or hyperplasia of the soft tissue around the rehabilitation, and chipping or fracture of the veneering material, which requires repair, maintenance, time, and cost to both the clinician and patient.

The biomechanics of double full-arch edentulism and the effect of an implant-supported fixed prosthesis as opposing dentition is not known to a great extent, with few clinical studies addressing this issue.[6,8,27,28] It may be that an implant rehabilitation as opposing dentition constitutes a risk factor for late implant loss.[27] Studies addressing this finding in immediate function implants are nonexistent.

The aim of this retrospective cohort study was to compare the outcome of double full-arch versus single full-arch rehabilitations in long-term outcome. This study aimed to determine the influence of opposing dentition on the treatment outcome of immediate implant-supported fixed prostheses for rehabilitation of completely edentulous jaws. The null hypothesis was that there is no difference in the long-term outcome of implant-supported fixed rehabilitations, regardless of the opposing dentition.

MATERIALS AND METHODS

This article was written following Strengthening the Reporting of Observational Studies in Epidemiology (STROBE) guidelines.[29] This retrospective cohort study was performed at a private rehabilitation center (Maló Clinic, Lisbon, Portugal). This study was approved by an independent ethical committee (Ethical Committee for Health; Authorization no. 014/2010). The inclusion criterion was edentulous arches, or arches with hopeless teeth, in need of fixed implant restorations as requested by the patient. As exclusion criteria, patients presenting with emotional instability, and patients who were not followed at the rehabilitation center were excluded from the study. From January 2004 to December 2006, a total of 149 patients were rehabilitated with full-arch rehabilitations according to the All-on-4 treatment concept (Nobel Biocare, Göteborg, Sweden) in both jaws on the same day, and 311 patients were rehabilitated with one full-arch rehabilitation according to the All-on-4 treatment concept (maxilla: 153; mandible: 158). Fifty-five patients were randomly selected from the double full-arch rehabilitations (Group 1 [G1]; Fig 34.1) using a random sequence generator. The patients with single full-arch were selected based on the absence of an opposing dentition containing implant-supported fixed prostheses, and matching for age (±6 years of a double full-arch patient) and gender with patients from G1. Of the 169 patients with single full-arch rehabilitation who qualified in the matching procedure, 55 were randomly selected (group 2 [G2], 26 maxillae and 29 mandibles; Figs 34.2 and 34.3), resulting in a total of 110 patients (68 women and 42 men; average age = 55.5 years old [standard

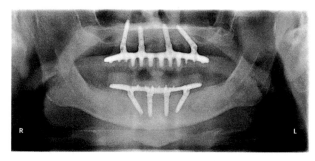

FIGURE 34.1   Orthopantomography of a double full-arch All-on-4 rehabilitation.

deviation: 8.9 years]; range: 38–80 years old) having received a total of 660 NobelSpeedy implants (Nobel Biocare AB, Gothenburg, Sweden). As opposing dentition, patients from G1 presented an implant-supported fixed prosthesis ($n = 55$), while in G2 there were 35 patients with natural teeth, and 20 had a removable prosthesis.

Sample Size Calculation

The sample size calculation was performed using a software program (power and sample size calculations, version 3.0.34, Dupont WD and Plummer WD Jr, Department of

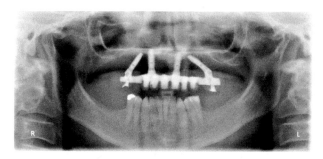

FIGURE 34.2   Orthopantomography of a maxillary single full-arch All-on-4 rehabilitation.

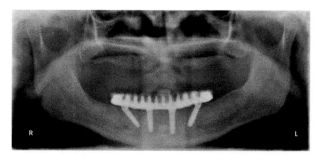

FIGURE 34.3   Orthopantomography of a mandibular single full-arch All-on-4 rehabilitation.

Biostatistics, Vanderbilt University, Nashville, TN). The authors planned a study with one control per experimental subject, an accrual interval of 6 time units (1 year = 1 time unit), and additional follow-up after the accrual interval of 3 time units. Prior data indicated that the median survival time on the control treatment was 6 time units.[13,30] If the true median survival times on the control and experimental treatments are 6 and 3 time units, respectively, it was deemed necessary to include 55 experimental subjects and 55 control subjects to be able to reject the null hypothesis that the experimental and control survival curves are equal with probability (power) 0.8. The type I error probability associated with this test of this null hypothesis was 0.05.

Surgical Protocol

The patients' medical histories were reviewed, together with clinical observation (treatment planning) and complementary radiographic exams with an orthopantomography (for bone height evaluation) and computerized tomography scan (for bone volume and evaluation of anatomical structures evaluation such as the dental nerve). The surgical procedures were described in previous reports following the All-on-4 treatment concept.[13,30]

Immediate Provisional Prosthetic Protocol

Implant-supported fixed prostheses of high-density acrylic resin (PallaXpress Ultra; Heraeus Kulzer GmbH, Hanau, Germany) with titanium cylinders (Nobel Biocare AB) were manufactured at the dental laboratory and inserted on the same day (G1: 110; G2: 55). Anterior occlusal contacts and canine guidance during lateral movements were preferred in the interim prosthesis. No cantilevers were used in the interim prostheses. The emergence positions of the screw-access holes at the posterior implants of the prostheses were normally at the level of the second premolar, and the prostheses were designed to hold a minimum of 10 teeth due to the favorable position achieved by the posterior tilting of the distal implants.

Final Prosthetic Protocol

Considering patient desires, a metal ceramic implant-supported fixed prosthesis with a titanium framework and all-ceramic crowns (Procera Ti framework, Procera crowns, NobelRondo ceramics; Nobel Biocare AB), or a metal-acrylic resin implant-supported fixed prosthesis with a Ti framework (Procera Ti framework) and acrylic resin prosthetic teeth (Heraeus Kulzer GmbH) was used to replace the interim prosthesis. In this definitive prosthesis, the occlusion mimicked natural dentition. The definitive prosthesis was typically delivered 6 months postsurgically.

Outcome Measures

Primary outcome measure was prosthetic survival and implant survival. Prosthetic survival (both interim and definitive) was based on function, with the necessity of removing the prostheses classified as failure. Implant survival was based on the Malo Clinic survival criteria:[13] (1) implant fulfilled its purported function as support for reconstruction; (2) it was stable when individually and manually tested; (3) no signs of persistent infection observed; (4) no radiolucent areas around the implants; (5) demonstrated a good esthetic outcome in the rehabilitation; and (6) allowed the construction of an implant-supported fixed prosthesis that provided patient comfort and good hygienic maintenance. The implants removed were classified as failures. Secondary outcome measures were marginal bone level, biological complications (periimplant pathology; fistulae formation, and abscess formation), and mechanical complications (loosening or fracture of any prosthetic component).

Marginal Bone Level

Periapical radiographs were made using the parallel technique with a film holder (Super-bite; Hawe-Neos, Bioggio, Switzerland). The holder's position was adjusted manually for an estimated orthogonal film position. A blinded operator examined all radiographs of the implants for marginal bone level. Each periapical radiograph was scanned at 300 dpi with a scanner (HP Scanjet 4890; HP Portugal, Paço de Arcos, Portugal), and the marginal bone level was assessed with image analysis software (Image J version 1.40g for Windows; National Institutes of Health, Bethesda, MD). The reference point for the reading was the implant platform (the horizontal interface between the implant and the abutment), and marginal bone level was measured to the first contact between implant and bone. The radiographs were accepted or rejected for evaluation based on the clarity of the implant threads: a clear thread guarantees both sharpness and an orthogonal direction of the radiographic beam toward the implant axis. Calibration of the radiographs was performed using the implants' platform diameter. The marginal bone levels, evaluated on periapical radiographs, were registered at 5 years of follow-up. The bone levels were averaged per patient and presented using the rehabilitation as unit of analysis.

Statistical Analysis

Patient-related survival (using the patient as unit of analysis and considering the first incidence of implant failure) was computed using the Kaplan–Meier product limit estimator (SPSS 17.0; SPSS Inc., Chicago, IL) with comparison of survival curves between groups through the log-rank test. The incidence of mechanical and biological complications, systemic compromises, smoking habits, and bruxism between both groups was analyzed by the chi-square test. The marginal bone levels were compared between the two groups using the Mann–Whitney test after testing the variable for normality through the Kolmogorov–Smirnov test. The level of significance was 0.05. Statistics were computed using the Statistical Package for Social Science (SPSS 17.0).

RESULTS

A total of 26 patients presented at least one systemic condition (G1: 11 patients; G2: 15 patients, $p = 0.369$); 33 patients were smokers (G1: 19 patients; G2: 14 patients, $p = 0.298$), and 37 patients were suspected to be heavy bruxers (G1: 22 patients; G2: 15 patients, $p = 0.158$). No dropouts occurred in this study, and the patients were followed for 5 years. Five patients lost five implants (G1: 3 patients; G2: 2 patients), rendering an estimated survival rate of 95.5% (Kaplan–Meier; Table 34.1). All implant failures occurred during the first year of follow-up and were counted as early failures. No failures of the prostheses occurred, rendering a 100% survival rate. The estimated patient-related cumulative survival rates (CSRs) after 5 years of follow-up were 94.5% for G1 and 96.4% for G2 (Kaplan–Meier; Table 34.2 and Fig 34.4). Survival curves did not differ significantly between the two groups ($p = 0.645$, log-rank test). At 5 years of follow-up, 94 of the 110 patients had readable radiographs (86%). The bone level was on average −1.56 mm (SD = 0.89 mm) overall; −1.45 mm (SD = 0.77 mm) for G1 (maxilla: −1.44 mm [SD = 0.88 mm], mandible: 1.42 mm [SD = 0.82 mm]) and −1.67 mm (SD = 0.99 mm)

for G2 (Table 34.3; maxilla: 1.72 mm [SD = 1.03 mm], mandible: 1.63 mm [SD = 1.01 mm]).

The difference in marginal bone level between the two groups was nonsignificant ($p = 0.414$).

The incidence rate of mechanical complications (considering both interim and definitive prostheses) over the 5 years of follow-up was significant between the two groups with 0.16 [(45/55)/5] for G1 and 0.13 [(35/55)/5] for G2 ($p = 0.032$). For G1, the type of mechanical complications were fracture of the prosthesis (41 patients), abutment screw loosening (21 patients), and prosthetic screw loosening (6 patients), with 21 patients presenting more than one complication. While for G2 there were fractures of the prosthesis in 31 patients (23 patients with natural teeth as opposing dentition and 8 patients with removable prosthesis as opposing dentition), abutment screw loosening in 12 patients (11 patients with natural teeth as opposing dentition and 1 patient with removable prosthesis as opposing dentition) and prosthetic screw loosening in 2 patients (both with natural teeth as opposing dentition), with 9 patients presenting more than one complication (all with natural teeth as opposing dentition). For G1, the majority of complications occurred in the interim prosthesis ($n = 29$ patients; fractured prostheses = 28 patients) compared to the definitive prosthesis ($n = 16$ patients; fractured prostheses = 13 patients), and 15 patients with complications in both prostheses; while for G2, the majority of complications occurred in the definitive prosthesis ($n = 19$ patients; fractured prostheses = 15 patients) compared to the interim prosthesis ($n = 16$ patients; fractured prostheses = 16 patients), and 2 patients with complications in both prostheses. Thirty patients (37.5%) suspected of being heavy bruxers experienced mechanical complications

TABLE 34.1 **Implant Survival of the Completely Edentulous Rehabilitations Using the Rehabilitation as Unit of Analysis (Kaplan–Meier Product Limit Estimator)**

Time (Months)	Status (0 = Nonfailure; 1 = Failure[a])	Cumulative Proportion Surviving at the Time		No. of Cumulative Events	No. of Patients at Risk
		Estimate	Std. Error		
Overall Rehabilitations					
0	0	–	–	0	110
3	2	0.982	0.013	2	108
6	1	0.973	0.016	3	107
7	1	0.964	0.010	4	106
10	1	0.955	0.020	5	105
12	0	–	–	5	105
24	0	–	–	5	105
36	0	–	–	5	105
48	0	–	–	5	105
60	0	–	–	5	105

[a]Failure was defined as the first implant to fail in one patient.

TABLE 34.2   Implant Survival of the Completely Edentulous Rehabilitations Using the Rehabilitation as Unit of Analysis (Kaplan–Meier Product Limit Estimator); Survival Distribution Between the 2 Study Groups

Time (Months)	Status (0 = Nonfailure; 1 = Failure[a])	Cumulative Proportion Surviving at the Time		No. of Cumulative Events	No. of Patients at Risk
		Estimate	Std. Error		
Group 1 (Double Full-Arch Rehabilitations)					
0	0	–	–	0	
3	1	0.982	0.018	1	54
6	1	0.964	0.025	2	53
7	1	0.945	0.031	3	52
12	0	–	–	3	52
24	0	–	–	3	52
36	0	–	–	3	52
48	0	–	–	3	52
60	0	–	–	3	52
Group 2 (Single Full-Arch Rehabilitations)					
0	0	–	–	0	
3	1	0.982	0.018	1	54
10	1	0.964	0.025	2	53
12	0	–	–	2	53
24	0	–	–	2	53
36	0	–	–	2	53
48	0	–	–	2	53
60	0	–	–	2	53

Difference between groups in survival was not significant ($p = 0.645$, log-rank test).

[a]Failure was defined as the first implant to fail in one patient.

(18 patients in G1, 12 patients in G2). The prosthetic planning for patients who presented mechanical complications was adjusted in an attempt to resolve the complications. The loosening of prosthetic components was addressed by retightening the prosthetic components; the prosthesis fracture was addressed by mending the prosthesis (acrylic resin) or repairing the ceramic (metal ceramic prosthesis). The common strategy addressing both complications (prosthetic

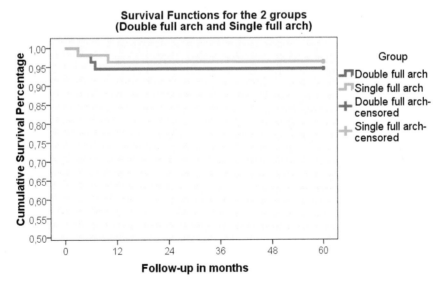

FIGURE 34.4   Survival estimation for both groups using the patient as unit of analysis and calculated through the Kaplan–Meier product limit estimator. No significant difference was registered between the two survival curves ($p = 0.645$, log-rank test).

TABLE 34.3 **Marginal Bone Level, Situated Apically to the Implant Platform, After 5 years of Follow-up with the patient as Unit of Analysis in Groups 1 and 2**

	Group 1: All-on-4 Double Full-Arch		Group 2: All-on-4 Single Full-Arch	
Average (mm)[a]	1.45[b]		1.67[b]	
Standard deviation (mm)	0.77		0.99	
Number	46		48	
Frequencies (mm)	N	%	N	%
0	0	0.0	1	2.1
0.1–1.0	15	32.6	15	31.3
1.1–2.0	24	52.2	17	35.4
2.1–3.0	4	8.7	9	18.8
>3.0	3	6.5	6	12.5

[a]Overall marginal bone level was 1.56 mm (0.89 mm).
[b]Difference between groups in marginal bone level was not significant ($p = 0.414$).

components loosening and fractures) was the adjustment of the occlusion and manufacture of a night-guard.

The patient-related incidence rate of biological complications over the 5 years of follow-up for the two groups was 0.06 [(16/55)/5] for G1 and 0.05 [(14/55)/5] for G2, with no significant differences between the groups ($p = 0.669$). For G1, there were 15 incidences of periimplant pathology and one fistulae formation ($n = 16$ implants, 7.2%); while for G2 there were 12 incidences of periimplant pathology, one of suppuration and one abscess formation ($n = 14$ implants, 6.4%). Thirteen of the patients (G1: 7 patients; G2: 6 patients) with biological complications were smokers. Eighty-one percent of the patients (13/16) in G1 and 86% (12/14) of the patients in G2 presenting biological complications also presented mechanical complications.

DISCUSSION

The difference in survival rate between the two groups (G1: 94.5%; G2: 96.4%) was not significant; however, a significant difference was registered between both groups concerning mechanical complications. Therefore, the null hypothesis stating that there is no difference in the experimental and control group survival curves could be partially rejected. The overall 95.5% (patient-related) CSRs at 5 years for the immediate loading protocol in double full-arch rehabilitations and the overall marginal bone level of 1.56 mm apical to the implant platform after 5 years (group 1: 1.45 mm; group 2: 1.67 mm) was within the limits of previous reports on the rehabilitation of edentulous jaws using the same protocol in single full-arch rehabilitations.[13,19,30] In a longitudinal study on the survival of implants in the rehabilitation of the edentulous mandible using the All-on-4 treatment concept, a CSR of 94.8% at 5 years using the patient as unit of analysis was reported.[30] Another study evaluating the 5-year outcome

of the same concept in the maxilla reported a 93% CSR using the patient as unit of analysis together with −1.95 mm of marginal bone level.[13] An additional study evaluating the 5-year outcome of immediate function implants in completely edentulous maxillary rehabilitations with different degrees of bone resorption (low-to-high bone resorption) reported an 88.6% CSR using the patient as unit of analysis.[19] There were also no significant differences in marginal bone level or the incidence of biological complications between the two groups.

There was a significantly higher incidence of mechanical complications in double full-arch rehabilitations (occluding with implant-supported fixed prostheses) compared to single full-arch rehabilitations (occluding with natural teeth and removable dentures). A previous study reporting the long-term outcome of up to 10 years of a retrievable metal ceramic implant-supported fixed prostheses with milled titanium frameworks and all-ceramic crowns registered a twofold increase in the probability of crown fracture in the presence of a metal ceramic implant-supported fixed prosthesis opposing dentition.[31] A retrospective analysis of porcelain failures of implant-supported metal ceramic crowns and fixed partial dentures (FPDs) investigating patient- and implant-specific predictors of ceramic failure reported that metal ceramic prostheses (single crown or FPDs) had approximately 7 times higher odds of porcelain fracture and 13 times greater odds of a fracture requiring either repair or replacement when in occlusion with another implant-supported restoration, as compared to opposing a natural tooth.[32] Nevertheless, the explanation for this result cannot rule out other variables including not only a lack of proprioception by the patient and/or the lack of shock-absorbing capacity by the prosthesis, but also relating to technical failure in the manufacturing process, occlusion failure in controlling the occlusion following predetermined guidelines, or parafunctional movements by the patient, all these variables acting independently or in association.[31–33] In our study, 84% of the patients with mechanical complications were either suspect of being heavy bruxers or presented an implant-supported fixed prosthesis as opposing dentition. This implies that these patients may benefit from a prosthetic protocol including periodic clinical maintenance appointments in short intervals for occlusion evaluation and the use of a night-guard prescribed from the initial stage of implant rehabilitation to decrease the probability of mechanical complications. Nevertheless, these mechanical complications did not affect the long-term survival of the prostheses or the implants, demonstrating that those procedures are safe and effective.

The biological complication incidence rate, mainly peri-implant pathology, affected patients at a similar rate in both groups. These biological complications seemed to cluster in a determined number of patients, as 13 of the 16 patients in G1 (81%) and 12 of the 14 patients in G2 (86%) also presented mechanical complications, suggesting a synergetic effect between mechanical and biological complications, a situation that has been previously described in a systematic review investigating the effect of occlusal overload on periimplant tissue health in the animal model.[34] Furthermore, biological complications occurred in 44% (7/16 patients) and 43% (6/14 patients) from G1 and G2, respectively, who were smokers. These results find parallels in the literature, where a recent systematic review reported smoking, together with history of periodontitis and poor oral hygiene as risk indicators for periimplant pathology.[35]

The limitations of this study include: the retrospective design being performed in a single center, which implies further validation in different social and cultural backgrounds; the different subgroups in G2 (single full-arch patients occluding with removable prostheses or natural teeth) as the amount of forces that can be generated by denture patients versus dentate patients is different; and the possible differences on the occlusal concept followed for the different subgroups, as these were chosen according to the specific conditions and treatment plan performed for the patient and not according to a specific inclusion criteria as a prospective study would imply. The strengths of this study include the long-term follow-up of 5 years and the use of a control group in the study design. Randomized controlled trials should be performed to confirm these results and investigate the effectiveness of using a controlled prosthetic protocol on the long-term outcome of double full-arch rehabilitated patients.

CONCLUSIONS

Rehabilitating double full-arch or single full-arch patients did not yield significant differences on implant survival and marginal bone level in the long-term follow-up; however, the incidence of mechanical complications registered was significantly higher for double full-arch patients than for single full-arch patients.

ACKNOWLEDGEMENTS

The authors thank Miss Andreia de Araújo and Mr. Sandro Catarino for all the help in data management.

REFERENCES

1. Cooper LF: The current and future treatment of edentulism. *J Prosthodont* 2009;18:116–122.
2. Brunello DL, Mandikos MN: Construction faults, age, gender, and relative medical health: factors associated with complaints in complete denture patients. *J Prosthet Dent* 1998;79:545–554.
3. MacEntee MI, Nolan A, Thomason JM: Oral mucosal and osseous disorders in frail elders. *Gerodontology* 2004;21:78–84.
4. Douglass CW, Shih A, Ostry L: Will there be a need for complete dentures in the United States in 2020? *J Prosthet Dent* 2002;87:5–8.
5. Zarb GA, Schmitt A: Implant therapy alternatives for geriatric edentulous patients. *Gerodontology* 1993;10:28–32.
6. Randow K, Ericsson I, Nilner K, et al: Immediate functional loading of Brånemark dental implants: an 18-month clinical follow-up study. *Clin Oral Implants Res* 1999;10:8–15.
7. Tarnow DP, Emtiaz S, Classi A: Immediate loading of threaded implants at stage 1 surgery in edentulous arches: ten consecutive case reports with 1- to 5-year data. *Int J Oral Maxillofac Implants* 1997;12:319–324.
8. Schnitman PA, Wohrle PS, Rubenstein JE, et al: Ten-year results for Brånemark implants immediately loaded with fixed prostheses at implant placement. *Int J Oral Maxillofac Implants* 1997;12:495–503.
9. Maló P, Rangert B, Nobre M: "All-on-Four" immediate-function concept with Brånemark System implants for completely edentulous mandibles: a retrospective clinical study. *Clin Implant Dent Relat Res* 2003;5:S2–S9.
10. Fazi G, Tellini S, Vangi D, et al: Three-dimensional finite element analysis of different implant configurations for a mandibular fixed prosthesis. *Int J Oral Maxillofac Implants* 2011;26:752–759.
11. Fermergard R, Astrand P: Osteotome sinus floor elevation and simultaneous placement of implants—a 1-year retrospective study with AstraTech implants. *Clin Implant Dent Relat Res* 2008;10:62–69.
12. Agliardi EL, Pozzi A, Stappert CF, et al: Immediate fixed rehabilitation of the edentulous maxilla: a prospective clinical and radiological study after 3 years of loading. *Clin Implant Dent Relat Res* 2014;16:292–302.
13. Maló P, de Araújo Nobre M, Lopes A, et al: "All-on-4" immediate-function concept for completely edentulous

maxillae: a clinical report on the medium (3 years) and long-term (5 years) outcomes. *Clin Implant Dent Relat Res* 2012;14 Suppl 1: e139–150.

14. Hsu Y, Fu J, Hezaimi K, et al: Biomechanical implant treatment complications: a systematic review of clinical studies of implants with at least 1 year of functional loading. *Int J Oral Maxillofac Implants* 2012;27:894–904.

15. Wood MR, Vermilyea SG: A review of selected dental literature on evidence-based treatment planning for dental implants: report of the Committee on Research in Fixed Prosthodontics of the Academy of Fixed Prosthodontics. *J Prosthet Dent* 2004;92:447–462.

16. Gross MD: Occlusion in implant dentistry: a review of the literature of prosthetic determinants and current concepts. *Aust Dent J* 2008;53:S60–S68.

17. Maló P, de Araújo Nobre M, Lopes A, et al: Preliminary report on the outcome of tilted implants with longer lengths (20–25 mm) in low-density bone: one-year follow-up of a prospective cohort study. *Clin Implant Dent Relat Res* 2015;17 Suppl 1: e134–142

18. Maló P, Rangert B, Nobre M: All-on-4 immediate-function concept with Brånemark System implants for completely edentulous maxillae: a 1-year retrospective clinical study. *Clin Implant Dent Relat Res* 2005;7:S88–94.

19. Maló P, Nobre MD, Lopes A: The rehabilitation of completely edentulous maxillae with different degrees of resorption with four or more immediately loaded implants: a 5-year retrospective study and a new classification. *Eur J Oral Implantol* 2011;4:227–243.

20. Friberg B, Jemt T: Rehabilitation of edentulous mandibles by means of five TiUnite implants after one-stage surgery: a 1-year retrospective study of 90 patients. *Clin Implant Dent Relat Res* 2008;10:47–54.

21. Kim KS, Kim YL, Bae JM, et al: Biomechanical comparison of axial and tilted implants for mandibular full-arch fixed prostheses. *Int J Oral Maxillofac Implants* 2011;26:976–984.

22. Bevilacqua M, Tealdo T, Pera F, et al: Three-dimensional finite element analysis of load transmission using different implant inclinations and cantilever lengths. *Int J Prosthodont* 2008;21:539–542.

23. Francetti L, Romeo D, Corbella S, et al: Bone level changes around axial and tilted implants in full-arch fixed immediate restorations: interim results of a prospective study. *Clin Implant Dent Relat Res* 2012;14:646–654.

24. Ogawa T, Dhaliwai S, Naert I, et al: Impact of implant number, distribution and prosthesis material on loading on implants supporting fixed prostheses. *J Oral Rehabil* 2010;37:525–531.

25. Gross MD: Occlusion in implant dentistry: a review of the literature of prosthetic determinants and current concepts. *Aust Dent J* 2008;53:S60–S68.

26. Papaspyridakos P, Chen C, Chuang S, et al: A systematic review of biologic and technical complications with fixed implant rehabilitations for edentulous patients. *Int J Oral Maxillofac Implants* 2012;27:102–110.

27. Balshi TJ, Wolfinger GJ: Immediate loading of Brånemark implants in edentulous mandibles: a preliminary report. *Implant Dent* 1997;6:83–88.

28. Esposito M, Grusovin MG, Achille H, et al: Interventions for replacing missing teeth: different times for loading dental implants. *Cochrane Database Syst Rev* 2009 21 (1): CD003878.

29. von Elm E, Altman DG, Egger M, et al: STROBE Initiative. The Strengthening the Reporting of Observational Studies in Epidemiology (STROBE) statement: guidelines for reporting observational studies. *J Clin Epidemiol* 2008;61:344–349.

30. Maló P, de Araújo Nobre M, Lopes A, et al: A longitudinal study of the survival of All-on-4 implants in the mandible with up to 10 years of follow-up. *J Am Dent Assoc* 2011;142: 310–320.

31. Maló P, de Araújo Nobre M, et al: Retrievable metal ceramic implant-supported fixed prostheses with milled titanium frameworks and all-ceramic crowns: retrospective clinical study with up to 10 years of follow-up. *J Prosthodont* 2012;21:256–264.

32. Kinsel RP, Lin D: Retrospective analysis of porcelain failures of metal ceramic crowns and fixed partial dentures supported by 729 implants in 152 patients: patient-specific and implant-specific predictors of ceramic failure. *J Prosthet Dent* 2009;101:388–394.

33. Kim Y, Oh TJ, Misch CE, et al: Occlusal considerations in implant therapy: clinical guidelines with biomechanical rationale. *Clin Oral Implants Res* 2005;16:26–35.

34. Chambrone L, Chambrone LA, Lima LA: Effects of occlusal overload on peri-implant tissue health: a systematic review of animal-model studies. *J Periodontol* 2010;81:1367–1378.

35. Heitz-Mayfield LJ: Peri-implant diseases: diagnosis and risk indicators. *J Clin Periodontol* 2008;35:S292–S304.

INDEX